TO MY BEST ~~FRIENDS~~

Born in Hampshire, Sam Baker studied politics at Birmingham University. She has been editor of *Just Seventeen, Minx, Company* and *Cosmopolitan* in the UK, and is now editor-in-chief of *Red*. She lives between Winchester, Hampshire and central London with her husband, the novelist Jon Courtenay Grimwood, and has one stepson.

Praise for *The Stepmothers' Support Group*:

'I really, really loved it'   Marian Keyes

'Sometimes, a book can be such a brilliant idea you can't believe no one has done it before . . . Stepmothers, stepfathers, stepchildren: all will find amusement and comfort in its pages'   Nigella Lawson

'This funny, touching novel by *Red's* editor is *The First Wives Club* meets *Sex And The City* – with stepchildren . . . Fast paced and unexpectedly moving'   *Red*

'The narrative is well thought out with a great plot and likeable characters. Writing from the point of view of the Wicked Stepmother makes for an interesting and different read'   *Daily Mail*

'In this feisty female-support fiction, each of her group of five women – Eve, Clare, Mel, Mandy and Chloe – has her own way of managing the complexities of 21st-century family life – living with the ghosts of dead wives, looking after the little ones, and nursing the big ones' egos'
Good Housekeeping

'This hilarious novel addresses an inevitable question for step-parents: what if you didn't get on with your partner's children?' *Hot Stars (OK!)*

'A great read with characters you can sympathise with'   *Woman*

'Her cracking novel is a stylish tale about what to do when you love him but don't love his kids. Rather cleverly she lays the old myth of the wicked stepmother to rest, or so we hope. Either way it's a super-sassy read'   *The Lady*

'Baker charts the lives of four very different women, each embroiled in a family crisis, offering us a compelling, honest and moving view of motherhood, in all forms'   *Psychologies*

'I loved it . . . all the women's stories [are] really engaging and entertaining . . . a really good read'   Jane Fallon

Also by Sam Baker:

The Stepmothers' Support Group

SAM BAKER

To My Best Friends

HARPER

Harper
An imprint of HarperCollins*Publishers*
77–85 Fulham Palace Road,
Hammersmith, London W6 8JB

www.harpercollins.co.uk

A Paperback Original 2011
1

A catalogue record for this book
is available from the British Library

ISBN: 978 0 00 730554 4

Set in Meridien by Palimpsest Book Production Limited,
Falkirk, Stirlingshire

Printed and bound in Great Britain by
Clays Ltd, St Ives plc

Mixed Sources
Product group from well-managed
forests and other controlled sources
www.fsc.org Cert no. SW-COC-001806
© 1996 Forest Stewardship Council
FSC

To my *best friends*
Nancy, Clare, Catherine
Jude
Shelly
And, above all, Jon

PROLOGUE

That navy Prada suit, the one with the nipped-in waist
you wished you'd never bought? Trust me, get the skirt
taken up two inches and wear it with my red Marc
Jacobs mary-janes. The ones with the blue trim. They
always fitted you better than they did me, anyway.
You'll look a million dollars . . .

Slipping the lid back on the cartridge pen, Nicci dropped it
on the duvet beside her and let her head fall back onto
plumped pillows. She closed her eyes and felt the bedroom
spin. It was a familiar sensation now, almost comforting, in
a sick sort of way.

Three and a half lines of writing. Five sentences. Fifty-five
words. How could fifty-five measly words be so exhausting?
They weren't even the important words. Those were still to
come. These were just the preamble, the housekeeping. Nicci
risked opening her eyes and the room sped up.

Damn it, she thought, and let her lids drop, feeling the
spinning recede. This wasn't her. Illness didn't suit her. Nicci
Morrison didn't do sick, just as she didn't do sitting around
at weekends, chilling or downtime. And she didn't do lying

1

in bed in the middle of the afternoon. At least not since she was twenty-one and had met David. Then they'd done nothing much other than lying in bed all afternoon when she should have been writing a ten-thousand-word dissertation on the way clothes reflect women's place in society in nineteenth-century literature. Well, not so much lying, but bed had figured prominently. Bed, the floor, the bath . . .

Nicci smiled at the memory. Half sad, half glad they'd had that then, and the rest.

Come on, she urged herself. *Get a grip. One down, three more letters to go.*

The trick was catching her morphine at the right stage: long enough after her injection for the pain to have eased, but not so soon the opiates dulled her capacity to think straight. Pulling herself up, Nicci rummaged around her for the pen while trying to find her train of thought. Light shimmered at the edge of her vision, brighter than she could stand.

Jo wouldn't refuse, Nicci was sure of that. Especially not when she opened the parcel containing the red mary-janes, which David would deliver with the letter. How could she – how could any of them – when Jo knew only too well what Nicci had been through in the past year? Biopsies, mastectomy, chemo and radio. None of which, ultimately, had worked. Wasn't wearing an old navy-blue suit the least a girl could do for her best friend?'

Looking at the sheet of thick cream paper resting on a magazine on her knee, Nicci smiled. She would have the last laugh. And her business partner would thank her for it. In the weeks to come, the last thing her friend would want to think about – the last thing any of Nicci's friends would want to think about – was what to wear.

Now, that's the outfit sorted. And don't argue, Jo. Remember, on the wardrobe front, Nicci knows best!!!

2

Just think of it as one less problem to worry about. After all, you're going to have enough on your plate with Capsule Wardrobe once I've gone.

But that's not the point of this letter. No, what I'm really writing about are my twin babies, my darling girls, my Charlie and Harrie, your goddaughters. And you've been such a good godmother, Jo, the very best. Which is why I want you to be more . . . .

ONE

There were few things in life Nicci Morrison had not been able to control. But being buried on a dank, drizzly day in February was one of them.

It was not yet two o'clock, and the dirty grey cloud hung low over the church, obscuring the spire, making the hour seem closer to dusk.

'There you are!' Jo Clarke called out as a tall thin woman, hair frizzing from the bun at the nape of her neck, picked her way along the muddy path. She was clad head to toe in black – hardly unexpected at a funeral – but her spike-heeled ankle boots would have looked more at home in a bar.

'Let me guess,' Jo laughed, eyeing the Jimmy Choo boots. 'The person responsible for you buying those in the first place is to blame for you wearing them now?'

Mona Thomas raised her eyebrows and looked pointedly at the red mary-janes on Jo's feet. 'Takes one to know one,' she said.

'Typical Nicci, huh?' Jo hugged Mona hard to distract herself from her tears. Nicci had known outfit-planning would be the last thing on anyone's mind, and so, unable to break the habit of a lifetime, she had done it for them.

'Hello, Si.' Mona reached over Jo's shoulder to pat his cheek. 'Am I the last?'

Shaking his head, Si moved aside to make way for a group of unfamiliar faces waiting impatiently in the mizzle behind his wife and her friend.

'Lizzie and Gerry are inside. Well, Lizzie is. Gerry dropped her off at the gate and went to park the car. You on your own?'

'Yep. I thought I'd spare Dan. I know he was fond of Nicci – and he adores David – but, y'know . . . kids and funerals . . .' Mona's voice trailed away, and Jo and Si nodded. They knew. Adults and funerals, too.

'You guys go on in,' Si said. 'I'll wait for Gerry. The, erm, the . . . hearse will . . . you know . . . be here soon.'

Jo nodded gratefully and took Mona's arm. Si knew she wouldn't want to see her best friend arrive that way.

'So have you told Si yet?'

'Told him what?' Jo whispered, leaning across the pew so she could be heard by Lizzie and Mona, but not the random mixture of family members, customers and distant friends who had gathered to pay their respects.

'About the letter, of course,' Mona hissed.

Jo's eyes bulged. 'Of course I bl—' she stopped herself, remembering where she was. Jo wasn't religious, but even so. 'Of course I haven't! What was I supposed to say? "Hey, Si, after the last three years, all the money we've spent, all the . . ."' she swallowed, focusing on her hands until Lizzie's freckled arm reached over and squeezed one of them, "'. . . all the disappointment, guess what. It doesn't matter now if we can't have kids because we've been left shares in someone else's?" You can imagine how that would go down.'

Actually, now she thought of it, Jo didn't have the first

clue how that news would go down with Si. It was months, longer, since they had even talked about it.

'You don't have to put it quite like that,' Lizzie whispered gently. 'After all, it's not as if it's that straightforward.'

'It's not remotely straightforward.'

Closing her eyes, Jo leant back in the pew. Centuries-old oak dug uncomfortably into her vertebrae and the organ music was giving her a headache. Whatever Nicci's instructions for the funeral, and, Nicci being Nicci, there would have been plenty – the flowers for a start; the church was awash with blue and yellow, not a lily in sight – Jo was sure they hadn't included a wheezing, clunking rendition of 'Dido's Lament', or anyone else's lament come to that.

'I've told Gerry,' Lizzie coloured as she rushed the words out. She couldn't help herself; never had been able to. If there was a crease Lizzie had to iron it out. A silence – awkward or not – she had to fill it.

Jo's eyes flicked open. 'About our bequests?' she asked, her voice tight. 'Didn't we agree to keep that between ourselves for now, just while we work out what to do? Whether we have to, you know, comply with Nicci's wishes.'

'Not yours and Mona's, just mine.'

'Oh,' snorted Mona. 'That's hardly the same, is it? At least Nicci left you some*thing*—'

'Just out of interest,' Jo interrupted, hearing Mona's voice rise and seeing Lizzie's lip quiver, 'what *did* Gerry say, about your bequest, I mean?'

Lizzie's mouth twisted. 'What d'you think he said?'

'Let me guess,' Mona said. 'I bet it had something to do with cheap labour.'

Lizzie's laugh burst out over the hush of voices and the wheeze of the organ. She clapped a hand over her mouth, but not before earning a scowl from an elderly woman sitting on the other side of the aisle. 'That's about the sum of it.

Gerry said . . .' she put on his voice. It was posh Yorkshire. He used being northern when it suited him and hid it when it didn't, '. . . "Don't you usually have to pay someone to do that?"'

Jo and Mona exchanged glances. They loved Lizzie but, despite years of trying, they still didn't get Gerry. If he hadn't married one of their dearest friends their paths would never have crossed. Nicci had barely tolerated him, declaring him smug and materialistic, and nowhere near good enough. But once Lizzie announced a date and flashed a rock that – as Nicci muttered later – cost a fortune and still looked as if it belonged in an Argos sale, she backed off. If Gerry was what Lizzie wanted then, like him or not, he was what they wanted for her too.

As 'Dido's Lament' segued clumsily into Albinoni's 'Adagio' Mona mimed sticking her fingers in her ears. 'Clearly there are some things even Nicci's ghost can't control. *Now That's What I Call Funerals.*'

'Still,' said Lizzie, 'what are the alternatives? Westlife? Celine Dion? Bette Midler?'

'That, and the self-invited guests,' said Jo. 'Guess it's what you get for being popular.'

'Yeah,' said Mona. 'Can you imagine having loads of people you hardly know turn up for your wedding?'

'I did,' Lizzie said. 'Remember? My mother insisted on inviting a bunch of aunties and cousins three times removed.'

'Nicci did too,' Jo said. 'But weren't they all distant relatives of David that he said he hadn't seen since his christening?'

A sudden hush cut them short. The organ music had died and all around them people were getting to their feet as the pallbearers entered the church. Si slid in beside Jo, Gerry behind him.

'Here we go, love,' Si said, slipping his arm around Jo's shoulder . . .

'Ready or not,' she agreed, reaching for Lizzie's hand . . .
'Not,' Lizzie whispered, squeezing Mona's hand in turn . . .
'Never will be,' Mona replied, squeezing it back.

'Nicci had to be first at everything,' said Jo, trying to raise her quavering voice so it was audible at the back. The flowers seemed to muffle it, each petal, leaf and stamen cushioning the sound. Who knew flowers buggered up your acoustics? Not even Nicci could predict that.

Think of this as a business presentation Jo coached herself. Imagine those red eyes and puffy faces belong to financial backers, not fellow mourners at your best friend's funeral.

Her best friend's funeral.

How had she got landed with this? She hadn't known Nicci any longer than the others. Well, no longer than Lizzie. A day, maybe a week, certainly no more. Why did Jo always have to be the grown-up?

Gripping the lectern to steady herself, she took a deep breath. 'You name it,' Jo continued, 'Nicci beat the rest of us to it. She was the first to meet *The One* – her lovely David.' Jo ventured a smile at where Nicci's widower sat in the front pew, two tiny blonde girls in mini-me coats held close on either side of him, confusion on their small faces. David's parents sat either side of the three, creating a protective barrier around their son and granddaughters.

'The first to marry, the first to have children . . .' Jo swallowed. That last bit wasn't strictly true. Mona had had her son long before the others even started thinking about kids, but they'd discussed it the night before and agreed that simply didn't count. Mona had gone away, and when she came back there was Dan. It was different. They didn't really know why, it just was.

'. . . her adorable and much-loved Harriet and Charlotte.

Harrie and Charlie to their besotted godmothers – Mona, Lizzie and, of course, me . . .'

Did David know about the bequest, Jo wondered. Of course, he knew about the letters; he'd delivered them. But was he aware of their contents; that he was handing over grenades? He had to, didn't he? Nicci wouldn't have done that without telling him . . . would she?

Seeing a hundred faces gazing up at her, Jo forced herself on.

'She was the first of us to have it all. To juggle her new family, her beloved husband and our little business: her other baby, Capsule Wardrobe. And now . . .' Jo tried to concentrate on the neat capitals printed on the index cards in front of her. It wasn't as if she didn't know the words off by heart – poor Si had listened to this speech a dozen times in the last couple of days – but her eyes filled with tears, and the neat letters doubled and tripled until she couldn't even see her words, let alone recall them.

'And now, our beautiful Nicci . . .' she heard Lizzie prompt gently from the front row.

Jo blinked away her tears. 'And now, our beautiful Nicci,' she repeated, 'our best friend, the love – I know he won't mind me saying – of David's life, is the first of us to die.' Looking up, she pasted on a smile. 'Taking this number-one thing to extremes a bit, I think.'

A ripple of laughter echoed around the small church and Jo risked catching David's eye. Misery, exhaustion and disbelief at finding himself in this place, for this unthinkable, unimaginable, reason . . . all her own emotions were in his gaze but ripped raw. He squeezed his daughters tighter. Was it her imagination, or was he sending a signal?

Stop it, Jo told herself. *Concentrate.*

'I met Nicci,' she continued, 'on my first day at university. She took me under her vintage-store-clad wing and I never looked back. Soon after, she found Lizzie and, for want of a better word, adopted her too. Then, by sheer fluke, Mona found us. And together we found David. The poor thing didn't know what he was letting himself in for . . .' Another ripple of laughter.

'Nicci wheedled her way into David's life, and his wardrobe!' More laughter, louder now. 'As she did for so many of us here.'

Jo let her gaze roam the front pews where Nicci's influence bloomed. How had Nicci known they would all be so obedient? Or were they all just too exhausted, too heartbroken, to greet Nicci's instructions telling them what to wear to their best friend's funeral with anything other than gratitude?

Lizzie's taupe cardigan was loosely belted over a beautiful floral Paul Smith tea dress that Jo knew for a fact had cost as much as half a month's mortgage; the Burberry trench coat that had cost the other half lay over the back of the pew behind her. Mona wore a slick black Helmut Lang trouser suit, which just about made up for the four-inch heels Nicci had convinced her 'cost per wear' would be a bargain. At the last count, 'cost per wear' those boots still stood at six months' Council Tax. David's scuffed Church's brogues, identical to the ones Nicci had bought him their very first Christmas together, already showed signs of missing Nicci's care. And Jo's own navy suit was nowhere near as frumpy as she remembered now the skirt was taken up, as per Nicci's instructions.

As ever, Nicci had been right. It might be her funeral, but her friends still looked a million dollars. In a subdued, funeral-appropriate, style.

'I know this isn't the done thing,' Jo said, deviating from her script, 'but I'd like to do a straw poll.'

A bemused murmur rippled through the congregation. Lizzie glanced at Mona, who shook her head. This wasn't planned.

'How many here today are wearing outfits, or at least items of clothing, that Nicci picked out for us?' Jo raised her own arm. She felt like an idiot. And from the way half the congregation stared at her, she knew she looked like one too.

Widening her eyes at them, she willed Lizzie and Mona to join her.

Mona raised her arm, then Lizzie. A second later, David joined them. Harrie and Charlie's arms were raised by their granny and grandpa. Then, as if in a Mexican wave, arms rose around the church, rippling right to the back where, Jo realised now, Capsule Wardrobe's most loyal clients stood, the pews too full to hold them.

Laughter burst from her. Jo couldn't help it; didn't even try to suppress it. The sound of the first genuine laugh she'd managed in the two weeks since Nicci's death pealed up into the apse.

'How much would Nicci love this?' Jo said. 'She made clothes her life, she believed that what we wore spoke volumes more than anything words could say; that a T-shirt, or a dress, or a pair of shoes, really was a statement. That woman contributed in some way to the outfits of what must be over a hundred people here.

'My friends . . . all of whom, like me, loved and trusted Nicci, there can be no better affirmation of her life. Because if there's one thing I know Nicci would have wanted it's this: no frumps at her funeral.

'Nicci, we love you, we miss you, and we don't yet know what we will do – how we will even begin to cope – without

12

you. But you are forever in our hearts . . .' Jo paused, locking wet eyes with Lizzie and Mona, strengthened by their tearful smiles.

'. . . And in our wardrobes.'

TWO

'Isn't David going to wonder where we've got to?' Lizzie asked, as she fumbled with the lock of the shed. In the fading light, she misjudged the distance and the key landed in the sludge at her feet. Bending, she noticed her high-heeled loafers were now crusted with mud. 'Anyone got a tissue?'

Mona shrugged, and Jo shook her head.

'Where is David, anyway?' Jo said. 'I haven't seen him for at least half an hour.'

'Hiding, probably,' Mona said. 'Who can blame him? House full of total strangers feeding their faces at his expense. Anyway,' she added, 'it's not as if it matters. It's Lizzie's shed now.'

Lizzie didn't look convinced. 'I know that, but does David? Does David know any of it?'

'Look,' Jo said, turning back to the house. Every window in the Victorian terrace was ablaze and the kitchen was crammed with people. 'It looks odd, doesn't it? Wrong, somehow?'

The others followed her gaze.

'It's not that the house is full – ' Lizzie said – 'it was always full – it's *those* people. Who are they? Does anyone know?'

'Someone must,' said Mona. 'David probably.'

'Come on,' Jo said, 'you must recognise some of them? The girls from Capsule Wardrobe, some suppliers, a few clients. David's mum and dad, his brother and his wife . . .'

'There was an awful lot of family at the church for someone who didn't have any,' Lizzie said.

Jo shrugged. 'David's, I suppose, like the wedding. And there are some old friends of Nicci's from the drama group at uni.'

'I can't believe none of Nicci's family bothered to show up,' Lizzie persisted. 'You'd think some would have wanted to pay their respects.'

'You don't know they didn't,' Jo said. 'There were plenty of strange faces in that church. Not inconceivable one or two of them belonged to Nicci.'

'You pair of romantics,' said Mona. 'Nicci didn't have family, you know that. She was always saying so: "You're my family. You, David and the girls. You're the only family I need."'

'That doesn't mean she didn't have one. No one comes from nowhere,' said Lizzie. 'Much as they might want to.'

'She fell out with her mum, we know that,' Jo went on as if Lizzie hadn't spoken. 'I remember her talking about it one night – when we were pissed, of course. You must remember?' Jo grinned. 'Whisky night.'

'Not sure I remember much from whisky night.' Lizzie grimaced.

Jo never forgot anything. It amazed Lizzie, and annoyed her slightly. Jo and Nicci always could riff off events, jokes and incidents she barely remembered at all. Most of her time at university was a blur. A blur then, and a blur now.

'Think that was the only time she mentioned it. And you know how she always spent every holiday at uni, working in Sainsbury's, when the rest of us went home. Said someone had to look after our house. Like we were going to fall for that.'

'We did, though, didn't we?' Lizzie said.

'Her dad left when she was a baby, didn't he?' Mona said, tucking her hands under her arms in a bid to keep warm. The fine wool suit looked good but it wasn't much use against the damp chill that hung in the air.

'So Nicci said that night. You know how she was: all ears where our problems were concerned, but always playing her own cards close to her chest.'

Having wiped the muddy key on her hem, Lizzie pushed it into the lock, turned it but found the door wouldn't open.

'Come on,' said Mona. 'My toes are going to drop off if you don't let us in soon.'

Lizzie looked puzzled. Turning the key back the other way, she felt it click and reached for the shed's door handle. The shed had been unlocked all along.

'Here we go,' she said, pushing open the door, and stopped . . .

Lizzie could hear breathing. There was someone in there. As her eyes adjusted to the dimness, the toes of a scuffed pair of shoes came into view. Church's brogues.

'D-David,' she asked, 'is that you?' Her mind raced through their conversation. Had they said anything he shouldn't have overheard?

'Yes,' said a familiar voice, and she felt her shoulders sag. 'It's me. Sorry. I didn't mean to make you jump, I just had to . . . you know . . . get away for a bit. I couldn't think where else to go. Every room in the house is . . . and Nicci always . . .' David stopped, unable to go on. After a careful breath, he said, 'She came down here when she wanted peace, you know. Said it was the only place she could think. Away from the house, with the sounds of the garden.'

'And the A3 in the distance,' Mona said wryly.

David flipped a switch and Nicci's shed came into focus. It was larger than Lizzie expected. The light came from two small lamps. They were the kind of lights her gran might have had: dark wood sculpted base, lampshades of faded chintz. Lizzie wouldn't have given them houseroom. Typically, here they looked somehow stylish. The one nearest David sat on an old sideboard, which doubled as a worktop, a kettle, glazed brown teapot and assorted mugs, plus a couple of boxes of herbal tea, piled haphazardly on its surface. In the far corner was an old-school Victorian sink. It appeared to be plumbed in.

One of the mugs Lizzie recognised: she'd bought them all 'I ♥ NY' mugs back from her honeymoon. The chair David sat in was from his and Nicci's first flat. A battered old thing that had been more holes than leather when they'd bought it for a tenner in a junk shop. Nicci had restored it.

'I always wondered what happened to that chair,' Lizzie said. 'And those cushions . . .'

'What did she need a kettle for?' Mona said. 'I know it's a big garden, but it's not *that* big.'

'Mona,' Jo said crossly.

'What?'

'Think about it.'

An awkward silence fell. Lizzie and Jo were thinking the same thing: a couple of hundred feet is a long way when you've had chemo.

'Like I said,' David got to his feet, 'Nicci used to spend time down here thinking. Until the last few weeks. Then the state of the garden made her feel too guilty. She hadn't been well enough to put it to bed for winter, and she felt bad about that. Said it wore its neglect like unloved clothes.'

Yes, Lizzie thought, that sounded like Nicci.

David looked wrung out. Anyone who hadn't known him

with a purple Mohican would have thought the same hairdresser had cut his short brown hair in the same style since he was a toddler. His brown eyes were bloodshot, his face puffy. His mouth, usually ready with a quiet smile, was set in a tense line, as if one wobble would bring his composure crashing down.

'I'm sorry,' Lizzie said. 'We didn't realise . . . I mean, if we'd known you were here we wouldn't have intruded.'

'OK,' he said, brushing off his trousers, even though there was nothing on them. 'I should get back anyway. After all, it's my party . . .'

'And I'll cry if I want to,' the women finished for him.

'David,' Lizzie said, 'I'm so sorry.'

'I know,' he said, his voice almost inaudible. 'But not as sorry as I am.'

'He knows,' Mona said, when David had shut the shed door firmly behind him. 'About the letters. He knows.'

'What makes you say that?' Lizzie asked. 'He'd say something, wouldn't he? If he did.'

'We know,' Jo pointed out. 'And we haven't.'

'Of course he knows,' Mona said. 'When has it ever been that awkward with David? He's known us as long as he's known Nicci. It's never been awkward. If you'd asked me a couple of weeks ago I'd have said I was closer to him than my brothers, by a mile. Dan certainly is. I've seen a lot more of David in the last fifteen years than I have of them.' She grinned. 'Hell, when we lived in that dive in Hove he probably saw us naked almost as often as Nicci.'

A memory of David walking in on her in the bathroom came to Mona and her grin slipped as fast as it had arrived. His appraising glance, before embarrassment hit them both. Nicci's forty-eight hours of coolness, David's mumbled apology in Nicci's presence, and the wariness with which she watched David and Mona for a few weeks after that. It was unnecessary. Even if Mona would have, David wouldn't. 'Damn it,' she said. 'He knows.'

'The awkwardness could be coming from us,' Lizzie said. 'I know I've never felt uncomfortable around him before, but look at what we just did. We barged in on him in his own shed – a shed to which I now have the key – like we owned the place.'

'Which you do,' Mona said. 'If those letters mean anything. Which is a whole other conversation.'

'Look,' Jo interrupted, 'suppose Mona's right?' She'd been standing at the small window watching David's back recede in the darkness. His drooping shoulders and scuffing walk radiated anguish. 'And given that we just let ourselves into his shed – with his wife's key – and he didn't bat an eyelid, I think she is, then he's waiting for us to make the first move.'

It took a while to sink in.

'What did he say?' Lizzie turned to Mona. 'When he delivered your letter, I mean. How did he look?'

Mona shrugged. 'Rough as hell. Like he hadn't slept in days. Which he probably hadn't. And he didn't say anything much. Certainly wasn't up for a cup of tea and a chat. He just handed me the envelope and said something like, "Nicci wanted me to give you this." We hugged, just barely, now I think about it. He definitely wanted to get away as quickly as possible. Said he had the girls in the car.'

'Which he did,' Jo pointed out.

'I found this,' she said, pulling a crumpled piece of paper from her coat pocket. 'After I'd read the letter – about a hundred times – I went up in the attic and dug out the copy of *The Bell Jar* Nicci gave me for my birthday.'

Mona and Lizzie groaned.

'She was obsessed with that damn book for a while,' Lizzie said.

'Bloody depressing,' Mona added. 'I'm pretty sure I binned mine years ago, before I went to Australia.'

'Anyway,' Jo interrupted them, 'this fell out. I must have been using it as a bookmark and forgot all about it.'

Smoothing the square of paper flat with her hand, Jo held it up. The picture was faded where the flare of the flash had turned pink. Blu-Tack stains still speckled its back.

'I remember that night!' Mona exclaimed. 'It wasn't long after I moved in with you.'

Jo glanced at her friend anxiously. She knew the fact that Mona had joined their little group a year after the others still smarted, but if Mona was thinking that it didn't show.

The photograph was of the four of them, just before a party. Snarls and pouts and grins for a camera on self-timer and balanced on a bookshelf. All with that early nineties hair, which was still really late eighties. Except for Nicci, of course. She had a bleached crop, the kind that looked like she'd cut it herself, which she had.

'Look at you!' Lizzie laughed, and Jo was embarrassed to see she was hoisting her boobs for the camera. As if they weren't big enough already in those days. She wore a towel and nothing else. Lizzie was all wild red hair, in an over-large man's shirt and Levi's 501s, a look she adopted in their first term at university, under Nicci's tuition, and wore for years. As ever, her hair hid her face.

Mona was in the hippy phase that presaged her wander-lust. A long Indian skirt and a mirror-beaded waistcoat over a puffy shirt. On anyone else it would have looked like a sack, but she looked as lean as always. Only Mona would hide the slim-hipped, long-legged figure of a model under that outfit.

And Nicci? She was channelling Courtney Love.

20

Doc Martens, with her original sixties biker jacket, over a peach satin slip, her hair spiky. A bottle of vodka in one hand and a cigarette in the other. Jo was pouting, Mona was inscrutable and Lizzie was grinning, more or less. As for Nicci, she had a rock star snarl and that wildness in her eyes. The wildness that had only started to fade when she met David.

Lizzie's sniff broke the silence. 'Still no tissues, I suppose?' she asked, glancing around the shed. Her gaze fell on the remains of a kitchen roll. She tore off a square and passed the roll to the others.

'Nicci lived in that leather jacket,' Lizzie said. 'She was wearing it the very first time I met her.'

THREE

The Sixties Vintage Biker Jacket
Sussex University. Brighton, 1992

Lizzie barely opened her mouth in the Hardy seminar. It wasn't that she didn't know what she thought; she'd read Jude the Obscure *three times to be sure. But why would anyone care what Lizzie O'Hara thought? And anyway, she was too intimidated by the peroxide blonde in the charity-shop nightie and battered motorbike jacket who'd been holding court for the last ten minutes. Where did she get her self-confidence, Lizzie wondered. At least she wasn't afraid to express her opinions, even if Lizzie wasn't convinced they were entirely accurate.*

When the blonde came up to Lizzie as she waited for a lift after the seminar, Lizzie couldn't have been more amazed if Damon Albarn had asked her out. 'I'm Nicci Gilbert,' the girl said. 'Don't know about you, but I'm gasping for a coffee. Fancy one?'

Dumbfounded, Lizzie just nodded, and found herself walking beside – well, slightly behind – the coolest and fastest-walking person, she'd ever seen, let alone spoken to, in her entire eighteen years of small-town life.

They looked like chalk and cheese.

Despite her best efforts, Lizzie's long reddish hair was frizz

22

rather than curls. Her skin was white and freckly, what little of it could be seen beneath her floor-length black jersey skirt, which bagged at the knee where she'd crossed her legs in the tutorial. An over-sized man's shirt was meant to disguise her pear-shaped – and much-loathed – size fourteen body. In Lizzie's eyes, it did the job adequately.

Apparently not . . .

'I don't mean to be rude,' said Nicci, sliding into a corner table in the Students' Union café, laden with plastic cups of nasty, luke-warm machine coffee. Allegedly black, the liquid looked more like a murky brown. 'But that skirt . . . it really doesn't suit you. You should try men's jeans with a big belt. Or leggings, they'd work. The shirt's great, by the way. But a baggy top and a baggy bottom just make you look . . .'

At the expression on Lizzie's face, the conclusion trailed away.

'I didn't mean . . .' Nicci said. 'What I meant to say was, you've got that amazing body, and I'd kill to have curves.' She ran one ring-laden hand down her birdcage-like chest to reveal a Jenga of ribs under her slip. 'No such luck. If I had boobs – even small ones like yours – and a bum, I'd make sure everyone knew about it.'

Lizzie was mortified. Where did she get off, this stranger slagging off her clothes and calling her fat? The way Lizzie was brought up, if you couldn't say something polite, you didn't say anything at all. One reason why she didn't tell Nicci where to stick it, crap coffee and all. Plus, she didn't have the nerve. Her instinctive reaction was to crawl under the table and stay there until Nicci had gone. Instead, she just nodded sheepishly and stared hard at the brown plastic cup in front of her.

So that's what I am, she thought as she stomped back to halls half an hour later, a charity case. And a fat one, at that. Well, bugger off. I can find my own friends. And I can dress myself without your help too.

But somehow next day, without intending to, she found herself the centre of Brighton, in a second-hand shop in The Lanes, fingering a ripped up pair of 501s, washed and worn to soft.

The following week, after their seminar Nicci was waiting for Lizzie by the lift, a battered paperback copy of A Pair of Blue Eyes in her hand.

'Cool jeans,' she said, when she spotted Lizzie. 'Vintage too.' She nodded approvingly. 'They're perfect on you. You look sexy.'

Lizzie flushed, embarrassed. In spite of herself, she was pleased. Nicci grinned. 'I didn't mean to be rude last week,' she said. 'I'm sorry if I upset you. I can be clumsy like that. I need to learn to keep my trap shut.'

Smiling cautiously, Nicci slid her arm through Lizzie's. 'I just thought you'd look better in jeans – and you do. Come on,' she added. 'I'm meeting my friend Jo in the Union. I think you'll like her. She lives in the room next door to me in halls. She's the first friend I made here.' She grinned again, taking Lizzie by surprise. 'And you're the second.'

It was supposedly the first day of the rest of Jo's life. The day life really started to happen. But sitting on a yet-to-be-made-up mattress in a single room on the third floor of halls, Jo had never felt so out of her depth.

Her parents had left an hour earlier and she hadn't moved since. So she sat surrounded by black bags, cardboard boxes and a new John Lewis suitcase bought especially for the occasion. Her worldly goods, such as they were. Sat and stared at the detritus of the room's last occupant: Blu-Tack stains freckling the walls where once a montage of photographs had been, fading gig tickets still pinned to a corkboard, smiley-face stickers obscuring the window, which wasn't big to start with. Proof, if proof was needed, that room 303's previous inhabitant had been 'popular'. All the signs so far suggested that Jo was going to be the opposite.

To judge by the blank stares, uninterested glances and irritated

24

sighs as she'd lugged her bags into the lift, Jo was sure friends whose photographs might paper those walls would be in short supply.

Feeling like nothing so much as her eleven-year-old self, Jo allowed herself a few minutes to wallow. She knew absolutely no one here, and didn't have a clue how to go about changing that. She'd probably be back home in Watford by the middle of term; friendless, grade-less and with a queue of people who couldn't wait to tell her how much too big for her boots she'd been for wanting to do a degree in the first place.

Ten minutes and then she'd get it together.

Jo had just hurled herself face down on to the bed when there was a sharp rap at her door. Precisely the knock her mother used when she was making a show of respecting Jo's privacy but intended to come in regardless.

Before Jo could shout, 'Hang on a sec,' let alone blow her nose and wipe tears from her eyes, the door had swung open and a small, pointed face with huge kohl-rimmed green eyes topped with spiky white-blond hair appeared around it.

'Hi. Not interrupting anything, am I?'

Without waiting for an answer, she clambered over Jo's bin bags and propped herself against the wardrobe, arms folded. One foot beat impatient time to the bass line of 'Smells Like Teen Spirit' rising from the floor below. She wore a beaten-up leather jacket over a faded floral minidress and her skinny tanned legs disappeared into eighteen-hole Doc Martens that reached almost to her knees. The boots were ostentatiously battered.

Tugging her Hello Kitty T-shirt down over her too-big boobs, Jo wished her hair wasn't mousy brown and held out of her eyes with a pink scrunchie. She had never felt so square in her life.

'I'm Nicci Gilbert,' the girl said. 'We're neighbours. I thought I'd brave the bar, but, I didn't really fancy walking in on my own. To be totally honest,' she said disarmingly, 'you're the only person I've met here, so I thought we could give each other some moral support.'

FOUR

'That's what these are meant to be,' Jo said, pulling a letter out of her bag. The once-pristine vellum was now scuffed, the midnight-blue ink smudged by tears.

She might have expensive highlights and a three-figure haircut where once the mousy-brown split ends and pink scrunchie had been. She might even have a five-times-a-week runner's body where once puppy fat had reigned, but right now Jo needed Nicci's moral support more than ever.

'Moral support?' Mona snorted, pulling her own letter, minus its envelope, from her jacket pocket. 'Only Nicci would do this and expect us to call it moral support.'

Ignoring Mona's comments, Jo stretched out her hand. 'Swap?'

'Hey, what about me?' Lizzie said, pouting. 'Just because you two think my bequest is a joke.'

Leaning over to hug Lizzie, Jo handed her letter to Mona and reluctantly took Lizzie's from her. It was true, though. She didn't really want to read Lizzie's letter. It was Mona's she wanted to get her hands on. Mona had to be mistaken, she just knew it.

Mona dropped into the leather chair vacated by David, while Jo perched on the edge of the sideboard and Lizzie sat on a crate. For several long seconds, the women read in silence; the shed was so quiet they could hear voices coming from the kitchen at the far end of the garden.

'Lizzie!' Jo snorted, breaking their concentration. 'I don't want to be mean, but leaving her garden to you – a woman who famously reduced a cactus to an explosion of dust – what was Nicci thinking?'

'I know.' Lizzie's laugh was mirthless. 'How did she put it? "I can't trust anyone else with it"? She might as well have said I'm the best of a bad lot!'

'Cheers,' Mona muttered without looking up. 'What does that make me, then?'

'That's not true,' Jo said, as if Mona hadn't spoken. 'Listen to this:

> 'I need to make sure the things I love, the people I love, look after one another . . . So I'm leaving you my garden. The most nurturing of my friends. I know you'll lavish on it the care that I tried to.'

Lizzie smiled. That much, at least, was true. She would try. But she couldn't guarantee she would succeed, not if her own garden was anything to go by. The twenty-by-twenty square of concrete (inappropriately and not entirely honestly described by the property developer as a 'private terrace ideal for outdoor entertaining') was lined with the corpses of slaughtered plants. Not even last summer's dead plants: most were relics from the summer before, when Lizzie had still believed her green fingers were in there somewhere, their potential just waiting to be discovered.

Returning her attention to Mona's letter, Lizzie gasped. 'Oh, Mo! This is excessive, even by Nicci's standards.'

'Told you,' Mona shrugged. 'Mind you,' she waved Jo's letter in the air, 'talking of excessive . . .'

Jo rolled her eyes. 'Tell me about it.'

'But if I read this right,' Lizzie continued, 'Nicci's left David to you because you're "too self-sufficient". Is that Nicci-speak for lonely?'

Avoiding her gaze, Mona shrugged.

'Let me see,' Jo held out her hand for the letter. 'It can't be that basic. That doesn't sound like Nicci at all. There must be some mistake.'

'There isn't,' Mona rounded on her. 'I know what that letter says – how many times d'you think I've read it? How many times have you read yours?'

'OK, OK.' Jo held up her hands in defeat.

'It is,' Lizzie said. 'Listen . . .' And she began to read aloud.

'The thing is, I worry about you. You're so . . . self-sufficient. Dan's growing up fast and I worry you're both alone. I know Greg broke your heart and then Neil stomped on it, but it's like you've given up. You're not interested in anyone else, in finding anyone new. It's over two years now. You have to stop mourning the loss of – don't hate me, but I have to be honest, it's not like you can kill me, after all! – the loss of something that never really was. You *must* move on. For your sake and Dan's. And I want to help you.'

'Help?' Mona spat. 'Interfere, more like.'

Jo threw her a look, but she didn't disagree. How could she?

'Well,' Mona said. 'Honestly, only Nicci could interfere from beyond the grave. And I don't know why *you're* sticking up for her. I mean, take a look at this.'

'I have,' Jo said. 'Believe me, I have.'

'Let me finish this first,' Lizzie interrupted. 'She says it. I can't believe she actually says it: "So I'm asking you to take care of David . . . the love of my life. The man I've been with my whole adult life . . . until death us do part."' Lizzie looked up, her eyes wide and glittering.

'Lizzie,' Mona said, 'did you think I'd made it up?'

'No, no. It's just . . . I . . .' Lizzie started reading again. "I can't believe I'm writing this, but I have to – death is about to part us. It will have parted us when you read this, and so I'm bequeathing my beloved David to you."'

'Give me that.' Jo snatched the letter and the others watched her eyes speed down the page.

'What the fuck?' she murmured as she reached the end. 'What. The. Fuck. Nicci, Nicci, Nicci, you can't just go leaving people to other people. What were you thinking?'

'Perhaps . . .' Lizzie put in cautiously, '. . . perhaps she wasn't? Perhaps . . . the drugs?' Her voice faltered.

'No!' Jo said fiercely. 'Don't say that. Much as we don't want this to be happening, Nicci *wanted* it. We have to . . . we have to try to find a way to cope with it.'

'And you?' Mona said, suppressing a shiver. The shed had not got any warmer in the half an hour they'd been sitting there. If anything the temperature had dropped. 'What are you going to do to "cope with it"?'

'No idea,' Jo said, heaving herself off the sideboard and perching on the arm of the chair beside Mona so she could see her own letter over her friend's shoulder. Not that she needed to. She knew the damn thing by heart. She'd read it so many times it was a wonder her eyes hadn't worn away the words.

'"You've been such a good godmother, which is why I need you to be more,"' she read aloud.

'More? What does that mean, "more"?' Lizzie asked.

'Read on.' Jo nodded to Mona.

Mona did, the words sounding wrong through the remnants of her Aussie twang.

'I've watched you over the years struggling to be a good stepmother to Si's boys, trying and not managing to have children of your own. Harrie and Charlie are going to need a mummy. And I'd like her to be you. Not literally, of course! But their emotional care I leave in your hands. Under your watchful eye my two girls will find the confidence to grow into fearless, talented, wonderful young women. The women I know they can be. The woman you are. The woman I always strove to be.

'But what's she asking, precisely?' Mona asked, when she'd finished reading. 'Surely she's not leaving you custody of Charlie and Harrie over David?'

'No,' Jo laughed. 'No,' she said again, with less certainty. 'At least . . . I don't *think* so.

'I think what she's saying, in her clumsy, bossy, Nicci way is, since, so far, I've been unable to have children of my own,' Jo paused and swallowed hard, 'I can have first dibs on hers. You know, Christmas, Easter . . . As if I don't have enough other people's children to keep me busy on public holidays with Sam and Tom.' Her smiled dropped. 'Not that I don't love Si's boys, because I do.'

'We know that, Jo,' Lizzie said gently. 'Don't we, Mo?' Mona nodded.

'She meant well,' Jo said at last. 'I'm sure of it. Nicci was a control freak but she was a good person. She meant well.'

Mona looked up. 'Did she, Jo? Do you really think so?'

Silence filled the shed and cold crept under the door and through the tiny gaps in the window frame. It was as cold now inside as out.

'I feel . . .' Lizzie said, looking around, taking in her friends sitting side by side and feeling inexplicably left out, '. . . like I hardly knew her at all. There were hundreds of people at church I didn't recognise, friends, maybe even family, I didn't know existed. And this, two hundred yards from the kitchen where we spent so much time.' She gestured at the shed. 'I didn't even know this was here, did you?'

'I thought it was all dirty pots, plastic trays and bags of compost,' Mona said, swiping her eyes with the back of her hand. 'Not another little world.'

'It's like she's gone off,' said Jo, getting up and brushing ineffectively at her skirt, 'and taken the map.' She sounded lost.

'She left us the letters,' Lizzie said.

'They're not a map,' Mona said crossly, stamping her feet against the cold. 'They're hardly even a clue.'

FIVE

It has to be done, Jo told herself. Someone has to sort through Nicci's clothes and that someone has to be us. David isn't in a fit state to do it.

The high street was gridlocked: a snarl-up caused by the usual mix of road works, double parking, plus an icy drizzle so depressing it felt like it had been falling for eight weeks straight.

Checking her watch, Jo sighed. Six thirty. Too early and too late. When she left work she'd thought she had plenty of time to spare. That was before it took forty-five minutes to drive less than a mile.

She wasn't due at Nicci's house until seven – it would always be Nicci's house to her – but the way the traffic dragged, one car crawling through the lights at a time, there was barely any point going home at all. Only she'd promised Si she'd put in an appearance because it was Wednesday, his night to have Sam and Tom. Si's sons from his first marriage stayed every Wednesday night, every other weekend and exactly half of all school holidays. That was the deal.

Supper wasn't an issue. Wednesday night was pizza night. The same order every week: chicken dippers, followed by medium, stuffed-crust pizzas with some unimaginably disgusting meat combo on top, and brownies and a tub of Ben & Jerry's Phish Food to finish. Cardiac arrest delivered on the back of a motorbike. Jo had long since stopped trying to force vegetables down the boys, although Si had taught her all his little tricks for concealing them. Domino's could set their clock by Sam and Tom's order. It didn't thrill their mother, but that was Si's battle. Jo had learnt that over the years. All Jo knew was carbs oiled the wheels of domestic harmony. Plus pizza straight out of the box seriously reduced the washing-up.

At what point did it become better not to show at all than to sprint in, wave to the boys and sprint out again? If she dropped home now, she would be late to Nicci's, and Jo had been the one who promised David they'd sit Charlie and Harrie, get them to bed, so he could have a night out without worrying.

It was hardly a night off if the sitters turned up half an hour late. Mind you, it was hardly a night off if you suspected one of the sitters had been left joint custody of your children.

Too late Jo noticed the news had finished and been replaced by one of those annoying comedy news programmes. Flicking through the channels, she found something classical she didn't recognise on Radio Three and something dance-y she didn't recognise on Radio One. She turned off the radio and groaned into the silence. When had she got so *old*?

But the silence was worse. It let her thoughts crowd back in.

Capsule Wardrobe *was* Nicci. That fact had smacked Jo in the face in the few short weeks since Nicci's death. In every meeting, phone call and email, all Jo could see was Nicci's absence. It showed in the eyes of the loyal customers;

in the pity of the suppliers tiptoeing around her, in their concern.

Oh, the company couldn't run without Jo, there was no question of that. Jo was the organiser, the administrator, the accountant. She was the person who kept the show on the road, day in, day out. But it was Nicci's innate sense of style that made Capsule Wardrobe what it was. Jo didn't begin to know how to keep it going without her. And yet she had to keep telling the others it was going to be all right. The internet business was thriving. The name was strong, their reputation excellent, these things would live on.

Kelly, Nicci's right-hand woman, was trying – trying really hard – to fill Nicci's shoes. Sitting up late into the night on her laptop, scouring the ready-to-wear shows look by look, noting the key pieces she thought would work for Capsule Wardrobe's loyal core of customers. Items that nodded to the new season's trends but would last far longer than that, making their three- or even four-figure price tag vaguely justifiable, cost per wear. Kelly was there each morning, hovering in Jo's doorway like a puppy desperate to be stroked. Wanting praise for her list of looks, her trend notes, her buying suggestions. And every morning Jo praised her, and saw relief soften Kelly's face. But the truth was, Jo wasn't convinced.

She couldn't put her finger on the problem. She certainly didn't know how to solve it. But despite Kelly's enthusiasm and hard work, she just didn't have Nicci's taste; Nicci's ability to sling on a moth-eaten leopard-print coat, belt it tight, and look like Liz Taylor in her golden years, not Bet Lynch in her Rovers years.

Kelly just didn't have it. Worse, Jo was pretty sure she couldn't learn it.

When Nicci was there, Kelly could take her cues from her, but Nicci wasn't there now, was she?

And then there were Si and the boys, and the attention they deserved, but that she knew they hadn't been getting from her lately. Not since it became clear how ill Nicci was.

And then there were Charlie and Harrie.

Nicci had meant well, Jo was convinced of that. Until the cancer took hold, Nicci had watched helplessly her friend's growing anguish as first one, then two, then three attempts at IVF failed. And now . . . what? Who knew? Not Jo, and not Si. They'd both steered well clear of the subject since Nicci's cancer was declared terminal.

Jo adored her goddaughters, but seriously . . . ?

Behind her some jerk leant on his horn. Lifting her head, she saw the four-by-four in front had rolled forward a few feet, leaving a patch of rain-darkened tarmac. There were still four cars between her and the red lights. Big whoop. What difference did it make if she moved now or in five minutes?

In her rear-view mirror, the middle-aged guy in his BMW made a show of drumming his hands impatiently on the steering wheel. It was too dark to see clearly, but she just knew that his expression screamed 'women drivers'.

Tosser, she thought as she eased her foot off the brake to allow her Golf to close the gap between it and the car in front.

Charlie and Harrie . . . Three weeks had passed and still Jo hadn't said a word to Si, let alone David. She didn't know where to start, with either of them.

Si was a good guy. A keeper, Nicci called him. The kind of guy who knew what to do on a long, empty Sunday. Hardworking, reliable and unfailingly kind. Still sexy at forty-five, twice-weekly swimming sessions ensuring his body was firm. Plus, he still had his own hair, and lots of it. She loved him, baggage and all.

He knew there was something going on. 'What's wrong?'

he'd asked, a couple of nights ago after they'd made exhausted love, when the lights were out and she hoped he'd fallen asleep. She let him think it was work; that she was worried about what would happen to Capsule Wardrobe. That was true, as far as it went. All their savings were in the company: big money, by their standards. And no pension. Capsule Wardrobe *was* her pension. But that wasn't all. Far from it. The IVF had gone on a backburner when Nicci became sick, but now she was dead there was no excuse not to get back on the wagon. Or not. Three strikes, they'd promised themselves. Three strikes and then they'd stop. But neither of them had expected it to come to that. Not really.

And then there was the other madness. The *Mona and David* thing.

What the hell had Nicci been thinking?

In her darker moments, when Jo woke at three or four or five and couldn't get back to sleep, she wondered whether Nicci had been thinking at all; whether the cancer and chemo . . . but no, that was too hideous to consider. And yet, even for Nicci – and Jo had a high tolerance for Nicci's plots, seeing them as endearingly hare-brained rather than Machiavellian – this whole letter thing was extreme.

The traffic lights changed and the Golf rolled forward. Beyond the lights a comparatively empty road beckoned. One more car and she was on her way.

If she were honest, Jo was dreading this evening. Not just because she hadn't seen David to talk to since the funeral, but also because the idea of sorting through Nicci's clothes felt wrong. The mere thought of it made Jo feel like an intruder. It was so . . . final. If Nicci was letting them touch her clothes there was no escaping it. She was gone.

The first time she'd read Nicci's letter Jo hadn't noticed the P.S. tacked on the end. The enormity of the rest of the letter had overshadowed it. But then David called and asked her when she wanted to start dealing with Nicci's clothes, and it dawned on her – not that if he knew about the clothes, he might know about everything else too – but that every item, and there were thousands, had to be sorted into one of three lots.

CHUCK: Far from being junk, these were the valuable but dispensable pieces – and there were plenty – that should be sold to raise money for the girls' futures.

CHERISH: The pieces with sentimental value to be kept for the girls as a kind of wearable memory box.

CHARITY: Where the rest went. Nicci, being Nicci, had specified charities: Oxfam, the NSPCC, Macmillan Cancer Support, Refuge, Safe Shelter; those specialising in children and cancer, mainly. Although Jo had been surprised by the inclusion of Refuge, and had never even heard of the last.

Well, now that task was upon her and there was nothing for it but to gather her strength and face it.

SIX

'Not early, am I?' Lizzie asked. The confusion on David's face when he opened the front door made her wonder if she had the wrong time, or even the wrong day. Instinctively, she glanced at her watch: ten past seven. That was Lizzie, always early or late. Try as she might, she could never just be on time.

Usually she would have thrown her arms around him, hugged him hello. But since letter-gate it felt wrong. Instead, she stood on tiptoe to peck his cheek and stepped back when he took a second too long to respond.

'No,' David said, eventually. 'You're not.'

He looked, if anything, worse than the last time she had seen him. His usually pink skin was sallow, the bags under his eyes tinged with grey. 'It's just . . . I was expecting Jo first.'

'She isn't here yet?'

Before he could answer, a shriek came from the far end of the house, followed by a crash and a wail.

David glanced over his shoulder. 'I better go and see . . . Come in.'

Before Lizzie had a chance to ask how he was coping,

David had vanished into the kitchen. Not that she needed to ask. One look told her he wasn't.

'Why don't I take over?' she offered when she reached the kitchen, and the full chaos Harrie and Charlie had wrought on their bedtime milk and cookies became clear. Crumbs and puddles splattered the oak table. The solid wood worktops were thick with dirty dishes, open cereal packets and the debris of an earlier meal – or two. And the toddlers were hardly to blame for that.

Lizzie headed purposefully towards the sink. 'I'll start on this while I wait for Jo,' she said. Anything was better than this awkward hovering.

David made to protest but Lizzie waved him away. 'I thought you were going out,' she said. 'Why don't you get off and let me sort this?'

David hesitated. 'I was . . . am . . . it's just . . .'

Still he loitered. Surely he wasn't planning to stay home after all?

'Off you go then,' Lizzie said, channelling her mother in the days when her mother could still strike the fear of God into cold callers, and hoping he couldn't hear the panic in her voice. This evening was going to be hard enough without David here. 'The reinforcements have arrived.'

At least one-third of the reinforcements was lurking around the corner, sheltering from the rain.

'Hurry up,' Mona muttered, adjusting her inadequate umbrella so the drips stopped soaking her back and spattered her boots and jeans instead. It was only five minutes since she'd seen Lizzie park and go inside. But, thanks to the cold and the wet, it felt far longer.

Through the downpour she stared at the solid Victorian end terrace and felt a familiar sense of isolation. Nicci and David had bought the house as part of a probate deal eight years earlier, soon after Mona returned from Australia. 'In need of modernisation,' the estate agent had said. Understatement of the year. 'Buy it while it's still standing,' Mona had muttered the first time the proud new owners showed their friends around. That was before the builders and plumbers and electricians had transformed it into the twenty-first-century family home of Nicci's dreams.

Mona had spent endless Sundays and bank holidays there in the intervening years, but still she felt like an outsider. It was entirely her own fault, she knew. Nicci, Lizzie and Jo had been such a tight-knit group when she'd answered their ad for a fourth person to share their student house that she'd never felt totally part of it. She hadn't helped herself, of course, by heading off to satisfy her wanderlust as soon as graduation forced everyone to decide how they were going to live their lives. It was in Australia, as far away from home as possible, she hoped to find the person she wanted to be.

Instead she found heartbreak. Although it hadn't looked that way at first.

Temping by day, Mona learnt yoga by night, which was where she met Callie, the instructor. And through Callie, her brother, Greg. Tall, blond, oozing confidence. As unreconstructed as it was possible to be. One look and, for the first time, Mona fell in love and lust so hard she barely caught her breath. Pregnancy and marriage, in that order, took her by surprise, followed, almost as rapidly, by rumours of Greg's 'hook-ups'. At first, she refused to believe the man she loved would do that to her; at second, she turned a blind eye for the sake of their baby boy.

Until he left her.

He. Left. Her. For a blonde waitress called Justine. Just one of many things she omitted to tell Nicci and Jo and Lizzie. Instead, she returned to London, aged twenty-eight, and with nothing to show for her travels but a newfound passion for yoga and a wide-eyed five-year-old boy with a *Star Wars* rucksack, who looked nothing like her and everything like the man the memory of whom she was running away from.

Glancing irritably at her watch, Mona stamped her feet against the damp, spraying water on to her jeans. Seven twenty – what the hell were they doing in there? And, come to that, where was Jo?

The rain had slowed, but by now the bottom half of her jeans were soaked. Mona knew she should just go in, face David, get it over with. But she couldn't make herself. Just as she hadn't been able to make herself tell Nicci about Neil. Though there were many times she'd wanted to.

Neil Osborne. If she'd felt distanced from her friends before, it was Neil who sealed her alienation.

'Because Sunday afternoons were family time, which, for Mona and Dan, meant long lazy roast lunches around Nicci's big oak table. And for Mona Thomas's lover meant roasts at home. With his wife, Tracy (although Mona did her best not to give the woman a name, just as she didn't want to see her face). Tracy, she forced herself to think, and his three teenage daughters.

So it was always just Mona and Dan. Mona's lover was never there to top up her glass or squeeze her knee under the table at some private joke; never there to kick a ball around David's back garden or talk sport in the kitchen.

But then, to be fair, Neil had never been invited.

It wasn't that Nicci and David excluded him, more that they didn't know he existed. None of them did.

They knew he *had* existed. To begin with, they'd even managed sisterly empathy. 'He wants to have his cake and eat you,' Jo said, thrilled at her own witticism. Mona had just confessed she'd fallen for a married man, with all the usual qualifications: *I didn't know to begin with . . . She doesn't*

41

understand him . . . He's not happy . . . They're only together for the sake of the children . . .

'Mona,' Nicci said, as Jo and Lizzie rolled their eyes.

And they all chorused their favourite line from their all-time favourite movie, 'He's never going to leave her.'

Mona's mouth had twisted as it always did when she was a little bit hurt, a little bit guilty, but didn't want to show it.

'You're right,' she said, forcing a smile and channelling Carrie Fisher as she knew she was required to do. 'You're right. You're right. I know you're right.'

But that was three years ago. More. What they didn't know was that he was still around. They thought Mona had dumped him because that was what she'd told them. It wasn't a lie, exactly; more a lie of omission. She'd intended to end it, putting it off each time she saw him, but then, out of the blue, he dumped her, and to her surprise and horror she'd thought her heart was going to shatter all over again.

In the end, it was easier to let the others think she'd been the one to do the dumping. And when they'd been so pleased they cracked open a bottle of Nicci's favourite pink Laurent Perrier to celebrate, Mona knew she'd been right. Better by far than telling the truth, which was that she'd do anything – anything at all – to have him back.

Despite the fact she'd been on the receiving end of a cheating husband herself, and knew precisely how it felt to be left.

So when Neil turned up at the fashionable organic restaurant where she was manager, claiming he couldn't live without her – literally, that was what he'd said: 'Mona, I can't live without you' – well, Mona just 'forgot' to mention it the next time she saw her friends. And the next time, and the next. And because there'd always been a part of herself she'd kept private, the deception hadn't even felt that unnatural. And then it felt too late, like she'd missed her chance to tell them the truth. And now . . . well, now she had.

The sound of an engine igniting brought Mona to, just in time to step back into the shadow of a six-foot garden wall as David's people carrier appeared, indicated and turned in the opposite direction. Nearly seven thirty. And still no Jo. Lizzie was going to be livid.

SEVEN

'Where the hell have you been?' Lizzie had barely opened the front door before she started in on Mona. 'It's nearly half-past!'

'You want the honest answer?' Shaking the rain from her umbrella, Mona leant it against the wall of the porch.

'Would I like it?'

'Doubt it,' Mona said.

'Then forget it.' Turning her back on her friend, Lizzie marched back to the kitchen. Charlie and Harrie were charging around in increasingly small circles, but they were now washed and wearing pyjamas. The kitchen table still looked like a battle in a biscuit factory, but the washing-up was done and the wood worktops were, at least, visible.

'I was hiding round the corner like the pathetic coward I am,' Mona said, pointing to the drenched lower half of her jeans, 'waiting for David to leave. I just didn't bank on a monsoon.'

'Shhhh.' Lizzie's gaze flicked towards two pairs of small but flapping ears. 'You could have texted me; at least waited somewhere dry. I'd have let you know when the coast was clear.'

'Where's Jo?' asked Mona, hanging her damp jacket over the back of one of the mismatched kitchen chairs.

'Stuck in traffic, she said. And she had to nip home. Should be here any minute.'

'Probably avoiding you know who too,' Mona concluded, turning her attention to the tiny hands now clinging to her wet legs. 'Hello, my lovelies.' Sweeping Charlie and Harrie up, one under each arm, she spun them around until their squeals pierced Lizzie's ears.

'When did you get so big?' Mona groaned, setting them down with a kiss each.

'Again!' Harrie insisted.

'Don't. You'll make them si—'

'Just one,' said Mona, spinning on the spot.

'Mo . . .' Lizzie protested.

'Shouldn't you two monsters be in bed?' Mona asked when she'd stopped.

'Nooo!' Harrie shrieked.

'No bed!' That was Charlie. 'Auntie Lizzie say no bed.'

'That doesn't sound like Auntie Lizzie to me.' Mona raised an eyebrow.

'Did!'

'It's true.' Lizzie waved an open bottle of Sauvignon Blanc at Mona.

'Just a small one.'

Lizzie raised her eyebrows. 'No small glasses in this house.'

'As it comes then.'

'We agreed, remember? It's for them, after all. They should be there for the ceremonial opening of the wardrobe.'

'Wardrobe!' Harrie and Charlie shrieked, running around the kitchen again. 'Wardrobe!'

'Do you feel weird?' Mona asked half an hour later when they had transferred to the large bedroom that took up the

45

entire front half of the first floor, where Nicci had spent most of the last six months of her life, when she hadn't been in hospital.

'Not *weird*, exactly,' Lizzie lowered her voice. 'Just, you know, empty. Like a piece is missing.'

'I do, really weird.'

'Well, you would, wouldn't you?' Jo said, walking in with a bottle of pink Laurent Perrier and three fresh glasses. She set the glasses on the bedside table, slit the foil and began unfurling the wire.

'Why me more than anyone else?'

Jo smiled grimly, although she didn't feel much like laughing. If a year ago someone had told her they'd be standing here, the three of them . . . *Three* . . . She shook herself.

'Pot-kettle,' Mona said. 'And anyway, isn't it about time you mentioned your little bequest?'

'Stop it, you two,' Lizzie said. 'Little ears.'

But the little ears were shut. Their owners fast asleep, curled up, their dark blond heads like inverted commas on the pillows of David's bed. Thumbs firmly in place.

'Anyway, I didn't mean that,' Mona replied, prowling the room, unable to settle. 'I meant this whole scenario. Last time we were here . . .'

Nobody needed to say it. The last time was the night before Nicci was moved to the hospice. The night she said her real goodbyes.

Easing the cork from the champagne as silently as possible, Jo poured three glasses and handed one each to Mona and Lizzie. 'I thought we should do this properly . . . for Nicci and for the girls,' she said. 'But I think we've already lost our audience. I'm sorry I missed them awake. How did they seem?'

'OK. A bit hyper. But I guess that's better than the alternative. Better than David, anyway.' Lizzie stared pointedly

46

at Mona, but her friend was making a show of rearranging the large cardboard boxes lined up along the bedroom wall. Each had a scribbled yellow Post-it note attached: the first 'Chuck', the second 'Cherish', the third 'Charity'.

'Do you want to do the honours?' Lizzie pointed to the mirrored double doors that led to the walk-in wardrobe.

'No, it's OK,' Jo said.

'I'm not doing it,' Mona put in, too hastily. 'It's all yours.'

Anyone would have thought they were opening a long-sealed family crypt, not the spot-lit inner sanctum that housed Nicci's fashion collection, Lizzie thought.

She sighed, but she didn't move. She didn't want to do it. Didn't see why she should. It wasn't as if she was Number One Friend, anyway. That was Jo's domain. But Lizzie had always been the tidier-upper, the smoother-over, the peace-maker. Where Nicci had been the leader, forging ahead with plans and ideas, Lizzie had always trailed at the back, shutting doors behind them, unable to come up with a good reason not to be the one to clean up after the others. She even helped mop up the trail of emotional devastation a much younger Nicci had left in her wake.

'Looks like it's down to me then,' Jo said. Positioning herself by the double doors, her right hand on the handle, she lifted her glass stiffly. 'To Nicci,' she said, raising it higher and pulling the door open.

'To Nicci,' Lizzie and Mona echoed.

Ceiling-set spots had come on automatically as the doors opened, lighting the eight-by-twelve room lined with rails, one row of full height on the right, two of half height on the left. A wall of drawers faced them, and a double row of shoe shelves skirted the room from floor level. More shelves piled high with bags and hatboxes lined the top. There, any suggestion of order stopped. The room was stuffed.

'I had no idea it was such a mess!' Lizzie gasped. 'I was

47

expecting, you know, neat colour-coded piles. The law of the wardrobe, copyright Nicci Morrison.'

'Are you telling me,' said Mona slowly, 'that when it came to her own clothes the queen of clean was the world's biggest hoarder?'

Jo shrugged. 'Looks that way.'

'How the hell did she collect so many?'

'It was her life's work,' Jo said, 'her passion. You know that. Her job and her hobby. Some people collect books or works of art, Nicci collected clothes. This isn't even the whole lot. David says there are about eight suitcases in the attic, maybe more. He reckons there's nothing of value in them; Nicci was too worried about moths and damp for that. We should have a quick sort through just to be sure. But I reckon those can go straight to the charity shop.'

'The question is,' said Mona, putting her glass on Nicci's dressing table and joining Lizzie in the doorway, 'where the hell do we start?'

'Knowing Nicci,' Lizzie said, 'there's an arcane filing system. Nothing as straightforward as "what goes with what".'

'Alphabetical by designer?' Mona suggested.

Jo scanned the wardrobe. The air was far cooler in here than in the bedroom. On the wall beside her, just inside the door, a thermostat was set at fifteen degrees Celsius. Typical.

'Good guess,' Jo said. 'But I don't think so. It's too much of a mishmash. If all the McQueen, for instance, was in one place, the Prada in another, the rails would look more uniform.'

Mona frowned. 'By style?'

'I've got it!' Lizzie announced loudly, glancing over her shoulder at the sleeping girls almost before the words were out of her mouth. 'It's autobiographical!'

'Don't be daft,' said Jo. 'That would be chaos.'

'And your point is?' Mona laughed. 'Lizzie's right. Look.'

In the left-hand corner, tucked at the back, was a pair of

beaten-up Doc Martens, the fluro-pink that graffitied them now almost invisible. Above them hung a familiar cracked and faded leather jacket.

Jo blinked and stared hard at the thick-pile carpet, determined not to let the others see her cry. Tears rolled down the side of her cheeks, dampening her neck.

'I guess we start at the beginning then,' Lizzie said, taking charge. Pulling a small wooden stepladder from its place at the back of the closet, she lifted a yellowing hatbox from the uppermost shelf, set it on the floor and removed the lid.

'Omigod,' she said, wrinkling her nose as she stepped back from the box. A piece of something unquestionably dead was suspended between her thumb and forefinger. 'Gross. Can you believe she kept this?'

'What is it?' Mona asked.

'Dead bunny,' Lizzie said. 'It was dead as a doornail then, and it's even deader now. And it smells rank.'

'Bin!' Mona wretched. 'Where it should have gone long ago. Why haven't we got an option for bin? I'll go and get a black bag.'

'You can't,' Jo said. Taking the rabbit fur shrug from Lizzie's hand, she laid it carefully on the bed and stood in front of it, as if guarding it from Mona's malign intent. 'It's cherish, definitely cherish. Is there a peach satin slip in that box, too?'

Peering through folds of aged tissue paper, Lizzie nodded.

As soon as she saw the slip she remembered exactly what Jo had known the second she saw the shrug. Almost reverentially Lizzie handed the delicate fabric to Jo, who folded it neatly and put it on top of the shrug.

Mona watched, her expression one of revulsion. 'If you apply the principle to everything,' she said, 'that if-Nicci-kept-it-it's-significant, then the chuck-stroke-sell pile and the charity shop pile are going to be non-existent.'

'It won't apply to everything,' Jo said. 'But if it's twenty years old and has no obvious value – like, it's not the first piece of McQueen she saved up for, or those original Vivier shoes she bought in a junk shop on The Lanes in our second year, or her Helmut Lang suits – then it has a different value. A sentimental value. Like this.'

'Why that particularly?' Mona asked.

'You must remember?' Jo said.

She could still see Nicci in the living room of their rundown student house, drumming her newly graffitied docs impatiently while they waited for Lizzie to decide what to wear. 'It's what she was wearing the night we . . . The night she met David.'

EIGHT

The Rabbit Fur Shrug
Sussex University, Brighton, 1994

The evening hadn't got off to the best of starts.

'Lizzie, c'mon!' Nicci bellowed up the stairs. 'We're gonna be late.'

Silence.

Late wasn't Nicci's thing. She affected casual insouciance but she was scrupulously punctual. Lizzie was always late, a reaction to her mum, who would always rather arrive two hours early than be two minutes late. And this involved clothes. Clothes and Lizzie just didn't go together.

'Just wear the bloody 501s!' Nicci yelled.

More silence.

'I don't know why you're bothering.' Mona stuck her wet head, her arm and a single shoulder around the bathroom door. 'You know how she gets.'

Nicci did. They all did. Lizzie was at war with her wardrobe.

'Why don't you just go and style her?' Jo suggested.

Jo sat in the doorway between the hall and living room, a plastic cup of cheap white wine between her knees. She was wearing jeans. Mona and Jo both were. All three of them did, usually. Only Nicci

51

refused, claiming they made her look even more like a boy. They didn't, but who were Jo, Lizzie and Mona to argue? Nicci understood clothes in a way no one else did. Jo liked them – sometimes – more than clothes liked her, but she didn't know how to play them. How to make them do her bidding.

Nicci was wearing her beaten-up DMs, with torn fishnets and one of the many vintage underslips she'd bought from a local flea market, topped off with a rabbit fur shrug she'd brought home earlier that day. The row about how disrespectful Nicci's dead jacket was to Mona's vegetarian sensibilities had just finished, only to segue into this.

If I didn't love Nicci so much I'd be eaten up with jealousy, Jo thought. But she did. Nicci was Nicci. Whatever 'it' was, she had it. She could pull it off, black bra showing beneath the slip and all. That was just how life was.

'Finally!'

Jo looked up at the sound of Nicci's voice. Lizzie was hurrying down the stairs in her usual uniform of 501s and outsized man's shirt.

'You look great,' Nicci said.

But Lizzie obviously didn't feel great. She looked defeated. In the battle of Lizzie vs. her wardrobe, Lizzie had lost. Again.

They were so late they decided to skip the pub altogether. They'd drunk a bottle of the cheapest white table wine Tesco had to offer before they left the house, and had another two bottles in their bags so they went straight to the house party. The thud of the bass met them before they could turn the corner into the right street, and pissed students were already spilling onto the pavement.

The girls were so far behind everyone else on the alcohol-and-illegal-substance front that they almost kept walking.

It was Lizzie who saw him first. Not that his old-school purple Mohican was easy to miss. But in the dark, with the fug of B&H

and dope smoke clouding the ceiling, and the pulsing beat of The Prodigy destroying the bits of her concentration alcohol hadn't already wasted, it was a miracle she noticed anything at all.

Lizzie found him in the kitchen, beside a keg of Dutch cooking lager, set up on the draining board.

If she was honest his look intimidated her, but between the fierce hair and torn leather jacket were kind brown eyes.

'Want some?'

After glancing over her shoulder to make sure he really was talking to her, Lizzie nodded. 'Four cups, please.'

'The party that bad?

She grinned. 'I've been to worse.'

He grinned back. 'Me too.'

When Lizzie fought her way back to Nicci's corner, plastic cups of something warm and flat balanced between her hands, she looked different, somehow. Glowy.

'You look different. Have you been smoking?' Nicci asked, extracting one of the cups from Lizzie's hands.

'No!' Lizzie yelped. 'You know I don't.'

But Nicci was right. She felt different too.

'What is it then?' Jo said. 'You met someone? Fast work, O'Hara. You've only been gone ten minutes.'

'Maybe,' Lizzie said, but even in the dark they could see her blush.

'You left one behind.' The voice behind them made Lizzie start. She jumped, knocking Nicci's hand and sending warm lager sloshing across her peach satin slip. 'Bollocks,' everyone said in unison.

'Shit,' said the guy with the purple Mohican. 'I didn't mean to . . . I mean, I was just trying . . .'

'Yeah,' Nicci said.

'I'm David,' he added helplessly.

His face was in direct contrast to his hair. If his hair was all aggression and sharp edges, his face was round and friendly, his eyes

53

soft and brown. He looked genuinely mortified. 'Whose is this?'
He held up the final plastic cup and Jo claimed it.

'I'm Lizzie,' Lizzie said. 'And these are my housemates, Jo,
Mona and Nicci.'

In the time it took her to give their names Lizzie saw it happen.
She'd seen it before. She was used to it. They all were. So used it,
she didn't even mind any more. Not usually. It wasn't as if Nicci
did it on purpose.

David smiled warmly at the others but his gaze returned to
Nicci, who was staring back, her mouth slightly open. Lizzie started
to say something, anything, to capture his attention, but it was
pointless. She could have jumped up and down between Nicci and
David and neither would have noticed. She knew the warning signs,
but this wasn't just a sign, it was hazard lights and sirens and all
the makings of a ten-car pile-up.

'You're not at uni, are you?' Mona asked. 'I mean, I haven't
seen you around.'

'I know Phil, the guy whose party it is,' David said, dragging
his attention away from Nicci.

'Mad Phil?' Lizzie said.

David nodded, his gaze never leaving Nicci. 'I'm doing archi-
tecture at King's. Just finished my placement. And just broke up
with my girlfriend. Phil said there'd be some fit birds here so I
should come down.'

'They must have left already,' Jo said. Boom boom!

Lizzie rolled her eyes and stuck her elbow in Jo's ribs. Not funny,
she mouthed.

'What course do you do?' David was saying, but it wasn't a
general question.

'Eng lit. No idea why.' Only Nicci answered.

'What's wrong with English?' he asked.

'Nothing. I'm just more interested in fashion.'

'C'mon,' Jo said, grabbing Lizzie's elbow, 'let's go and steal someone
else's bottle.'

'But I just got—' Lizzie protested. She knew it was futile.

'Lizzie,' Jo hissed as Mona took Lizzie's other elbow. 'We. Are. Not. Wanted. Here.'

And imperceptibly, Lizzie drooped.

One of them met a bloke, then the bloke met Nicci and that was it. It wasn't that Nicci was a babe. Mona had the model body, Jo had better boobs and Lizzie had the wild Pre-Raphaelite curls. But whatever it was Nicci did have, men wanted it. The path to their student house was littered with the broken egos of Brighton's straight male population. And some of the gay ones too.

NINE

Seven fifty-five p.m. Mona glanced at her mobile, double-checked the clock on her DVD and sighed. Whichever clock she looked at it was still seven fifty-five.

She wasn't sure which made her more tense: the fact Neil said he'd phone between seven and eight, and it was now precariously close to being clear that call was not going to come at all (oh, there'd be a good reason, there always was); or that in five minutes Jo would be knocking on David's front door and doing what they'd all reluctantly agreed had to be done. Asking him the big questions. Had he had a letter too? If so, what did his say? Had he been in on this crazy plan all along? And if not, what was he going to do about it now he did know?

'Daniel!' Mona yelled. 'Have you done your maths homework?'

Silence. If you could call the drone of computer-generated gunfire and the grinding gears of video-game tanks, silence.

'Daniel!'

Silence, literal this time.

'*What?*'

'Homework? Have you done it?'

'Yes, Mum. Ages ago.'

'When, *ages ago*?'

Dan, all five foot ten and counting, filled the doorway. The flat was too small for them now. Too small for him, certainly. Barely fourteen and already four inches taller than Mona. Every inch his father's son. Physically, at least.

'After tea and before now. Maths *and* physics. Do you want to see it?'

It was a dare, not a question. He knew she wouldn't; especially not physics. English or history she might have taken him up on. Funny how his homework was never English or history.

She shook her head and watched his back – spookily familiar and scarily alien – return to his boxroom.

Once *Coronation Street* was finished, Lizzie dabbled with a documentary about obese babies on Channel 4 and now she was trying to care about *University Challenge*.

When Jo first volunteered to talk to David, Lizzie had to admit she'd been relieved. But now . . . she felt . . . what did she feel? Guilty, she supposed, for copping out. But also a bit excluded. This affected her too. All right, so Nicci had left her a patch of land (albeit right outside David's kitchen window). But still, it wasn't the same. The others had been left *people*.

'Picasso,' Lizzie guessed. Just as the boy onscreen said, 'Van Gogh.'

'No, it's Picasso.'

Lizzie high-fived the air. Still got it.

No matter how many times Lizzie looked at her mobile, balanced on the arm of the sofa, it refused to ring. Jo should be there by now. She'd promised to call as soon as she could, but that might not be for ages.

Idly, Lizzie flicked through the channels, ending back at *University Challenge*.

Gerry had gone straight to squash from a late meeting; he wouldn't be back until gone ten, maybe eleven. Perhaps if she texted Jo now she could go with her, be her wing woman. Lizzie could be at David's in ten minutes if she left now. Snatching up her mobile, she found Jo's number and clumsily typed, *Want some moral support?* She pressed Send, before she could think better of it.

Eight ten p.m.

David wouldn't mind Jo being ten minutes late. Since Jo hadn't warned him she was coming, he wouldn't even know. She hadn't told him because that way she could still chicken out. And he couldn't pretend it wasn't convenient.

She'd come straight from Capsule Wardrobe's offices, taking advantage of Parents' Evening at Si's school to get in some extra hours. She was knackered, and worried about last month's profits. The new season had been in full swing for two months now, but business was still slow. Part of her wanted to put it down to the weather, but who was she kidding? They'd had a sub-zero spring before; it hadn't affected sales then.

Smoothing down her sweater dress and tucking the hems of her skinny jeans into her ankle boots, Jo tried to gauge her reflection in the door's glass panel. Her hair had been thrown into a ponytail hours ago, her roots were long overdue and, apart from red lipstick reapplied in the rear-view mirror two minutes earlier, her makeup hadn't been retouched since breakfast. She knew she didn't look great.

It was now or never, she decided. Do it, or go home and beat yourself up for the rest of the evening. As she raised her hand to ring David's old-fashioned bell, Jo felt her mobile vibrate in her pocket. Damn. She was tempted to ignore it, but just in case it was Si she turned away from the front door and checked her screen.

Want some moral support?

Jo sighed. She didn't know which was worse, Mona not attempting to disguise her relief when Jo volunteered, or Lizzie's indecision. *Come or don't come,* she had wanted to say, *but make your bloody mind up*. The fact was, Lizzie didn't want to be there. She just didn't want to not be there either.

It had to be a charity, the local MP canvassing or a neighbour looking for a lost cat/apologising for noisy teenagers/wanting to borrow a parking permit. Nobody else knocked unannounced at quarter-past eight on a Monday night around here. If he ignored them, David decided, they'd probably go away. He couldn't be bothered with being neighbourly tonight. It had been one of those days. Another one of those days. He just wanted to sit in the dark and wait for it to end.

The doorbell rang again. Its ancient chords hitting precisely the right note to pierce his low-level headache. Another ring like that and the girls would be awake.

'Fuck off,' David groaned aloud.

Could his day get any worse? The girls had taken for ever to go down tonight, demanding story after story and then complaining in unison that he didn't do the voices the way Mummy did.

To which there was no answer. Parent fail.

David knew they weren't saying it to hurt him. They weren't even three years old, for God's sake. And they were hurting too. They didn't understand where Mummy had gone. Even though, as coached by the child psychologist his mother had insisted he consult ('She's an expert on child bereavement, you're not'), he'd taken Harrie and Charlie to the funeral. And, to be honest, he didn't understand why Mummy had gone away either.

The bell rang again. Whoever it was had no plans to go

away. It was a miracle it hadn't woken Charlie and Harrie already.

'All right,' he muttered as he dragged himself from the kitchen table. 'You win. I'm coming.'

'Look, just—'

David was in full flight as he flung open the front door. He stopped, as if looking for someone else behind Jo. 'Jo . . . I . . . you didn't . . . I wasn't expecting you.'

He didn't exactly look thrilled to see her.

From the far end of the hall she could hear the low buzz of voices competing for airspace. Someone in the kitchen. She strained to hear . . . someone in the living room, too.

'I'm sorry,' Jo said. 'I haven't seen you for a week or so. I dropped by on the off-chance. I should have called first, to check you didn't have visitors.'

'Visitors? I don't . . . ?'

Pushing gently past him, Jo went to investigate. The door to the living room was open and a documentary was on the TV. In the kitchen a poet was saying something she clearly thought profound on Radio Four. An iPod played softly from the dining table.

The kitchen was a mess again. One of the spotlights over the sink had blown since her last visit. It looked like the washing-up hadn't been done in days. And there were still bunches of dead flowers from relatives David claimed not even to know on the windowsill.

'Oh God.' She turned to him. She wanted to take him in her arms and hug him, but everything about his manner said no.

'That bad?' she said.

'Worse.'

Shoulders sagging, David shoved his hands in his pockets. He looked about twelve. Boyishly handsome, utterly lost.

There was a splosh of wine on the front of his work shirt. It didn't look recent.

'I can't stand the silence,' he said finally. 'Before Nicci . . . when she was here, her constant racket used to drive me nuts, all the music and chat – you lot always here, and when you weren't you were constantly on the phone. Never a moment's peace, never just us. You have no idea how hard it was to get that woman on her own. But now . . .' he shrugged, looking helpless. His eyes brimmed, the long lashes that Jo had always thought wasted on a man, glistened. 'Now I can't stand it, Jo.'

'You should get an au pair.' It sounded pointless even to her.

'A *what*?'

She could see David thinking, *How did we get from there to here?*

'I just mean it might help having another person around. With the girls, I mean, and . . .' Jo couldn't help glancing at the washing-up, a pile of clothes sprawling on the floor by the washing machine . . .

'You mean the mess?' He forced a grin. 'I have a cleaner. I just gave her a few weeks off. I couldn't, you know, cope with all her . . .' he grimaced, '. . . sympathy. The nanny's bad enough.'

Jo nodded, waited for him to continue.

'I don't think I could stand having someone around full time,' David said eventually. 'An au pair, I mean. Living here, with us. Not yet, anyway. It would be too much.'

'Tea?' Jo waved the kettle at him. 'Or something stronger?'

David grimaced again. 'Better be tea. I already tried something stronger. It just gave me a headache.'

The phone rang just as the kettle began to boil. Instinctively, Jo reached for it, as if it were her own. *Sorry*, she mouthed, seeing the expression that flashed across David's face, and held it out to him.

61

He shook his head.

'Hello?' she said, and paused. 'Hello? Hello?

No one there,' she shrugged a few seconds later. 'Must have been a wrong number.

'That's odd,' David said. 'Had a few of those lately. Wonder if it's a call centre or there's a problem at the exchange. Anyway,' he added, watching her move around his kitchen as if it were her own, 'I'm guessing you didn't just drop in on the off-chance. What is this? Project check-up on David? Or something else?'

'Does it matter?' Jo said.

David said nothing. Instead he waited for her to turn to look at him. He'd been wondering when she'd come. And he'd known it would be her. Jo was the doer, the efficient one. Lizzie was too beaten down by that idiot she'd married to volunteer for a confrontation. And Mona – the bolter, his mother called her – she'd run to the other side of the world to get away from her family, and then run all the way back to get away from her cheating husband. And poor Dan, the evidence of that marriage, had packed his little rucksack and come with her.

No, when it happened, it was always going to be Jo.

'You do know, don't you?' Jo said, after she'd dragged out the tea-making as long as possible.

Know what? David wanted to say. But he didn't have the energy.

'Of course *I know*.'

Even as he felt his anger rising, he tried to suppress it. This wasn't Jo's fault. There was no way she'd have come up with a stunt like this: four letters; life divided like a pie. No, there was only one person who could have come up with this.

Of course, Jo had been enabling Nicci for years. So had

62

he. Every little thing Nicci wanted to do he'd tried to help her with, from the moment he'd fallen for the peroxide pixie.

'What?' Jo asked.

David shook his head. 'Nothing.' How did you explain your heart just twisted?

Nicci hadn't been peroxide for a decade now, more, but the memory of that meeting was burnt in his brain. That was how he thought of her. Even now he felt bad about using Lizzie as an in. But from the moment Nicci had walked into the party, he'd known – like in some dodgy rom-com – she was his one, and he would do anything to get her.

'David?' Jo was standing in front of him. 'Are you OK? I mean, I know you're not . . .'

'I'm fine,' he said. 'Just thinking.'

'So did she tell you about the letters?' Jo ventured. 'Consult you, I mean?'

'You mean, did I *choose* Mona?' Amongst the confusion and disgust, despite himself David could feel his fury take hold.

Jo stepped backwards. It was instinctive; she couldn't help it. 'I'll take that as a no.' Her voice was full of sympathy.

'I'm sorry . . . I didn't mean . . .' David's anger was gone. Dragging out a chair, he slumped at the kitchen table, his head in his hands. 'No, Jo, she didn't tell me. She didn't consult me. She left me two letters. The first was instructions for delivering your letters; the second, to be read after I had, told me what she'd done. That she'd planned my future for me. Because she didn't trust me to do it myself. Like an idiot, I did what she asked, it didn't occur to me not to.'

'It wasn't like that,' Jo said. 'I'm sure it wasn't. Nicci adored you. She loved us all. She was just worried what would happen when she . . . when we found ourselves where we are now.'

'Maybe,' said David, hoping he could keep the bitterness from his voice. 'Or maybe Nicci just wanted to make sure we did it her way.'

Perhaps he should have been the one who went to the bereavement counsellor. Were you allowed to be furious with your wife for dying on you? She'd wanted the house, she'd wanted children, she'd wanted the business, she'd wanted their life. Then she'd left it. Was he allowed to be angry about that? Because he was. So gut-wrenchingly furious that thinking about it brought tears flooding to the surface.

'She left my garden to Lizzie, my children to you, and me – her husband – to Mona. What the fuck, Jo? I mean, seriously, *what the fuck* was she thinking?'

Pulling out the end of a bench, Jo sat next to him and slid her arm around his shoulders. And felt, rather than heard, him begin to sob. She didn't know what to say. So she held him tight and let him slip down and weep against her.

The house was quiet now, but alive with sound the way old houses are: pipes creaking as they heated and cooled, floorboards moaning with memories of past footsteps. Jo had circled the house, turning off the countless lights and electrical appliances, before returning to the kitchen to collect her bag.

'Will you start coming back now?' said David. 'The three of you? And Si, and Gerry, and Dan? You still eat Sunday lunch, don't you?'

'Wild horses wouldn't keep us away,' Jo said. 'Except maybe Mona.'

She smiled, to show she was joking, and he forced a laugh.

Now she'd gone, David punched 1471 for the fifth time in as many days, only to be greeted with the same message: *number withheld*. Despite what he'd said earlier, David didn't think it was a call centre or a fault on the line, not really.

In his darkest nights he'd started to fear Nicci had been keeping more from him than he'd realised. That she'd even – he could hardly bring himself to think it – been having an affair. No, he knew she wouldn't do that. Not his Nicci.

In an attempt to calm his brain, David made himself sit and listen to the quiet. Many, many times he'd yearned for this silence. Well, now you've got it, he thought. This is it. Better start getting used to it.

Outside next-door's tabby tortured the last drop of life from a small undeserving rodent, a car passed the end of the road, music so loud he could almost hear the words, teenagers shouted abuse as they made their way home from the town centre. He forced himself to listen to it all.

Floodlights came on suddenly, triggered by a small creature using his garden as a shortcut. Almost April, and still the soil was cold and bare, the grass straggly, beds bedraggled and neglected, the remnants of last autumn's leaves rotting where they'd fallen. It had been this way for months.

When the lights turned themselves off again two minutes later, he was grateful. It had been like looking inside himself, and finding nothing there.

TEN

Sunday lunch didn't happen. David knew it wouldn't.

'It's Mona, isn't it?' he said when Jo called on Friday night and suggested they take a rain check. 'She nixed it.'

'No,' Jo said. 'It's Lizzie. Something's come up with her mother. She needs to go and see the staff at the care home.'

'What about her sister?' David asked, already knowing the answer.

'What about her?' Jo's shrug was almost audible. Lizzie's sister, Karen, lived in the States and was conspicuous by her absence at the best of times, particularly when there was a mother-related issue.

'Look, David, I promise, it's nothing sinister. Nobody's avoiding you. Not even Mona. Lizzie does have to go to Croydon and she doesn't know how long it will take. But next weekend, Easter Sunday, if you're free, it's a date. I'll shop, Lizzie will cook. You get the booze in. And Mona can bring desserts that come out of a packet.'

He'd had to be satisfied with that. He understood; after all, they hadn't even begun to resolve the 'what to do about Nicci's bequests' problem.

Common sense said the whole thing was ridiculous.

Everyone agreed on that. You can't go leaving people to other people. Clothes, yes. Patches of garden, at a push. Even the shed, but not *people*.

Emotionally, though, it wasn't that straightforward. Emotionally, morally, ethically . . . Put like that, the less he saw of Mona the better. And he tensed every time he thought he heard Lizzie unlocking the side gate. Only the idea of Jo mothering his girls, for now at least, didn't bother him. After all, somebody had to.

The sound of Peppa Pig sloshing through the muddy puddles echoed from the sitting room. Harrie and Charlie were happy, sitting side by side on the floor in front of the TV, clutching their blankies. But it wasn't yet 9 a.m. The whole day stretched ahead.

If not going to the park or on play dates, Nicci would have baked cakes, done potato prints, or made dresses for their dolls, applying the same focus to making and baking on Saturdays and Sundays as she did to her other baby, Capsule Wardrobe, during the week.

'No one ever regretted time not spent cleaning the house,' she'd been fond of saying (about pretty much anything she didn't like doing), which was why they'd got a cleaner. 'But if I don't spend time with the girls, I'll regret that.'

As it turned out, Nicci was right. Of course, they hadn't known then just how little time with the girls she had left.

David once asked where Nicci had learned it all, the sewing and cooking and making, hoping she'd tell him about her childhood, but she just shrugged. 'I taught myself,' she'd said. Now he wished she'd taught him too.

Wandering back to the kitchen, David flicked the radio on, then off again. He'd promised himself he'd dispense with the white noise, but it was instinctive. Another weekend stretched before him. Another weekend of not doing the

67

right voices, of eating shop-bought cookies. He had to do *something*.

'You know you can always come to us,' his mother had urged, from the very first weekend, and his father had clapped him on the shoulder in silent agreement.

He knew. He'd been to his parents five out of the last six weekends. The last time, Charlie had announced, as he lifted her from the car, 'Not Granny's *again*!' in a voice that carried all the way to his mother standing beaming on the doorstep. She sounded so much like Nicci, he barely held it together.

There was always the swimming pool. Si might be there, with his boys. Although last time David had tried getting Charlie and Harrie changed and into the baby pool, he'd lost Harrie for a full minute and nearly had heart failure. And he'd been able to see what all the mums were thinking: typical weekend dad, can't be left alone for five minutes. The ones who recognised him were worse. There were days he feared he might drown in other people's pity.

Then it dawned on him: Whitstable. The beach hut had been one of Nicci's favourite places, especially in the winter. ('Fewer tourists, more personality,' she'd said, neatly side-stepping the fact that owning a beach hut in Whitstable didn't exactly make her a local.) They hadn't been since the end of last summer. Once the chemo started, and the radio, Nicci wasn't well enough to go back.

'Let's go to the beach!' he announced, tiggering into the living room in his best children's TV presenter manner.

Two small blond heads turned to watch him, two pairs of brown eyes gave him a look of withering contempt, usually reserved for idiots who thought they might eat green stuff.

Harrie cocked her head on one side, Charlie the other. 'But, Daddy,' they said, 'it raining.'

* * *

68

Angry waves lashed the shingle just short of the row of weather-beaten huts. There was no horizon that David could see. The unforgiving grey of the North Sea merged with a steely, rain-laden sky. Only the occasional tuft of green showed where feisty blades fought their way through spits of land, only to wonder what the point was when they got there. The usually cheerful pastel pinks and blues of the beach huts failed to inject any joy into the landscape.

He tried to see what Nicci would have seen if she'd been here. Spirit! Nature! A challenge! Without her to show it to him, all David could see was a cold beach; nature in the grip of the meanest of mean reds.

He'd come here looking for comfort. But there was nothing comforting on this bleak stretch of shingle.

The beach was empty in both directions. Not so much as a dog scavenging for scraps. Even the oyster stalls weren't open, not that David would be using them if they had been. The memory of trying to force-feed the girls oysters – working on Nicci's theory that they should get them used to everything early – and the look of disgust on their faces as they spat five quid's worth of seafood across the table gave David his first smile of the day. 'Heathens!' Nicci had declared.

The only tourists dumb enough to brave the Kent coastline in the coldest March for thirty-one years had taken refuge in Nicci's favourite café, Tea & Times, nursing steaming mugs and the papers. This was where David and the girls had been, eating cheese on toast and drinking hot chocolate until half an hour ago. And where, it was painfully clear, they should have stayed.

His was the only beach hut open, and David was rapidly wishing he hadn't bothered. The interior – which in his mind's eye was a stylish combination of nautical blue and white – was, in reality, drab and faded, the rattan sofa coated with grit that had crept through the cracks in the clapboard.

The Calor Gas heater was empty. And he hadn't thought to bring a new bottle. The beach hut was as desolate inside as it was out.

'Need a wee-wee,' Charlie announced.

David counted backwards from ten.

'Sweetie,' he said, when he reached zero, 'you just had a wee-wee in the café. Come and help me tidy Mummy's hut.'

'Need one now.'

'Right,' David said. 'We'd better go outside then.'

'Co-old,' Harrie said, plonking herself heavily on the gritty sand at his feet, as David helped Charlie crouch. 'Harrie need a wee.'

Any second now the grizzling would start. Who could blame them? The afternoon was cold and wet and, frankly, no fun at all. Given the chance, he would happily sit down next to them on the damp shingle and grizzle along with them.

'Come on, girls,' he said, trying to sound convincing. 'Let's go for a walk. It'll be fun.'

They weren't fooled. 'Cold, Daddy!' Their little faces looked pinched and blue.

David closed his eyes and prayed for help; for a hot-water bottle, thicker coats for the girls, a teleporter, brandy, anything to get him through this.

'Excuse me, are you OK?' A kind voice out of the blue.

The woman's trench coat was so wet it had turned dark grey, her cheeks were red with cold and her hair stuck to her face in tendrils. Not exactly the angel of mercy he'd had in mind.

'No . . . I mean, yes. Thanks. I'm just, erm, regrouping.' He forced a smile.

There was a yelp from behind. They both turned to see a black and white mongrel sniffing Harrie's Peppa Pig lunch

70

box, the only pink thing Nicci allowed houseroom, except pink wine.

'Stop it, Norman,' the woman yelled, tugging at the dog's collar. 'I'm sorry,' she added. 'He's such a piglet. He thinks there might be second lunch in there.'

David's smile was weak. 'Afraid he's out of luck. Nothing in there but dolls, clothes and KitKat wrappers.'

'You're David, aren't you?' she said. 'I thought I recognised you. Your girls have got so big.'

He racked his brains. The woman was vaguely familiar, but only in the way people you see in the street or on television are.

'Jilly,' she said. 'Three huts down from yours. Usually see more of you guys in the winter. How's Nicci? Seems like an age since you were here. Must have been what, September?'

'August Bank Holiday,' David said.

It was only seven months ago, but his mood could scarcely have been more different.

Back then, they'd known Nicci was ill. The cancer had been given a name and a stage. There was still hope. Not a lot, but it was there. The date for Nicci's operation was just days away. So this was their last family weekend away before the unavoidable weeks of treatment and, they hoped, recovery. This time, next August, they'd be back, they told themselves, drinking ice-cold rosé, David barbecuing Cumberland sausages, Nicci unpacking tubs of salad and olives, tearing crusty French bread into a basket. Far too much food for the four of them.

The girls had been crouching on the sand, wearing pants and Hello Kitty T-shirts, their shorts and crocs long discarded, faces comical masks of concentration as they built sandcastles for their Baby Alives, which Nicci had let David's mother buy them. She'd stalled at the accoutrements. Fortunately, Jo and Lizzie hadn't. The sky had been a perfect August blue, broken by a smattering of cartoon clouds the twins could have drawn.

Despite the Choos, and the Chanel, and the designer jeans that replaced her vintage frocks and Doc Martens, Nicci was the same girl he'd fallen in love with the moment he saw her. The knackered denim cut-offs with a hole in the bum where, if he looked hard enough, he could see a flash of black lace knickers, were gone. And so was the faded Stone Roses T-shirt – the one he'd bought her the first birthday after they'd got together. Although, knowing Nicci, it was folded in a box or bin bag somewhere. She'd worn it to grey and with sleeves rolled up to reveal slim tanned upper arms. The peroxide had been replaced by a pricey, professional dye-job, and the skinny tanned legs ended in orange toenails and clashing pink Havaianas, not the battered Docs she'd lived in when they first met. But she was still his Nicci.

He could see now that her face that day had been brave. With hindsight, her exhaustion and fear were obvious, but at the time it had been easier not to see. Kinder too. To both of them.

Too often he'd complained that they didn't spend any time alone. Never did anything together, just the four of them, as a family.

'The house is always full of your friends!' he'd snapped, more than once, when the twins had gone to bed, and Sunday was about to slip into Monday, when they'd both be back at work without a private word spoken. 'Why can't we be just us? If I'd known I was walking up the aisle with all four of you—'

She'd put her hand in front of his mouth and he'd let her shush him.

'They're not just my friends. They're my family,' she said, as she always did. 'You know that.'

And she replaced her hand with her mouth.

He missed her face and her smile. Her scent, the texture of her hair, the taste of her skin. She'd been what let him be him: David, the thoughtful one. He missed her body, and he missed feeling her naked skin as he fell asleep, and their hands clutching as they sometimes did when they both awoke.

The woman was staring at him, looking anxious. The rain was heavier now, slicking dark curls to her forehead.

He remembered her now. Well, he didn't. But Nicci was always striking up conversations. Standing up to the rims of her Hunters in the freezing surf, chatting with strangers, as if it was July. You never knew who you might meet, she said. Better to waste ten minutes talking to a dull person than miss a chance of meeting an interesting one. To her, three huts down was almost family.

Always open, always looking. His exact opposite.

Nicci collected: people, things, clothes . . .

'Oh!' The woman's face was ashen. 'I'm sorry. I've said the wrong thing, haven't I? You two haven't . . . you haven't split?' Mortification crossed her face. 'I can't believe it. You always seemed so, happy . . .' Her voice trailed away.

David shook his head, finally glad of the rain blurring his vision and trickling down his face. 'No,' he said. 'We haven't split.'

Oblivious to the rain, the girls sat at his feet petting the dog, content for the first time that day. 'I'm sorry,' David said. 'I told everyone I could think of. Everyone in Nicci's address book . . . I don't know how to say this . . . She had cancer. It . . . the end . . . was quick.'

Quick, but not painless.

The expression that crossed the woman's face was agonisingly familiar. He'd seen it before, many times, over the last two months. In the months before too, when the end became inevitable. But that didn't make it any easier, for either of them. As the woman hastily made her excuses and strode off down the beach, dog in tow, head down, into the rain, David decided he could hardly blame her.

Nicci's Dead. It was a hell of a conversation stopper.

They packed up soon after. There was no point staying. He'd come here looking for Nicci, but he hadn't found her. She wasn't here to be found.

ELEVEN

The only good thing about Croydon is leaving it, Lizzie thought, as she pulled her second-hand Renault out of The Cedars' car park.

It wasn't Croydon's fault. She didn't have anything against the place. In fact, it wasn't Croydon she hated at all. It was Sanderstead, and The Cedars in particular.

The Cedars had been Lizzie's mother's home for two years now and Lizzie's elder sister, Karen, had only managed to visit once. OK, so Lizzie lived an hour's drive away, and Karen's journey involved an eight-hour transatlantic flight, but even so, Lizzie thought, stomping her foot on the brake as a bus pulled out, would it kill her to visit her mother a couple of times a year?

'I only get two weeks' holiday,' Karen reminded her when Lizzie called from the car park to give her an update. 'And anyway, what would be the point of begging unpaid time off work? She wouldn't recognise me anyway.'

Lizzie'd had to resist the urge to hurl her mobile onto the gravel. She couldn't afford to replace it. 'You think she recognises *me*?' she said instead.

Before the home there had been the memory loss. The missing

door keys, the lost handbags, the returning from school to twenty-five voicemail messages from her mother, all checking she hadn't been killed in a car crash reported on the local news thirty miles away.

Doctors' appointments, specialists' appointments, MRI scans and CAT scans, had swiftly followed those calls. Lizzie handled it largely on her own. Gerry was in meetings. Entertaining important clients. Away on business/at a training course/being fast-tracked. Gerry was off being Gerry.

And then they had the care home row.

I wouldn't be any help, babe. What do I know about care homes?
'The same as me,' Lizzie had said. *Fuck all.*

She didn't add that bit. Just as she never gave her sister a piece of her mind. Just as she'd never properly quarrelled with her mother. The stand-up knock-down row she should have had at nineteen or twenty-one had somehow gone astray.

Instead she visited countless care homes, each more depressing than the last, and then found an estate agent to sell the family home to pay for her mother's care. Each step of the way she religiously called Karen in Brooklyn so she'd know exactly what was going on. And each time Karen had been too busy with work, with her husband and children, to come and help.

Eventually, after Lizzie threatened to give every last stick of furniture to charity, Karen took unpaid leave from her job on Wall Street. The forty-eight hours she stayed at the Gatwick Hilton and systematically tried to 'put right' every decision Lizzie had made were topped off by their mother's glazed lack of recognition. No, Lizzie was pretty sure Karen wouldn't be coming back any time soon. And who could blame her? Lizzie only wished she had the same option.

In a way, she was glad. Sometimes doing everything yourself was simply easier . . . As she pulled onto the M23 and put her foot down, she felt her spirits lift. It was done.

The Stone Roses went on, the early album with all the good tracks. Not even her music really, but an old boyfriend at uni's. Somehow she'd adopted his music taste as her own and had never really moved on.

Mum had been even worse today.

'Isn't it nice of Kathleen to come and see me,' she'd said, before lapsing into one of many long and intricate conversations with herself. It was ironic. Mum had never been chatty. Now you couldn't shut her up.

Janet, The Cedars' manager, had shrugged apologetically. As if to say, *What can you do?* Lizzie had shrugged back. If Janet didn't know, she certainly didn't.

Kathleen was her mother's cousin, dead for ten years. Lizzie had been Kathleen for months now. At first she'd thought Mum did it on purpose, to punish Lizzie for not being Karen. Now she knew it was the illness at work.

The next call to Karen was going to be grim. Lizzie needed to tell her The Cedars felt Mum needed specialist care. For which read *expensive*.

'What's wrong with the NHS?' Karen would say. And Lizzie would reply, 'They'll pay for Mum when we can't afford to any more.'

And Karen would say, 'We can't afford to now.'

So predictable. So pointless. So why bother? Because Karen was the eldest, that was why. It had always been that way, Lizzie's entire life.

Turning the corner into the cul-de-sac, Lizzie saw instantly that their three-bedroom house was dark, the only unlit house in the loop of *exclusive* three- and four-bedroom New England-style properties. Everyone else was in, doing whatever Lizzie's neighbours did in the evenings. Watching television, having dinner parties, drinking too much white wine.

Wherever Gerry's silver Audi Quattro was, it wasn't here.

She knew she should have felt cross, that she should have wanted Gerry waiting here to greet her. Instead she felt relieved. Pulling up in front of their glossy garage door, she grabbed her bag off the passenger seat and locked the car, watching lights blink as the alarm set itself. Wanting time alone – even on Sunday evening – wasn't necessarily a bad thing. She could indulge her secret passion for *Countryfile*, open a bottle of something cold and white, instead of drinking the Rioja that Gerry preferred.

She could drink white wine, hog the bathroom, use all the hot water. She could even make headway into the damn gardening books she'd taken out of the library.

Having drawn the curtains, she flipped on the television – in that order, always in that order – and peered in the fridge. So much for the wine choice: half a bottle of Pinot Grigio and two cans of Peroni.

One eye on the television, she settled onto the sofa and picked up Alan Titchmarsh's *The Gardener's Year*.

The phone inside began ringing precisely as David's house alarm started peeping. Thirty seconds and counting to disable the beeping, before all hell broke loose. The phone would have to wait. There probably wouldn't be anyone on the other end anyway.

By the time he'd keyed in the security code the phone had fallen silent and he felt his shoulders relax. Head down, he ran back to the car, hoisted first one child, then the other, and carried them into the house, depositing one on each sofa, before heading back to grab their bags and lock the car.

As he did, the phone started up again.

'Da-addy . . .'

'I'm here,' he promised them. 'Just let me get rid of this.'

'Hello?'

'I'm sorry to bother you on a Sunday. I'm looking for David Morrison.'

The voice belonged to a woman. Not old, but certainly not young. She sounded anywhere from fifty something upwards. What she didn't sound like was a cold caller.

'That's me,' he said.

'Ah, um, good. I mean . . . it's good that I've found you,' the woman said. 'It's taken weeks. And then I wasn't sure I had the right number.'

'Da-addy!'

Christ, David thought, *cut to the chase*. 'Well, you've found me,' he said. 'What can I do for you?'

'Well, um. You don't know me. But you might know my name. It's – well, it was – Lynda Webster.'

David racked his brains. He didn't know anyone by that name.

'Lynda Webster?' the woman repeated, her voice a question now.

When it became clear the name meant nothing to him, she cleared her throat and when she spoke again the nerves had been replaced by sadness. 'David, I'm Nicci's mother.'

David put down the phone. He didn't intend to. It was instinctive.

The telephone rang again almost immediately.

'Sorry,' he said. 'I don't know why I did that.'

'Nicci must have told you terrible things about me . . .'

'She didn't tell me anything,' David said. 'You weren't a welcome topic of conversation. I didn't even know you were still alive.'

Brutal, he thought. Before deciding he just didn't care. There was a silence at the far end of the line, as if the woman was considering that. And then a sigh.

'You did know she had a mother?'

79

'*Da-addy!*'

'Look, the girls—' David stopped; suddenly aware he was talking for the first time to his children's grandmother. 'I can't talk now. Give me a number where I can reach you and I'll call you back when they're in bed.'

A silence said the woman didn't believe him.

'I will, Lynda,' he said. It sounded weird; over-familiar. 'Look, Mrs Webster . . . apparently you know where to find me. It's not like I have a choice.'

He heard her mutter something.

'Give me your number,' he repeated. 'I'll call back. It won't be before seven, maybe later. Depends how long it takes to persuade them to go down.'

'What are their names?' the woman asked, tentatively.

David hesitated.

'Charlie and Harrie,' he said, before hanging up a second time.

TWELVE

Bedtime was a nightmare, as if all the stress of the day at Whitstable had seeped into Harrie and Charlie's pores, along with the salt, grit and tar. When the girls finally went down, after two stories and endless grizzling, David barely had time to pour himself a large brandy before the phone rang again. This time he knew there would be someone on the other end.

'I said I'd call you,' he said, without waiting for her to speak. 'The girls are, tricky, at the moment. It took a while.'

'Hardly surprising,' Lynda Webster said. 'They've not long lost their mother. I expect they're confused.'

'That's one way of describing it.' David took a slow sip of the Courvoisier and felt its warmth slide down his throat. 'Sad, mainly.'

'You've really never heard of me?'

'I knew you existed. But no more than that. She didn't tell me you were dead, if that's what you're asking.'

'It wasn't,' the woman said tightly. 'That's all?'

'You fell out before university. That's it.'

'That's the truth at least.'

'I'd like to be able to tell you something different,' David said. 'But Nicci *never* talked about you. It was one of her conditions, right from the start. She didn't know her dad, and you and she had a huge row in her teens and hadn't spoken since. End of subject.'

'End of subject?'

'That's what she said.'

'You didn't ask?'

'*Of course I asked!*' David struggled to hang on to his temper. Who did this woman think she was?

'I didn't mean to suggest—'

'You did,' he snapped, cutting her off. '*Of course I asked about her family.* I was married to her, for Christ's sake.'

Was. Tears threatened to burst through.

Am, he thought. *Am married to her.*

Closing his eyes, David took a deep breath and then another. 'I only asked a couple of times,' he said, when his voice was steady again. 'Near the start, before I learnt it was on Nicci's *Don't Go There* list.

'Don't go there . . . ?' The woman's shock was clear.

This wasn't like him, David thought. Why was he jabbing away at her? Whatever this woman was to blame for, Nicci's death wasn't on that list. But she'd asked, and for some reason he felt obliged to tell the truth.

'Listen,' David said. It wasn't quite an order. 'Once, at uni, when I asked, she got up, walked out of my room and wouldn't speak to me or even see me for a week. When she came back she told me it was on the condition that I never asked again. I thought I'd lost her. So I decided right there that it wasn't worth the risk. I didn't like to see her hurt, I loved – love – her.'

'And when you had your babies, she didn't . . . ?' The woman took a deep breath. 'You didn't ever . . . ?'

'I know what you want to hear,' David said quietly. 'But it would be a lie. Nicci never mentioned you. Not once. Not

82

when we married. Not when we had Charlie and Harrie. Not even when she was . . .'

He couldn't bring himself to complete that sentence.

'I guessed as much. That's why I called. When I read she'd died I thought . . . well, I'd wait to hear. I thought she might have left me something.'

David tensed, his fingers clenching the phone. It must have been somehow audible.

'Oh, not like that,' Nicci's mother said. 'I don't mean money. Although I know she was well off. By my standards, anyway. I don't want you to think that's why I called. I thought perhaps a letter, or something.'

'Something?'

'A brooch . . . ?'

It was not quite a question, and they both recognised she already knew the answer. Her voice had risen on the word more in hope than expectation.

David shivered at a memory of Nicci and he on the shingle near the beginning, in mid-winter. She'd pushed her hand into her pocket and pulled out a silver brooch. A very ordinary brooch. So ordinary, it could have passed for tin.

'What's that?' he'd asked.

She hadn't answered. For a moment, he'd thought she was going to hurl it straight into the cold grey sea. Instead she'd put it back into her pocket, almost as if deciding throwing it wasn't worth the effort. He wasn't meant to notice when she'd dropped it into a bin on their way back to his rooms. Another lover, he'd thought. And he'd kept thinking that, until now.

When David didn't say anything the woman sighed.

'The reason I'm calling . . .' she paused as if seeking the right words, '. . . I thought . . . I'd like to know my granddaughters.'

'Your granddaughters?'

'If you don't mind. I mean, obviously I understand you'll need time to think it over.'

In a way he'd been expecting this from the second the woman announced herself. But now she'd come out with it, he could hardly contain his anger. *If he didn't mind?* Of course he bloody minded. And, more importantly, Nicci would mind.

Nicci would mind violently. If Nicci had wanted Charlie and Harrie to know their grandmother, she'd have introduced them long before now.

'Oh, not right away,' the woman said, sensing David's mood. 'I wouldn't dream of asking that. I thought maybe you and I could meet, for a coffee or something, So you can see I don't have two heads. Or whatever Nicci told you I had.'

'You're missing the point,' David said curtly. 'Nicci never told me anything at all.'

Once he'd put the phone down on her for the third time that evening, Nicci's mother didn't call back. Or maybe she did. David pulled the jack from its socket so he didn't have to find out, refilled his glass and retired to the bedroom. Now he sat on his side of the bed, brandy long since drained.

Their room was lit only by the orange glow of the street-light through open curtains, and the nightlight's glimmer from the children's room next door. David didn't need any extra light to see the photograph he was holding. He'd looked at it so many times since he'd put down the phone, the image was imprinted on his brain.

Seven weeks Nicci had been dead. Seven weeks, two days and twenty-one hours. And already he knew more about her than he had in the sixteen years they'd been together.

The square lay in the palm of his hand, corners bent upwards from over-handling. It was a Polaroid, the white frame daylight-faded to creamy yellow, the image itself washed opaque.

Snuffling came through the baby monitor as Charlie – or was it Harrie? – turned over in her sleep. Nicci had deemed the monitor redundant almost a year earlier, but since her death David had reinstated it. He found it comforting. The sound of his daughters' slow breathing got him through most nights.

The photograph had been in her bedside cabinet all along.

He'd found it a couple of weeks back as he bagged up the last of her medicine to return to the hospital, unable to bear the sight of her cancer paraphernalia any longer. It had been at the bottom of the drawer, book-marking a page in one of the cancer memoirs that had become her favoured reading. Now they sat in a bag under the stairs waiting to go to Oxfam. Where the Polaroid would have gone too, if it hadn't slipped from the paperbacks as he carried them downstairs. He only knew who it was now because of a scrawl in an unfamiliar hand across the back.

Lynda and Nicola.

It was a very seventies Polaroid, Nicci's mum all Suzi Quatro hair and denim flares, standing beside a small girl – three years old, maybe four – squinting warily into the camera. Red gingham dress bunched up, revealing skinny legs, white socks and red T-bar shoes. The girl stood half on, half off a blue trike with a yellow seat and handlebars.

If only he'd known it was there before, he could have asked Nicci about it. Only Nicci wouldn't have told him. But now he knew someone who would. If he'd let her.

The other person in the photo.

THIRTEEN

'Marking homework?'

Lizzie jumped. She'd been so engrossed in her gardening books she didn't hear Gerry's key in the lock. She'd only just reached April and the things that should have been done by now already stretched to three pages of an exercise book.

'A gardening book?' He looked surprised.

With one sock-clad foot Lizzie kicked a half-eaten packet of chocolate HobNobs under the coffee table and out of Gerry's line of sight. Only that morning he'd grabbed her bum as she struggled into size twelve jeans – jeans that now cut into her middle, forcing a roll of flesh over the waistband – and made some comment about her 'filling her jeans'.

How had that happened? Only last autumn she'd been comfortable in her favourite size tens. Now she was on the verge of swapping the twelves for the fourteens she kept under her bed for just such emergencies. Some people, people who mostly didn't need to lose weight in the first place – Nicci, for example – responded to life's traumas by losing their appetite. The heartbreak diet.

Lizzie was the total opposite; her emotional history mapped out in junk food. Recently, this ran:

1) Mother with Alzheimer's – one packet of chocolate HobNobs.

2) Row with sister, over Mother – whole tube of Pringles.

3) Best friend's funeral – bottle of dry white and a bowl of peanuts with takeaway pizza chaser, repeat as necessary.

4) Fight with Gerry about giving up teaching to become a proper wife/mother; her timekeeping; what she/he was doing at the weekend* (*delete as applicable) – that happened so often it barely merited more than the bar of Sainsbury's cooking chocolate she'd hidden from herself at the back of the freezer.

Hunger had nothing to do with it.

Closing the gardening book, Lizzie stretched her cheek up to receive his kiss. Gerry had the kind of whiskers that meant if he shaved at 8 a.m., he had a beard by lunchtime. It was early evening now. There were days she felt she could get a rash just by looking at him.

'Pooh,' she said. 'You smell beery.'

Gerry winked. 'I am beery,' he said. 'Nineteenth hole.'

'Thought it was rugby today.' She didn't need to glance at her watch to know he'd spent far more hours in the clubhouse than he had on the course.

'Golf. Told you this morning. Anyway, I knew you'd be out so I went for a late lunch with the guys after.'

And drove home? Lizzie wanted to say, but didn't. Instead, she reached for her book, flicking to a boxout on compost.

What was the difference between peat, loam and ericaceous compost? Who cared and why would it matter? She couldn't believe Nicci had. Nicci had to be more of a 'shove it in and see what grew' type of gardener. Didn't she?

'How was your mum?'

'The same,' she said. 'Still thinks I'm Aunt Kathleen, though . . . Thanks for asking.'

Crouching down beside her chair, Gerry slipped both arms around her, fingers grazing her breast as they passed. His breath was yeasty on her ear. Lizzie forced herself not to tense.

'I'm glad you're not down,' he said, as his left hand crept back up, cupping her breast.

Lizzie wasn't in the mood, not really. Some people lost themselves in sex, used it as a release. Mona, for one. And Nicci too, when they were first at college.

Not Lizzie.

She'd always felt a bit out of it like that. A bit uptight – frigid, some git who played rugby had called her in sixth form – but that was just her. She had to feel close, loved and liked to want sex. And she had, with Gerry, in the early years, but now . . .

'Come upstairs?'

Closing her eyes, Lizzie emptied her mind, forcing herself to go with it as Gerry began kissing her neck, his free hand deftly unbuttoning her shirt. After all, you didn't get babies without sex and they hadn't 'done it' in almost a month.

They used to have the 'There's never a right time to have babies' row every second month. Back then, Lizzie was the one arguing to start a family. Gerry was too busy, he was in line for another promotion, he wanted to wait until next year when they'd be able to afford another, bigger, house . . . The only argument he never used back then was her job. Because he knew she'd throw that up in a second. It was a job – teaching at the local primary – and she enjoyed it, but it wasn't her life's work, not like her sister's career. Something she'd be willing to ditch when they started a family. Lizzie was positively old-fashioned like that. It was another thing she and Karen didn't agree on.

Then it changed. Gerry started talking about babies and she – Lizzie hardly dared say it – began to wonder if the time was right.

But she'd always wanted a family.

Lizzie could remember her elation the first time she'd mentioned babies over breakfast and he hadn't flinched. That had been a couple of years ago.

The other night, he'd made some comment about the pre-prep school his boss sent his son to. So now he was willing to talk babies; but the local school at which she taught was no longer good enough.

Gerry groaned as his hand eased into her bra and stroked her nipple until it stiffened. His other hand slipped inside her jeans.

No babies without sex, Lizzie reminded herself. And she did want to start a family . . . didn't she?

FOURTEEN

'Where's the roasting tin?'

'Same place as usual, I imagine.'

'Nu-huh.' Lizzie shook her head. 'I've looked there, and all the other likely places.'

The two women looked at each other and rolled their eyes.

Jo threw open the kitchen window. 'David,' she yelled. 'What have you done with the roasting tin?'

'What have I done with . . . ?' he shouted over the shrieks of two small girls. Having hunted Easter eggs, provided by Jo and hidden by David after they'd gone to bed the night before, Charlie and Harrie were on a carbohydrate high, taking turns to be pushed on the tyre hanging from the old apple tree.

'Higher, Daddy, higher!'

'In a sec . . . Nothing. Haven't touched the damn thing. Do I look like a man who'd know what to do with a roasting tin?'

'More than Gerry does,' Lizzie muttered, looking for a cupboard she hadn't yet searched. 'Who else would move it? The kitchen ghost?'

She caught Jo's eye. Jo raised a quizzical eyebrow.

Jo looked tired, Lizzie thought, nothing like herself. The roots were visible in her usually flawlessly highlighted hair and her fringe kept falling into her eyes. She was dressed as if for a ramble: battered biker boots; knackered, not-for-going-out jeans; and what looked suspiciously like one of Si's fleeces. A fleece? Nicci would have had something to say about that. Maybe that was the point. Nicci couldn't see them. For the first time in years Jo was at liberty to wear whatever she wanted. They all were. But it was Easter Sunday and the first time they'd all been here, together, since Nicci's funeral. Lizzie had assumed that meant they'd make an effort. But no.

She felt painfully overdressed. Glancing down at her floral dress and heels, she wondered if there was time to nip home and change.

'You OK?'

Lizzie snapped back to see Jo looking concerned. 'Yeah, fine, just spooked myself with the ghost comment,' she lied. 'But I didn't mean it like that. Anyway, if it *was* Nicci – which it isn't, obviously – at least she'd have put it back in the right place.' Jo started to laugh, and after a moment Lizzie joined in.

It was shaping up to be a beautiful Easter weekend, exactly as Jo had hoped. Late April sunshine crept round from the front and in through south-facing windows to throw a strip of gold across the oak table Nicci and David had lovingly sanded and varnished. The Chinese slate floor beneath the table reflected a rainbow of bronzes and gilts. The kitchen was warm from the Aga, the scent of coffee lingered, and the Archers squabbled amongst themselves in the background. Everything was as it should be.

Almost.

When Nicci became too tired to cook Sunday roast for ten, back in the autumn, the others had taken over, with Nicci presiding over the proceedings, passing judgement on the consistency of their stuffing or the sweetness of the apple sauce. And they smiled and gritted their teeth and let her. It was better to go on pretending nothing had changed. All of them – friends, partners and children – had lunched there every Sunday without fail, unless Jo and Si had his kids for the weekend; then they'd appear in the late afternoon after dropping the boys back at their mother's. Usually just in time for pudding and to help with the third or fourth bottle of wine.

Jo shook the image from her head. 'Got it!' she said, emerging from under the sink, roasting tin aloft. 'Suspect kitchen ghost's offspring put it there.'

'Sorry I'm late,' Mona said, shouldering her way through the back door and kicking it shut with her heel. 'No reason,' she added, pre-empting the question. 'Just late.'

She had once been a year late for Lizzie's thirtieth birthday party, since when anything less was considered minor.

'Good to see you.' Tossing the roasting tin on the side with a clatter, Jo threw her arms around Mona, coat, bags and all; ignoring the look of surprise that flickered across Mona's face. 'It's been too long.'

It had only been a couple of weeks, but that was long by their standards. Lately they weren't sure which of them was meant to be holding it together. Jo was trying, but it didn't come naturally. She preferred to watch from the periphery: not so much outside looking in as standing on the edge, with both choices open to her. She wasn't Nicci; didn't have that magnetism, the sort that made others gravitate to her.

'Where's Dan?' Lizzie asked. 'I bought him a tub of Celebrations. He is coming, isn't he?'

He's there.' Mona jerked her head towards the back garden, where her son was already kicking a football. 'I got organic crumble, real custard, profiteroles and crème fraîche. And organic hot cross buns, just in case.'

'In case of what,' Jo laughed. 'Famine? Apocalypse? Terrorist attack? We've got enough food here to feed the entire street.'

Mona's inedible cooking was the stuff of myth. Since no one could remember ever tasting it, Jo suspected the myth was urban, created by Mona to avoid having to do any. Like Jo's brother's famously crap washing-up.

Dumping her coat on the back of a chair, to reveal an embroidered smock over narrow dark jeans and ankle boots, Mona began emptying the contents of her carrier bags into the fridge.

'What needs doing? More coffee?' The others shook their heads but Mona filled the kettle anyway. 'Peel spuds then?' she offered, and took up position at the sink overlooking the back garden.

For a few minutes the three women worked in companionable silence, Lizzie salting the pork for crackling and slicing apples for apple sauce, Jo chopping nuts for nut roast and Mona peeling a mountain of King Edwards. Bags of carrots, parsnips and broccoli were lined up beside her.

'Is it me,' Mona said suddenly, 'or is this weird?'

'Is what weird?' Lizzie said. Her tone made it clear she wished Mona hadn't put the thought into words.

'This . . . the three of us preparing Sunday lunch in Nicci's kitchen, as if nothing's changed. David and Si and Dan in the garden, Gerry . . .' Mona frowned. 'Where's Gerry?'

'Rugby. Be here later.' Lizzie didn't look up from slicing apples, but Jo noticed her back tense in preparation for the Gerry-related onslaught. Nicci might be gone but clearly Lizzie didn't think that was about to change.

Jo loved Lizzie. She just wished Lizzie had married someone different. Someone who deserved her.

Mona opened her mouth to say something – probably exactly what Jo was thinking. Jo shot her a warning glance. *Back off*, she mouthed.

'It's you,' Lizzie said testily. Mona looked at Jo and raised her eyebrows so they vanished into her hair. It was her party trick. Jo stifled a giggle.

'It's me *what*?'

'You said, is it me or is this weird? It's you.'

'You reckon?'

'Reckon,' Lizzie snapped. 'We're old friends having Sunday lunch together. What's wrong with that?'

'You know what Mona means,' Jo said gently. Where was this coming from? Lizzie was normally resident peacemaker, the one smoothing the sheets and making the tea, not the one lobbing rocks. Maybe Nicci's spirit *was* lurking around, hiding roasting tins and making trouble.

'Come on, Lizzie, you have to admit, it *is* a bit weird,' Jo said. 'Especially the Mona-David thing.' She glanced around, double-checking little ears – and big ears – were safely outside. 'I mean, what are we supposed to do about the letters?'

'Ignore them, that's what *I* plan to do,' Mona banged the potato peeler on the worktop. 'It's just another of Nicci's mad schemes.' She raised her eyes to heaven, and Jo could have sworn that if Mona had been Catholic she'd have crossed herself.

'We don't have to do it.'

'I don't know . . .' Lizzie sounded thoughtful. 'I feel like we do.'

'Lizzie!' Mona said. 'All you've got is a bit of gardening! If Nicci has her way, I have to, well, you know . . . with *David*!'

94

'Mo . . .' said Jo, but Mona was in full swing.

'C'mon, Lizzie. Admit it, you got away light.'

'It might be just a bit of gardening to you,' Lizzie said tightly, 'but Nicci knew I can't even grow a weed! And have you looked out there? It's a wilderness. How can I get it looking right for David, for Harrie and Charlie?'

Jo and Mona followed Lizzie's gaze.

It wasn't strictly true. Although Jo had to admit she'd seen Nicci's garden in better shape. Not that she could remember even noticing the garden since last September, when Nicci had sat her down in this kitchen, put a large glass of red wine in front of her and told Jo she had cancer.

Since then, the leaves shed in autumn had been swept aside, but not cleared, and were mouldering on the flower-beds. Occasional spring bulbs had fought their way through, but their leaves were straggly as if, with no one to appreciate their efforts, they'd given up trying. Even Nicci's beloved vegetable patch beyond the apple tree was little more than mud and blown-over runner bean tepees.

Jo was horribly afraid Lizzie was right. The garden looked as desolate as they felt. Somebody had to do something.

'And even if it wasn't a wilderness,' Lizzie's tone, now verging on hysterical, took Jo by surprise. She looked as panic-stricken as she sounded, 'I'm not Nicci. I'll never be Nicci. I don't know a bromeliad from a perennial.'

The others looked at her in astonishment.

'What's a bromeliad?' Mona asked. 'Just out of interest.'

'I don't know!' Lizzie wailed. 'That's the point. I got a book from the library, and then I got three more. And now I wish I hadn't. It might as well be Chemistry A level, for all the sense it makes. I mean, it has *charts, diagrams, tables*.' Lizzie looked at Jo – the mathsy one – as if she could make it all clear.

Jo had made sure the bills got paid at uni. She divided them up, told you what you owed and you paid. If not for her, the rest of them would have been sitting in the cold, probably in darkness.

'It can't be that hard,' Jo said.

'*Diagrams!*' Lizzie repeated. 'And *tables*. You should see the list of things Alan Titchmarsh reckons need to be done by April. Even if I did nothing but garden full time between now and June I couldn't catch up.'

Jo slid her arms around Lizzie and suppressed a laugh as Lizzie buried her head in Jo's shoulder. Over Lizzie's head she saw Mona stuff her hands over her mouth.

'I mean,' Lizzie's words were muffled, 'how did Nicci fit it all in?' She let out a wail and Mona, unable to contain herself, dissolved into fits.

'Come on, Lizzie,' Jo said, gripping Lizzie's shoulders and fixing her with an encouraging smile. 'It's just a *garden*. Do it if you want. Don't if you don't. But if you decide to do it don't try to do it Nicci's way. Otherwise you're setting yourself up for failure. Do it *your* way. You know Nicci, she probably just did the bits she wanted to and ignored the rest. That's how she did everything else. Get out there and scratch the surface and you'll probably find it's not as magazine-perfect as it used to look from a distance.'

They were sitting at the refectory table watching Lizzie tear off sheet after sheet of kitchen roll, blow her nose, and toss it aside. She was nursing a mug containing the lukewarm dregs of a pot of coffee. All three women jumped when the phone rang.

It rang three more times before Jo found the handset under a tea towel on the worktop. 'Hello?' she said. 'David Morrison's, erm . . .' Jo looked at the others but they just shrugged. 'Residence?' she finished.

Mona sniggered and Lizzie waved a hand to shush her.

'Hello? Hello?'

There was no answer, just a distant click at her third 'hello'. But just like last time she had a distinct feeling someone was there.

'Who was it?' Mona asked.

'No one. It sounded like there was someone there when I answered but the line went dead when they heard my voice.'

'Probably a call centre in India,' Lizzie said. 'You know how the line goes quiet for a minute or two after you answer, like it's waiting for a connection. Always freaks me out.'

'Didn't sound like that. More like there was someone there, then they hung up. It happened that evening I came round to see David about Charlie and Harrie, too.'

'David's got a mystery lover,' Mona laughed.

'In your dreams!'

'I heard the phone.' David was standing in the open back door. 'Who was it?'

'Oi, goalie!' Dan shouted. David let the door swing shut on Mona's son's protests.

'Nobody,' Jo said. 'I'd have called you.'

'Didn't they leave a message?' he asked, crossing the kitchen and checking the little red light.

'When I say nobody, I mean, literally, nobody,' said Jo, trying to hide her irritation as he checked there was no one on the line anyway. 'Like last time,' she said when he replaced the receiver. 'Remember? Probably just a call centre.'

'Are you expecting a call, David?' Mona asked pointedly.

'No,' he said, but he seemed on edge. 'Just had a couple of strange calls lately, bloody irritating.'

'God,' Jo muttered when he'd rejoined the game, 'what's

eating him? Perhaps you're right, Mona. Maybe he's being consoled by a nurse from the hospice.'

Lizzie sprayed her coffee. 'Stop it, you two!' she said. 'David wouldn't do something like that.' She pushed the coffee away. 'It must be wine o'clock by now, surely?'

'It is by my watch,' Mona said.

The cork was out of the bottle and three indecently large glasses filled with Pinot Grigio when the phone rang again. This time David was in the kitchen before Jo could pick up.

He listened and then dropped it back onto its charger. 'Sorry,' he said. 'I don't mean to be paranoid. It's just I keep having these nuisance calls. They're getting to me a bit.'

'You can report them, you know,' Lizzie said. 'There's a number you can call to get your number put on some list that means they can't cold-call you. I'll find out what it is, if you like?'

'Nah, it's fine, thanks,' he said, taking a swig from Jo's glass before heading back out into the garden. 'I'll do it.'

Only Jo noticed him pull the wire from the socket before he left.

'Nom nom,' Dan said, walking mud across the slate floor. 'Smells brilliant. What is it?'

'Roast pork, roast potatoes, veg, apple sauce, nut roast for Mum,' Lizzie reeled off without taking her eyes off the gravy. There were lumps. There were always lumps. Carefully she chased one to the edge and squished it against the pan with the back of her spatula. Cornflour blossomed white in the golden liquid and dissolved.

Dan was right. The food smelled amazing. The rosemary and thyme that had been tossed in olive oil with the potatoes mingled with the scent of succulent pork, which was now crisping in the oven. Broccoli, green beans and peas were set to boil on the hob, their steam condensing on the windows overlooking the garden.

'Talking of Mum, where is she? I thought she was in here.'

Jo looked up from the *Observer* in surprise. 'Didn't realise she wasn't. Where'd she go, Lizzie?'

'Loo, probably. Dunno, though. She's been gone for a while.'

'Typical.' Dan rolled his eyes and grabbed a handful of crisps from a bowl on the side. 'She's always doing that.'

'Doing what?'

'Vanishing,' Dan said. 'On her mobile a-*gain*, I bet.'

'Her mobile?' Lizzie and Jo exchanged glances.

'Yeah,' Dan crunched through a mouthful of crisps and grabbed another handful. 'She's always on her mobile or looking at her mobile waiting for a text or a call. Reckon she thinks if she makes calls in the bathroom I can't hear her. Like, duh . . .'

'Hey, love, what's up?' Si leant over the back of Jo's chair and wrapped his arms around her.

'Lunch is up, nearly. Want a drink?'

'Definitely,' said Gerry, coming in behind him. 'What have you got? Hey, Jo, if you don't mind me saying, you look wrecked.'

'Cheers, Gez.' Jo stuck out her tongue. 'You sure know how to make a girl feel good about herself.'

He was right, though. She did look wrecked. Looked wrecked, felt wrecked, *was* wrecked. But she'd been hoping to get away without anyone pointing it out. So far, the girls and David had been kind enough not to. Trust *Gez*.

'What haven't we got?'

'I'm going to open Chablis, if anyone's interested,' David said, opening the fridge. 'In Nicci's honour.'

Chablis was another of Nicci's favourites.

'I don't mind mixing my reds and whites if you don't,' Gerry said.

Over his shoulder Lizzie caught Jo rolling her eyes and muttering something under her breath. From where Lizzie sat, it looked like, *Surprise me*.

'Gerry's right, you know,' Lizzie said, laying her free hand on Jo's shoulder as they unloaded roast vegetables into a piping-hot serving bowl. 'I didn't want to say anything earlier, but you don't look yourself. You're not ill, are you?'

Jo picked imaginary bits off Si's fleece, deciding how to respond.

Lizzie's hand snaked down to the bowl and broke off a piece of roast potato, spiriting it into her mouth.

There were many things Jo wanted to say, not least of which was: *pot/kettle, Lizzie O'Hara. You must have put on a stone since Christmas*. But she didn't. It would have been cruel. Being cruel, even to be kind, wasn't Jo's thing. It was Nicci's.

A roast carrot followed the potato.

Someone would have to intervene. Lizzie was eating for England, just as Jo had reverted to the clothes she wore at seventeen (basically, whatever her older brother had discarded) and Mona, well . . . where *was* Mona?

'I just put on the first thing I found this morning,' Jo said noncommittally, rinsing the roasting pan and sliding it straight into the dishwasher. 'Forgot to collect my dry cleaning yesterday. You know how it is.'

'That's not what I meant. Although I'm not sure Nicci would approve of your, erm, *look*.'

Why hadn't she made more effort? Jo should have known

Lizzie would notice if she didn't, but Jo just hadn't felt up to it this morning.

'Yeah, well,' she shrugged. 'Nicci's opinion of my outfit is the least of my worries right now.'

It was meant to sound casual, but it came out bitter, opening more questions than it closed. Shutting off the conversation, she slipped oven gloves over her hands and carried the steaming bowl of roast vegetables to the table.

In the time it took to put the food on the table and deal everyone a plate, Mona had slid onto the bench beside Dan, and popped Charlie onto her knee. Harrie had already bagsied David's.

'Where've you been? Dan was looking for you,' Jo said, hoping her voice didn't sound as interested in the answer as she was.

'He found me, didn't you, hon,' Mona said, ruffling the top of his head and turning her attention pointedly to slicing nut roast. 'Anyone else for this, or am I the only one who doesn't eat dead stuff around here?'

Jo and Lizzie exchanged glances. They weren't convinced.

'Is it me, or was Mona odd today?' Jo yawned, her head resting on Si's chest. They were shrouded in darkness, the only light orange stripes from the streetlamp that bled through their shutters onto the white duvet.

Lunch had gone on till seven, when David remembered – somewhat belatedly – that it was past Charlie and Harrie's bedtime.

Helped by Pinot Grigio, Chablis, more Chablis and then brandy, the food had gone down well. Jo, for one, was glad they'd done it. There had been awkward moments, of course; and Mona and David had barely exchanged a glance, let alone two words, but still, it was a start.

'Mona was odd, Lizzie was odd, David was odd . . . everyone was odd,' Si said, 'except Charlie, Harrie and Dan.'

'Was I odd?'

'No odder than usual.'

She slapped his still-firm tummy. 'I'm serious.'

'Everyone was odd, love. We were bound to be. It was the first time we've all been together, in that house, since the funeral. Next time will be easier. You weren't especially odd, you're just knackered.'

Jo heard him take a deep breath.

'On the subject of which . . .'

Jo felt herself tense. She tried not to. She couldn't help it. 'Not now, Si,' she ventured. 'Like you said, I'm knackered.'

'We have to talk sometime,' Si said, kissing the top of her head. 'We can't go on pretending it hasn't happened.'

'Which particular it?' Jo asked, closing her eyes.

'The Nicci it,' Si said.

And Jo exhaled.

'But also the IVF it.'

'Please, Si . . .'

'And the business it.'

She knew he was letting her off the hook. For now. And she was grateful.

'You can't go on like this,' he continued. 'You need help with the business. You might have Kelly and the rest of the team, but it's not enough. You can't keep trying to do your job and Nicci's too. I know she left you in charge, but she would expect you to get help. The way you're going, you're setting yourself up for failure.'

His words rang with a distant familiarity.

Rolling onto his side, Si gently took her face in his hands so she had no choice but to look at him. *First things first*, his eyes said in the glow of the streetlight. *And then we'll tackle the other things. But we* will *tackle them.*

'Face it, love,' he said. 'I know you think Nicci's irreplaceable. But you *are* going to have to find someone to replace her.'

FIFTEEN

It wasn't difficult for David to get away from work. Being the boss, or one of them, he had nobody to answer to. His colleagues were used to his comings and goings, and he told them where they could find him as a courtesy. He'd always worked mainly from his office at home, and when he wasn't there he was on site. Either way, he was always on the other end of his iPhone. In fact, he'd only started going to the office regularly in the last few months, since he reached the point where too much time spent with his own thoughts made him want to hurl something. Like himself, off a tall building.

Even now he didn't know why he'd agreed to meet Nicci's mother. Most people meet their mother-in-law at the start of a relationship, not the end. It was the worst of all worlds, he thought: losing your wife and gaining a mother-in-law.

He certainly didn't know why he'd chosen Starbucks in Kingston-upon-Thames. It wasn't convenient for her, and it wasn't convenient for him. What it was, was *away*. Away from the home Nicci had made without her mother's love, support, interference or knowledge. Away from the grand-daughters Nicci never wanted her mother to know. As far away from Nicci's life as possible. Anonymous enough not to run into anyone he knew.

So, Nicci, thought David as he locked the door of the racing-green Mini Cooper he'd had restored for her thirty-fifth birthday, and headed across the second storey of an NCP car park, *if you're so clever, you thought you could leave everything nice and tidy – a place for everyone and everyone in their place – Jo and the girls, Lizzie and the garden, Mona and me . . . well, answer me this, Nicci Morrison. What the hell am I supposed to do about your mother? You didn't see that one coming, did you?*

Stopping in the middle of the multistorey car park, he cocked his head, as if listening for an answer. Traffic roared on the main road, kids shouted down on the street outside, electronic locks blipped, car alarms bleated, footsteps echoed down concrete stairs.

See, he said sadly, shouldering his way through a swing door into a stairwell. *You can't tidy her up now, can you?*

'How will I recognise you?' Nicci's mother had asked when he'd called to admit defeat. He had no choice. His nerves couldn't take the constant worry that she'd phone when he wasn't there and get one of the girls instead. Even if they didn't understand a word she was saying, he'd still have some explaining to do to the nanny.

Or worse, she'd call when Jo or Lizzie were there and he wasn't. That Easter Sunday had nearly finished him off. He knew he'd behaved suspiciously, jumping each time the phone rang, unplugging it from the wall when he thought no one would notice. Though he was sure Jo had. She didn't miss much at the best of times. And she'd been on high alert the rest of the afternoon, rarely taking her eyes off him. Knowing Nicci's friends, they probably thought he was having an affair.

Hardly. He couldn't imagine ever wanting a relationship again.

Not even with Mona.

Not even with Mona? Where had that come from? *Especially not with Mona.*

His shudder had nothing to do with the cold. Easter had come late. There had been a May shower first thing this morning, but it had long since blown over and the air was now soft and warm.

The kind of day Nicci loved.

How could he even think of Mona? What had Nicci been thinking, trying to manoeuvre her friends' lives like they were pawns in her personal game of chess? The friends who should have been his comfort blanket in the months after her death had become something to be wary of. How could Nicci be so cruel?

Why hadn't she talked to him? About the children, the garden . . . any of it? It wasn't that there was anything wrong with Mona. Other than that she wasn't his type. That incongruous mix of itchy feet, yoga and herbal tea, combined with dollop of in-your-faceness she'd brought back with her from Australia, discomforted him.

The whole New Age thing was put on. It had to be. That Mona would never have had anything to do with that married tosser she used to see.

David racked his brains for the man's name. It was bugging him out of all proportion by the time he reached Starbucks, bought a latte and found a table out of the main drag. 'Distraction tactics,' Nicci would have said, but who was she to talk? That name had been every other word that came out of Nicci's mouth at one point. She hated him even more than Mona's ex, Greg, and despite the fact she'd never met him ('and never wanted to') Nicci didn't have a good word to say about him either.

106

Truth was, David had never really warmed to Mona. Not back at uni and not now. There was something off about her, as if she was permanently hiding something.

Pushing the thought from his mind, David glanced around Starbucks at the nondescript bunch of students, tourists and office workers on lunch break. 'You won't recognise me,' he'd told Nicci's mother. 'There's nothing to recognise. I'm an average-looking, average-height, average-build bloke at the wrong end of his thirties, with scruffy brown hair and a wardrobe full of jeans. I'll look like every other bloke in there.'

Yes, that about summed it up. *I don't for the life of me know what Nicci saw in me*. He'd managed to stop himself saying that bit out loud. 'But if you look even slightly like my wife, I'll recognise you.'

She was small. Unassuming, at first glance. A beige water-proof jacket hung open to reveal a slither of dark blue jumper, a brown leather bag clutched protectively in front of her body. He noticed her anyway, the second the door opened to let in another wave of the lunchtime flow. She was not what he expected. And yet she was.

But she was not Nicci.

It was not, in some melodramatic way, as he had hoped – and feared – it might be: like looking at a Nicci he would never see. A Nicci who had passed her sixtieth birthday. This woman was different: Nicci put through a fairground hall of diminishing mirrors, having lived a different sort of life and come out the other side. Plainer than her daughter; her face pinched, her age etched in every line. The results of a life less fabulously lived. Her grey hair was cropped close, her features small and sharp. She was striking rather than attractive, the lines exaggerating her features.

A receptionist at David's work apparently took one look

at her new baby and shrieked, 'Oh my God, I've given birth to my dad.' When David first heard the story, he felt repulsed. Now he understood precisely. Nicci's mother looked like Charlie and Harrie in the hours after they were born: scrunched-up versions of Nicci. Although he hadn't know it, for those few short days, they'd looked exactly like Nicci's mother.

Sharp grey eyes skimmed the room and settled on his. Hardly surprising. He'd been staring so hard that, even if she didn't know who she was looking for, she couldn't have missed him. Something flickered across the weathered face. Not a smile, nor recognition; maybe relief.

For the first time, anxiety clenched David's stomach. What was he doing here? If not dining with the devil, then certainly about to share coffee with someone Nicci had hated so much no mention of her was tolerated.

But what was he supposed to do? Change his phone number and move? Oh, he'd considered it. But it wasn't easy just to pack up your entire life and vanish when you had children and an architect's practice to think about.

'David? David Morrison?' Her voice was deeper than Nicci's. Up close she seemed bigger, her small weather-worn hands brown and ringless, her handshake firm but the skin rough against his. If she was nervous she hid it well. 'I'm Lynda.'

He nodded and stood up, instantly shrinking her back to size. 'Mrs Webster,' he said, 'I'd better get you something to drink.'

By the time he got back with her order – strong, milky tea and a ploughman's sandwich couldn't be further from Nicci's order – the world had settled back on its axis. Sitting anxiously on the edge of her chair and without her coat and bag for protection, Nicci's mother looked like what she was:

a woman in her sixties, wearing a navy jumper, unfashion-ably cut jeans and designed-for-comfort ankle boots.

'Aren't you having anything?' She sounded worried, as she watched him place her sandwich and two mugs on the table.

'A panini,' he said. 'They're toasting it.'

'Ah,' she nodded, took a sip of her too-hot tea, and winced. Around them the clatter of cups and cutlery, shouted orders and chatter drowned out the muzak filtering through the speakers. Workmates bitched about bosses; old friends caught up; new lovers gazed into each other's eyes, leaving their food untouched; old lovers chewed stolidly and read books or papers in, mainly, companionable silence.

'I'm so . . .'

'I . . .'

Both decided to break the silence.

'You go first.'

'No, you.'

David took a sip of his latte and waited. Nicci's mother took another sip of her builder's tea and followed it with a deep breath. 'Thank you,' she said, clutching her mug as if it was keeping her afloat, 'for agreeing to meet me.'

'To be honest, you didn't give me much choice.'

She looked at him.

'Unless you expected me to go to the police and complain about harassment? And, believe me, I considered that.'

Her hands were shaking. He wondered if she smoked and decided she did. Up close she had the skin of a smoker; the little lines sketched around her tight mouth from years of sucking up nicotine.

'I was her mother.'

'So you've said.'

Should he ask for proof? David wondered. Only he didn't need it. At least, not that Nicci and this woman shared some genes. He could see that from her face.

Nicci had been the decision maker in their family. Well, Nicci was dead; had been dead three months. And as much as he might wish it, she wasn't coming back. He had to live his own life now.

Trying to look more certain than he felt, David smiled at the stranger-who-wasn't on the other side of the table and took his iPhone from his inside pocket. He tapped open Photos, then Camera and slid the iPhone across the table.

Blinking, Nicci's mother stared at him.

'Photos,' he said, gently pushing it closer. 'You want to see what my daughters look like, don't you?'

For one awful moment he thought Lynda was going to cry. He could cope with almost anything – he'd surprised himself these last nine, ten months how much he could cope with – but he wasn't sure he could deal with making a middle-aged woman cry in a coffee shop full of strangers.

'They're . . .' Lynda said finally, swiping at her face, '. . . they're so like Nicci.'

David nodded, and said nothing. Not wanting to tell the woman about the picture in the beside cabinet. The one that wasn't meant to exist.

'Look,' she said, pulling a faded envelope from her bag and spilling the contents across the table. 'Look how like Nicci they are.'

It was inevitable the picture she handed him first was almost identical to the one he'd already seen, the next frame in the sequence, perhaps, but the same woman and the same girl in the same clothes on the same day, squinting at a camera and at the person behind it, who David could only assume had been Nicci's father.

SIXTEEN

'We haven't got long. I need to be back at work by three.'

Why did Neil always have to do that? Mona wondered, pulling her grey sweater over her head and flicking it across the room as Neil began unbuttoning her jeans. She wasn't asking for candles and roses – their affair had been going on far too long for that – but some small attempt at romance wouldn't go amiss occasionally. A box of chocolates. Or even an 'I've missed you, babe' before he headed upstairs.

'Neil, I . . .' but her knickers were around her knees and he was lapping at her hungrily.

'Neil, for Christ's sake,' she groaned, feeling herself grow wet. 'It's broad daylight, let's not give the neighbours a floor show.'

Not that Mona knew why she bothered. Closing the curtains in the middle of the day when Dan was at school and she'd nipped home in a stolen late lunch hour, swiftly followed by a suited man in a blue BMW who just about made a pretence of parking around the corner, was equivalent to hanging a sign on the door saying, 'Good Seeing to in Progress'.

Sex was Mona's thing. She didn't do steady boyfriends at

sixth form or university, but she had more than her share of lovers. She liked sex. Really liked it. And she couldn't be bothered with the aggravation of going steady. Unsurprisingly, she saw now, boys at college had regarded that as a winning combination.

But good sex – great, amazing, scrape-yourself-off-the-ceiling sex – proved her downfall. It was good sex that landed her with Dan's dad. Although sex with him had been entirely different from sex with Neil; wholesome and athletic, the kind that went on all night. Her first experience of sex that mattered. Sex with love attached. What a disaster that had been. Not that she regretted Dan for a second. Greg was another matter.

Neil, on the other hand, didn't do wholesome. That had been one of his many attractions for Mona. With Neil, if it hadn't been for the sex she wouldn't have got close enough to become so entangled with him.

And entangled with Neil was not a good place to be.

In the beginning, seeing him for sex when they could both manage it had suited her fine. No love, no emotion, not really; nothing to complicate things as she tried to rebuild a life for Dan with no Dad in it.

The sex with Neil was usually quick and dirty. And it was still as good now as it had been the first time they did it in the back of his car, that first night. There was no point saying she wasn't that kind of girl, because she was. And, back then, she hadn't wanted him to see her any other way. It was just, usually she didn't come back for seconds, thirds or one hundred and fourths.

Neil wasn't interested in *making love*. He'd said as much outside the bar. He had a wife for that. (OK, he hadn't actually said that last bit, but Mona knew it all the same.) Mona was there to fuck. To do the things his wife wouldn't. Mona was under no illusions about that.

And she liked it. Looked forward to it. But she knew that the day she'd started to mind that it was months since he'd last bothered to pretend he would leave his wife for her, was the day she should have ended it.

The sex was quick, dirty and over. She knew it was over, but not because she'd come. That meant nothing. When she was in the mood and time was on their side, they could do it three, four times, in the space of one lunch hour, each coming harder and faster every time.

Their affair might have seen better days but the sex hadn't.

No, she knew it was over because she'd opened her eyes as the vibrations receded inside her and caught Neil flipping his wrist to glance at his watch. Less than half an hour since he'd walked through the door.

'Off already?' she said, hating herself as the words came out of her mouth.

Irritation crossed his face.

'What's with you these days? I said last night I only had an hour door-to-door. And, if memory serves me right, you said, "It only takes fifteen minutes to fuck."'

She flinched as her words came back at her. Yes, she'd said that . . . But it had been late, she'd been on the wrong side of two large vodka and slimlines, and they'd been having hissed phone sex, Mona locked in her bedroom, under the duvet so Dan wouldn't hear from his room.

'I just don't want you thinking I'm sitting here waiting to jump when you call.'

Grinning, Neil stretched across her and grabbed his shirt from the floor. 'You didn't seem to mind ten minutes ago.' Rolling back, he nipped at her nipple.

For a split second Mona was furious, and then she felt her nipple harden between his teeth and knotted her fingers in his hair, locking him against her.

She knew Neil could be a git. Christ, Nicci had told her often enough. If only he didn't make her feel so good. When he wasn't making her feel like shit.

Closing her eyes, Mona tried to push Nicci from her mind. If Nicci had known she'd gone back to Neil . . . If Nicci had known, then what?

I bet David's not a bastard in bed.

The thought occurred to Mona almost idly as Neil slid back inside her and she locked her legs around his. *There's no way Nicci would have put up with that.*

'There are a few things I need to tell you.' The quiet determination in Lynda's voice made David shudder, it was so familiar. She'd barely touched her sandwich, but the tea was long gone. 'It took courage to call you,' she said. 'I need to do what I came here for.'

David nodded and took another bite of his mozzarella panini, forcing himself to chew and swallow as he gathered his thoughts.

He knew he should feel sorry for her, this woman who only found her daughter again when it was too late. Who had just seen pictures of her grandchildren for the first time. But how hard had she tried? Really? How many letters had she written? How many calls had she made when her daughter was alive?

His anger surprised him. This was her own fault. If she'd lost her daughter, her grandchildren, what did it have to do with him? Whatever had happened between her and his wife, Lynda was the mother, the adult, the grown-up. The responsibility was hers.

You're not being fair, he told himself. After all, if Lynda *had* tracked her down would Nicci have told him? Would she have given her mother the time of day?

He forced himself to meet Lynda's eyes. What was he

supposed to do? Put an arm around her? Hug her? Tell her everything would be all right, as he would his own mother? But this woman couldn't have been less like his own mother, who had 'Granny' down to a fine art.

'I'm not being polite when I tell you not to call me Mrs Webster,' she said, dragging his attention back to her. 'I'm not really Mrs Webster, haven't been for years.'

'I'm sorry,' David said. He felt faintly stupid. Why would she be? 'I didn't know.'

'Of course not. Webster was my maiden name. I changed my name back, and Nicci's too, when her dad left. Her dad's surname was Gilbert. Cummings was my second husband's name. Nicci's stepdad.'

'Nicci had a stepdad?'

'She really didn't tell you anything, did she?'

Lynda Cummings, an utter stranger, stared at him. David tried to decipher the look then gave up. He wasn't sure he wanted to know what it meant. Just as he didn't want to think about the things Nicci hadn't told him. Nicci had secrets; he'd known that right from the start. Take it or leave it, that was the deal.

'I met Brian when Nicci was nine,' Lynda said. 'She was hostile from the start, but I just put that down to jealousy. I mean, we'd been on our own for five, six years by then. Nicci wanted me to herself. Said she couldn't see why I needed Brian when I had her.

'Brian wasn't the first man I'd dated since Nicci's dad left, but he was the first she met. Usually blokes run a mile at the first sniff of a kid. Well, they did then. It's probably different now, I don't know. Most things are.'

David shrugged. He didn't know either.

'But Brian didn't. He was good about it. Liked Nicci even, though she was a right little madam. Talked back to him, cheeked him. All the usual stuff: "You're not my dad, you can't make me . . ." And that just made me love him even more. I mean, he was nice-looking, had a decent job, bought me flowers *and* he was nice to my kid. Then he proposed. I thought I'd died and gone to heaven. Well, you would, wouldn't you?'

She looked at him for acknowledgement, so David nodded. He guessed you would, if you were a woman on your own with a kid in those days.

'I knew Nicci wouldn't like it, but I thought she'd come round. When I told her Brian and I were getting married she cried so loud you could have heard her the other side of Margate.'

'Margate?' David frowned

'You didn't know she came from Margate?'

David shook his head, closed his eyes for a second. That explained Nicci's obsession with Whitstable. So near, and yet so far.

'Assume, where you're concerned, I know nothing.'

Nicci's mother raised her mug to her lips thoughtfully, and then seemed to remember it was cold and empty and put it down again. David wasn't fooled. He knew she was using the empty mug as a shield. He was doing the same himself.

Taking a deep breath, Lynda resumed, 'We'd been married about a month the first time Brian hit me.'

David snapped back to full attention. 'He hit you? Did he hit—'

'No . . . Yes.' Shame flooded the woman's face. 'But not at first. He only hit Nicci much later, when she tried to stop him hitting me. That first time I thought it was a one-off. That's the way it is. You don't believe it's going to happen again.'

David stared at her, revolted and appalled in equal measure. Poor Nicci.

'I know what you're thinking. Only that's not why Nicci wouldn't have anything to do with me. I mean, it is, but not that time.'

David felt like someone had removed his oxygen. *Breathe*, he told himself, pulling the air up into his nostrils. *Breathe*. 'Not that time?' he asked finally.

Without raising her eyes from the table, Nicci's mother shook her head. 'It happened again. It always happens again,' she said, voice barely audible. 'He hit me and, very occasionally, he hit her. More of a slap really. But still . . .'

'Eventually – but not nearly soon enough – I found the courage to leave. Well, Nicci found it for me. She heard about a refuge, saved her dinner money until she had our train fare (I didn't know that, of course) and she persuaded me we had to go, as far away as we could. By then I was so beaten down I just went with it. Nicci could be forceful when she wanted.'

David smiled, he couldn't help it. Forceful wasn't the half of it.

'We waited for Brian to go to the pub one night and just walked out of the house. Took virtually nothing with us, just a change of clothing. Nicci insisted. She didn't want anything to slow us down. We got a train to London.'

'That's all very well, but it doesn't explain . . .'

When the woman before him raised her eyes from the table it was as if she'd aged ten years. The steel was gone. 'Could I possibly have another cup of tea?' she said. 'Two sugars this time, please.'

'You've guessed what happened, I expect,' Lynda said before David had even sat down. He hadn't, but he nodded in encouragement and slid the mug across to her.

'I went back to him. Don't think I haven't regretted it every day since. But I went back. And took Nicci with me.'

117

She took gulps of the hot sweet tea. It must have scalded her throat, seared her windpipe and burnt her chest but she didn't stop.

'Nicci persuaded me to leave a second time,' she said when the still-steaming mug was drained. 'She found another refuge, and after we'd been there a few months they helped her with the paperwork to get us a council flat. We started to build a new life together. I got a job in Tesco. Nicci started sixth form, doing A levels in English, History and Art; discovered a passion for clothes that I assume, from her business, she never lost.'

David didn't respond. It didn't look as if Lynda expected him to.

'And then one day I looked up from my till and there he was with a pint of milk, a box of cornflakes, a jar of Nescafé and a four-pack of Carling. I can see those items on the conveyor belt as clearly as if they were in front of me now.'

'Brian came looking for you?'

'That's the saddest thing of all. I don't think he had. In a funny way it might have been better if he'd been scouring London for us, but I think it was a total fluke. I looked up and there he was. Still handsome, still charming.

'He said, "Lynda, darling, I love you, I miss you. I'm so sorry I'm an idiot, please come back. Give me another chance." Just like that, right there in the checkout queue. And everyone around us thought we were in a film or something.

'The truth was, I was lonely and missed him. Bloody fool. He'd given me more bruises than I dare think about, even cracked my cheekbone one time, and some ribs. But I still loved him. If it hadn't been for Nicci I'd probably never have left him in the first place. I was his wife. Brian was my husband. I went back again.'

If even half of the emotions storming through David's head made the transition to his face, he could only imagine his expression: disgust, contempt, horror, loathing.

'I can see what you're thinking,' she said. 'And don't think I don't know what I did because I do. It cost me my daughter.'

David stared at her. He wanted to shout, to pick up the small, pinched woman in front of him and shake her until her joints popped. God help him, he wanted to hit her. And he'd never hit anyone in his life, apart from a couple of pissed-up fights as a student.

'How could you?' he started. 'How could you choose a man who hit you over . . . over *your child*?'

Lynda shrugged in defeat. Surely she didn't expect him to feel sorry for her? 'Things were different then,' she whispered. 'You made your bed, you lay in it. That's how I was brought up.'

David felt his fury bubble up and overflow. 'You might have given birth to Nicci, but you couldn't be less like her if you tried,' he said, not caring at the pain he saw ignite in her eyes. 'Nicci was brave and strong and smart. She protected her family, she would never – *never* – turn her back on them and walk away. And she didn't want us to know she had a mother who would.'

The scraping of his chair as he pushed it back set his teeth on edge. The couple on the next table stopped talking and openly stared until he glared and they turned away.

'I'm sorry, *Mrs Cummings*.' David almost spat the name, he couldn't help it. 'You insisted we meet. Well, now I insist you obey Nicci's wishes and leave me, and my family, alone.'

SEVENTEEN

Winter had been wet and spring even wetter, so Lizzie shouldn't have been surprised the side gate was swollen in its frame. It would take more than a week of unseasonably hot sunshine to dry it out.

She leant her shoulder against it and pushed, felt it give slightly, and then nothing.

Sliding Nicci's key – *her* key – into the side gate at David's house had felt wrong. Lizzie felt like an intruder, despite having called David a few days earlier to ask if she could come round this weekend, just to size up the enormity of the task. His uneasiness echoed down the line even as he assured her it was fine. When he'd called back fifteen minutes later to say he'd forgotten he was taking the girls to his parents for the weekend, would she mind letting herself in? Lizzie recognised it for the white lie it was and felt grateful. Bad enough to be snooping around David's garden, without him watching her do it.

But she could do with David now, if only to let her in. Taking a few steps back, feeling faintly ridiculous, she took a small run and barged the gate with her shoulder. The gate barely noticed. It juddered, gave a little more and then

120

bounced back. Another two runs and Lizzie finally managed to force it open.

Now, of course, the gate was impossible to shut behind her. Where was Gerry when she needed some muscle? Lizzie's laugh echoed around the silent garden. Where he always was: playing rugby/golf/cricket. Or watching someone else play it.

Leaning back, feeling the cool damp wood through her sweater, she gazed down David's garden. The bottom, beyond the shed, was barely visible. She'd had no idea there was so much of it. Had it always been this long?

A paved terrace, where she stood, formed a ten-foot frill along the back of the house. A large rectangular metal table and matching French café chairs were stacked to the side, terracotta pots still laden with the brittle corpses of last summer's geraniums clustered beneath it. Long summer evenings had been spent around that table, downing bottles of icy rosé and watching David's half-arsed attempts to get the barbecue going.

Something yellow caught Lizzie's gaze between the pots. Crouching, she wedged her hand in the gap. The tips of her fingers grazed something waxy. She flinched before realising it was just the stump of a candle. The citronella-scented ones Nicci bulk-bought in Carrefour, ten for a euro, one long ago Spanish holiday, and used to keep mosquitoes at bay.

Enough, Lizzie told herself, blinking away tears.

Beyond the terrace, the top third of the large garden was laid to grass, with wide flowerbeds on either side. Beyond that, apple trees hung with swings made from tyres formed a dividing line between the playing garden and the working garden. At the bottom, Lizzie knew, lay a large vegetable patch that, much like the rest of it, was long overdue some love.

The garden that populated Lizzie's head was bold and

flamboyant. Snowdrops, bluebells and daffodils died down to give way to the riot of colour Nicci loved in the summer, chrysanthemums and dahlias replacing it as autumn closed in. The terracotta pots dominating the terrace contained geraniums and begonias. Lizzie knew this; she'd looked them up. Lesser pots contained trailing things she could recognise but not name.

The garden in front of her could not have been more different.

The grass was short and neat, but only because David had cut it so Dan could play football at Easter. The same could not be said for the rest. The pots that Lizzie had so often tried – and failed – to emulate for her own terrace huddled in a corner, their soil compacted, last year's plants no more than dead sticks.

The flowerbeds were as bad. If not for the shrubs that grew all year, oblivious to the human trauma around them, and the daffodils that had come up willy-nilly, unaware their arrival would pass almost unnoticed, they were bare. The ten varieties of clematis that smothered the left-hand wall had run riot. Nicci had religiously pruned them, cutting them back so brutally that Lizzie was amazed they survived. Now she could see why. Turn your back for a few months and the clematis took over. Lizzie hardly dared look at what lay beyond but she knew she had to, if only to pull it all up.

At least the soil was drying out. There was no squelch underfoot as Lizzie traipsed across the turf in Converse that couldn't have been less appropriate. She felt spooked – watched, almost. Even though she knew she was completely alone.

But that, in itself, was wrong. Not just no Nicci, but no David and the girls, no Jo and Si and Si's boys, no Mona and Dan. It suddenly dawned on Lizzie that she had never been here alone before. She'd babysat Charlie and Harrie once or twice. Sat with Nicci at the big metal table drinking coffee while David took the twins for a walk in their double pram. But just her in a garden that was large enough for a five-a-side football match? A garden that was meant to be filled with people, laughter and love.

Glancing back, Lizzie almost expected to see everyone gathered on the terrace, laughing at her for taking Nicci's mad bequest so seriously.

The feeling became so overpowering that, despite herself, Lizzie took a second look. Nothing, of course. What did she expect? Just a bare lawn, barren pots and abandoned garden furniture. No boys kicking a football. No tiny girls swinging. No sunburnt men standing at a smoking barbecue with cold beers, making serious faces as they pretended to know what to do. And no Nicci leaning out of the kitchen window yelling, 'Anyone need a top-up?'

'I do,' Lizzie whispered.

She permanently needed a top-up these days. Jo, too, she'd noticed. Not yet midday and Lizzie would kill for a drink. What would her gran have said?

Rounding the apple tree, she was greeted by a circle of runner bean wigwams collapsed drunkenly in on themselves. Flanking these were rows of long-gone-to-seed cabbages.

Down here, the part of the garden the sun only reached in the height of summer, it was like crossing over to the dark side. Shrouded in shadow, it smelt dank, like woodland. Along the edge of the shed the blackberries had run wild and were choking the life from Nicci's gooseberry bushes.

Lizzie couldn't help smiling. Gooseberries were so deter-minedly old-fashioned, like rhubarb. Another Nicci favourite.

Nicci and Lizzie's granny were the only people she could remember cooking gooseberries. Horrible hairy, pippy things.

The jam was good, though. One of Lizzie's favourite memories was of watching her gran make gooseberry jam. Lizzie couldn't have been more than three, the age Harrie and Charlie were now. Standing on a kitchen chair beside the stove, stirring steadily, as her gran poured in seriously unhealthy quantities of sugar and made Lizzie promise not to stop, even for a second, or the mixture would stick and burn. Keeping the hot jam moving was her responsibility and Lizzie took her responsibilities seriously, even then.

She checked the greenhouse next. Expecting long-dead tomato plants and mould-coated windows, Lizzie shuddered. She could hardly bring herself to look, but still she pulled the brambles aside and squeezed past the shed to the long glass building tucked behind. Even through condensation and lichen she could see the greenhouse was bare. Plastic pots formed pyramids on the wooden workbench at one end. The parallel beds were empty. She understood immediately. Nicci had done this on one of her long sojourns 'thinking' at the bottom of the garden. As the cancer had sapped her strength she'd managed to put the greenhouse to bed, if nothing else.

A heap of potato plants lay mouldering beside a still-damp compost heap, along with rancid black plants Lizzie had a vague idea might be broad beans. She wished she'd paid more attention now. Paid attention? Lizzie wished she'd taken notes. After all, it wasn't like she could call her mother and ask for gardening advice.

'Not now,' Lizzie muttered. 'One trauma at a time.' Then caught herself. 'You're talking to yourself, Lizzie,' she said aloud. 'First sign of madness.

'Nu-huh,' she corrected, as she pushed the second key into the shed's lock and the door swung open. 'First sign of loneliness.' And she plunked herself into the battered leather armchair and began to sob.

Half an hour later Lizzie dug out Nicci's trowel, fork and secateurs, shoved her feet into Nicci's too small Hunters, and parked herself in front of a clematis, secateurs flashing in her gloved hands.

The floral gloves had thrown her. If she hadn't known Nicci better she'd have sworn they were Cath Kidston. But Nicci wouldn't be seen dead in . . . Lizzie caught herself. Nicci wouldn't have bought Cath Kidston.

It wasn't just the incongruity of the floral print. The intimacy of sliding her bare fingers into gloves where Nicci's own hands, smaller and quicker than Lizzie's, had been spooked Lizzie. Before her next visit she'd visit the garden centre and buy herself a pair.

She had to go anyway. There were plants to buy. Not that Lizzie knew anything about buying plants. But she didn't know anything about gardening either. And here she was standing in front of a clematis, preparing to attack it with a lethal weapon. Had she been a betting woman, Lizzie would have put money on the clematis to win.

'Tough,' Lizzie said, her voice so loud it made her jump.

Tough love had been Nicci's philosophy – in gardening as in life – and now Lizzie vowed to make it hers.

Hacking the plant back was surprisingly cathartic. After the first two or three nervous snips, long strands of green shoots coming away in her hand causing her a surge of panic, Lizzie gained confidence, working her way down the fence through the many varieties.

A clematis was a clematis, as far as she was concerned. She could see now each had different leaves, in different shades of green, some curved and pale, some spiky and dark, but she cut them all. Nicci had planted it so different varieties flowered as spring moved through summer into autumn. The fence was a mini masterpiece that would never go out of bloom.

Her brain was occupied by cutting, trimming and tucking. Something – not someone, she told herself, definitely not some*one* – telling her to go with her gut. It didn't matter if she snipped the wrong bit; the plant could take it. Soon, the off-cuts filled two recycling bags and, when she'd finished, the clematis looked, if not pretty, then at least tidy. No longer hellbent on world domination.

Emptying the pots was harder than Lizzie expected, physically at least.

Trying to remember what she'd seen Nicci do, she lugged each one to the bottom of the garden, working the dry soil out of the pot with her fingers before emptying it on the vegetable patch, then tossing last year's plants onto the compost heap. She wasn't sure that was right, but how bad could it be?

Four o'clock.

How could it be four o'clock?

Lizzie frowned and held her watch to her ear to make sure it was ticking. It was.

It felt little more than an hour since she'd finished pruning and dragged Nicci's gardening mat up to the flowerbeds and started to weed. Logically, it had to be far longer. Beside her a fourth recycling bag was full of debris and the sun had long since vanished behind the house. That meant she must have been gardening for almost five hours. Lizzie leant back on her aching haunches and surveyed the bed that lined the left-hand side of the garden. Five hours and so little to show for it: a wall of clematis pruned and only one bed relieved of its weeds. But it looked good: neat and green, weed-free and clear of debris. No longer starved of light by clematis above.

126

Lizzie felt the smile grow from deep inside her. The kind of smile that started in your stomach and reached all the way to your eyes. The kind of smile she hadn't experienced in a long time. For the first time in many, many months, Nicci's garden – a little bit of it at least – looked like someone loved it.

EIGHTEEN

Four o'clock?

How could it be four o'clock?

Jo tapped her watch to make sure it was working. It was, so she glanced at the digital clock on her computer to double-check.

Shit, four o'clock. How had she let that happen? Si was going to kill her.

He hadn't wanted her to go into the office at all. 'It's Saturday, for God's sake, Jo,' he'd grumbled as she rolled out of bed at half-past eight. 'When are you going to give yourself a break?'

His best grumpy-old-man impression. Although the truth was, at forty-five, he was not that old and he wasn't especially grumpy, either. This morning his eyes had been full of concern. He was worried. Well, so was she, just not about the same thing.

'Jo, honey . . .'

She finished wriggling into her jeans and turned to face him. He'd shuffled up onto one elbow and salvaged his glasses from the bedside table. He fixed her gaze with his own, making her shift uncomfortably. Glancing away, she twisted her ring on her finger for something to do.

'I'm serious,' he said. 'You need a break. You're exhausted, emotionally *and* physically. In the end it's just a job, and this is your health we're talking about. Can't you take one weekend off? Sleep, eat, stop pushing yourself? Just this once?'

The question was rhetorical. Or if it wasn't, Jo pretended to think it was, reaching into the clothes piled on the armchair for a clean-ish sweatshirt. Si knew it wasn't 'just a job'. It was business; *their* business, repository of their life's savings, such as they were, and currently running on half-empty. The talented half.

His hand worked its way up her spine, beneath her vest's thin fabric, and settled on the curve of her left breast as she sat beside him on the bed.

'I don't have to get the kids till two,' he mumbled, his face buried in her sleeve. 'Come back to bed.'

'You know I can't,' she said. 'There's too much to do.'

His sigh told her all she needed to know about what he thought of that. But she was grateful he spared her the lecture.

'I'll be home by the time you get back here with Sam and Tom,' she said. 'I promise. I know I haven't seen them properly for a while.'

He started to speak, to tell her it was fine, the boys were big enough to understand, she'd been under pressure . . . Jo put up her hand to silence him. 'You get some bad DVDs and I'll pick up some junk food on the way home. Right now, though, I've got to go.'

Removing his hand from her breast, she brought it up to her mouth and kissed the palm. 'You know I must.' And with that she headed to the stairs.

If she hadn't paused at the laundry basket to pick up a sock that had fallen wide she wouldn't even have heard it. The sigh, and the words that followed: 'We'll never make a baby this way . . .'

* * *

And there it was, Jo thought. Another thing they didn't/ couldn't/had stopped talking about. If she was honest with herself, *the thing*. The source of all their problems.

Baby making.

They'd tried for what felt like years. The trying had been fun at the start, until fertility charts, thermometers and mucus tests turned it into one more thing on the to-do list. There was nothing, Jo discovered, more guaranteed to put you off doing it than having to. Nothing more guaranteed to make someone who had never considered herself the maternal type decide she desperately wanted – needed – to make a baby than discovering she couldn't.

Doctors and specialists came next. A dozen visits to half a dozen experts. All of whom reached the same conclusion: it was her, obviously. It didn't take a genius to work that out. After all, Si had fathered two boys already. The good news was, their position wasn't hopeless. In fact, the specialist had suggested IVF might well work for them. Not that she was making any promises. Nobody was.

So Jo and Si made themselves a promise; went out for dinner and drank champagne to seal the deal. They would allow themselves three tries and if, after those three tries, they still didn't have a baby, either one of them could say the word and they would call it quits. How very grown-up it seemed at the time. How sensible. How much easier said than done.

Their third attempt failed just as Nicci's cancer was diagnosed and everything else – *everything* – was put on a back burner. Once or twice Si tried to slide it back to the front but Jo waved it away. She was tired, heartbroken, had too much on her plate. Even Si had to admit it wasn't the right time. Apart from anything else, whatever happened with Nicci, the business couldn't afford both her and Jo off at the same time.

Jo knew she should have told him her reservations before the stakes became so high, back when it might not have been such a big deal. Before the money was spent and the pregnancy tests failed and the tears shed. Before she started to feel such a failure. She should have told Si she hadn't even been sure she wanted a baby until she met him. In fact, Jo was horribly afraid she'd been behind the door when the maternal genes were handed out. But his boys were so sweet and she loved him so much that suddenly it seemed the most important thing in the world; to make their family complete.

She should have told him that, straight out.

Just as she should have told him Nicci had left her responsible for the love and emotional care of two small girls. On top of the two boys she already loved and cared for, who didn't really belong to her . . .

Groaning, Jo rolled her head back on her shoulders, trying to ease the tension that burnt in her neck, and flicked off her computer.

Si was right: she needed to give herself a break. Devote a bit of time to herself, and then devote a bit of time to them. If she didn't get to the chiropractor soon her neck would seize up altogether. Her roots were so overdue her hair looked almost two-tone. And as for exercise? Jo glanced down at her hard-won runner's body and closed her eyes. She wasn't naturally slim. This body took effort. That figure was one hundred per cent woman-made. How long could she neglect it before it slipped back the way it had come?

But it wasn't just her muscles that benefited from the exercise, so did her brain. Jo had always found sanity in running, but she hadn't slipped her feet into her Nikes and pounded the public footpath that stretched along the back of their house since before Nicci died. Weeks before.

Add it to the list, love, she thought, rolling back her desk chair and shrugging on a striped suit jacket. *Add it to the list.* Just one more problem on her ever-growing list of problems and, frankly, she had bigger things to worry about than slack muscles right now. Like Capsule Wardrobe's 'cruise collections' order. Cruise was tricky at the best of times. Falling between the coats, sweaters and party dresses of autumn/winter and spring/summer's lighter-weight fabrics, it was, Jo always felt, designed for those women who holidayed away the winter months in St Barts. Never having been one, she hadn't a clue where to start.

Jo sighed heavily.

The autumn/winter order had been done in February, right after Nicci died. And even if Jo had the faintest clue what their customers would want to be wearing in September she was in no shape to say back then. So she'd relied on Nicci's assistant, Kelly, who claimed to have been briefed by Nicci. The chasm between Nicci's instruction and Kelly's innate talent, Jo could see now, was vast, and she seriously regretted letting Kelly order. There was no way Jo would make the same mistake again.

Grabbing a biro from her desk, Jo rummaged for a Post-it note and scribbled on it 'FASHION MONITOR, JOB AD,' in scruffy capitals. Then she slapped the note in the middle of her computer screen where she wouldn't be able to miss it on Monday morning.

It pained her to admit it, but Si was right. Jo couldn't ignore it any longer. She – and Capsule Wardrobe – needed help.

The house was quiet when Jo tossed her keys on the hall table. No computer-generated gunfire echoing from the living room, no thud of ball on wall echoing from the back garden. This was not a good sign.

Nor was the sheet of notepaper hastily torn from an exercise book lying on the worktop in the kitchen, next to the plans for the extension that looked unlikely ever to happen.

'Gone to cinema,' it said in blue felt pen. 'Don't worry about food. Will pick up pizza on the way home.'

It was tolerant, considerate even. Si hadn't called, he hadn't pestered, he hadn't even sent a 'where the hell are you?' text. But Jo could feel the disappointment in his words and she didn't blame him.

She'd promised and, yet again, she hadn't delivered.

Nice work, she thought. *You let him down. Again. Worse, you let his boys down . . .* She pushed the heels of her hands into her eyes, making a kaleidoscope of coloured lights. It was the cardinal rule. Never make children a promise you can't keep. With luck – given her recent track record – Si had anticipated this and had known better than to pass on Jo's promise to Sam and Tom. Yes, she reassured herself, that's what would have happened. After all, he'd even known she'd forget to buy food on the way home. Again.

Opening the fridge, Jo pulled out a bottle of Sauvignon Blanc, took a large goblet from the cupboard and started to unscrew the top. The familiar click of metal separating stopped her in her tracks. It was 5 p.m. and still light outside. Two more hours of daylight at least, if the weather held. Si and the boys wouldn't be back for a while. If she started on the wine now she'd be halfway down the bottle when they got back. There had to be something else she could do. Something that would make her feel better, not worse.

Sliding the bottle unopened back into the fridge, Jo turned over Si's note and grabbed the same pen he'd used to write it. She should be back long before they were, but better safe than sorry.

'Gone running,' she wrote, singing off with a 'Jx.' It was

optimistic – right now the 'x' was unlikely to be returned – but suddenly she felt optimistic.

Now where had she last seen her trainers?

Even though it was not yet dark, light shone from the downstairs windows as Jo turned the corner of the alley that led from the footpath back into their street. Damn it, she must have been gone longer than she'd thought.

Either that, or the film was shorter.

Her calf and thigh muscles burnt, her punishment for not remembering to warm up properly. How amateur could you get? Sweat marbled her T-shirt, and her sports bra clung to the underside of her breasts. Undoubtedly, she looked like hell, but for the first time in months, Jo didn't feel it. For two hours, maybe more, she'd lost herself in the pull of her muscles, the pumping of her lungs and had felt her spirits soar as the endorphins that had been absent for so long began to flood her body. A long-forgotten wellbeing suffused her body, something approaching, if not calm, then a sense that her problems were not insurmountable. How could she have forgotten this sensation, how good it felt?

Slowing to a halt, Jo dropped forward from the waist to rest her palms on her Lycra-clad knees and watched the sweat drip from her straggly fringe onto the black and white tiled path. She was still in that position, letting her breath slow to normal, when she heard the front door open.

Warily, Jo straightened up, expecting to see annoyance, even disapproval in Si's gaze. Once again she hadn't been where she'd said she'd be, when she'd said she'd be there. Once again, she'd let him down.

'You went running!' Si cried, and his face split into a beaming grin that Jo realised she hadn't seen in months. He flung his arms around her sticky body. 'You went running!'

'Yes,' Jo said, returning his hug.

Pulling back slightly, Si raised his hand to push a damp tendril from her eyes. 'Yuck,' he said, 'you're soaked and you stink.' But he didn't let go. If anything he held her tighter. 'I'm so pleased, Jo.' He kissed her salty skin and she could feel his breath warm against her ear. 'I thought you'd forgotten how!'

Jo grinned and kissed him back, hard. 'I think maybe I had for a while.'

Over his shoulder a dark head appeared in the living-room door. 'Eugh,' said Sam. 'Dad and Jo are snogging.'

'That's not all,' she said, when they were sitting in the kitchen, with Jo unlacing her trainers. She could feel blisters threatening on the balls of her feet and the nub of her heels, warning of payment due for the months of laziness and lack of warm-up. 'Tomorrow I'll take the day off, come swimming with you guys. If that's OK and I can still move my limbs? And on Monday I'm going to advertise for a head buyer/ stylist. Maybe both, if Capsule Wardrobe can afford two new members of staff, but ideally just the one.'

A new Nicci, she thought, but didn't say.

Placing a large glass of cold white wine beside her, Si frowned and then started laughing. 'Who are you?' he said. 'And what have you done with my Jo?'

The evening sped past. Pizza and brownies were delivered and demolished while Sam and Tom watched their way through every inappropriate film Sky movies had to offer, sniggering and nudging each other at every swear word and gagging at the slightest suggestion of a sex scene. Occasionally one of them would glance up to see if Jo realised what they were watching and she'd pretend to be engrossed in the Saturday papers while Si marked homework at the other end of the room.

Grinning, Jo buried her head in the newspaper so nobody noticed. This was how family Saturday evenings were supposed to be. How they were before Nicci got ill and everything came crashing in. For the first time in months, Jo's mind was, if not quiet, then turning gently rather than churning like a washing machine on spin cycle. None of her problems had gone away, she wasn't kidding herself. The difference was they were waiting patiently for her to get to them, instead of jostling for her attention. But how long before the jostling started again? Not long, she knew.

'Si . . .' Jo said when the boys had gone to bed, Tom complaining bitterly that he was two years older and no way should he have to go to bed at the same time as Sam. *Life*, he proclaimed loudly from the top of the stairs, *was unfair*.

'. . . there are some things we need to talk about.'

Si raised his eyebrows and came to sit on the sofa beside her, sliding his arm along the back and resting his hand on her shoulder. 'Sounds ominous,' he said, leaning back to look at her. 'It's not ominous, is it?'

'Ish.' Jo shrugged. 'Yes, I guess. I mean, it is, a bit.'

Seize the day and all that. That was what she'd thought as she'd sat waiting for him to return from seeing the boys into bed, but now she was wondering what possessed her. A shit day had turned good. Was she really about to turn it back again?

'Jo,' Si said cautiously, 'tell me . . . What is it?'

When she'd finished, Si just stared at her for what seemed like minutes. He'd already removed his arm from the back of the sofa about halfway through. 'Si . . .' she started, but he held up his hand, his blue eyes distant.

'Just . . . give me a second,' he said. 'I need to process this.'

Jo nodded and swallowed her questions. Over the years she'd learnt her need for an instant reaction was at odds with Si's need 'to process'. But it still wasn't easy.

'So,' he said, after what seemed like hours. 'This letter. Tell me when it came again?'

'A couple of days after Nicci died. David brought it.'

'And where was I?'

'Swimming with the boys. Or football. I'm not sure. It was Sunday morning, you were out.'

Taking off his glasses, Si rubbed his eyes and put them back on again. 'And it didn't occur to you to tell me? That evening perhaps? Or the next day? Or the day after? You decided to wait three months to drop this bombshell? I thought we were better than that, Jo.'

Jo swallowed and bowed her head. He was right. It was unforgivable.

'We are,' she said. 'I promise we are. I just wasn't in any state to . . . I mean, with everything, I just . . . I'm sorry, I know it was stupid, but I was in shock. Nicci – my best friend – was dead and then . . . *this*. I mean, she'd left me – us – *people*. How could she? I just couldn't get my head around it. And . . .'

Now wasn't the right time to raise it, Jo knew, but she just couldn't see how else to explain her reticence.

'And what about Lizzie and Mona?' Si interrupted. 'They didn't think you should tell me? I presume you told them?'

Nodding, Jo kept her eyes firmly on the worn denim of her old jeans. She couldn't bear to see the hurt she knew would be in his eyes. Si and she were a team, they shared everything. Or used to.

'I called Lizzie as soon as I opened the letter. If you'd been here—'

'Jo, don't.'

'I'm not, I didn't mean that. I meant . . . well, I was on

my own. I got this letter. It was . . . *insane*, and I didn't know what to do so I called Lizzie. I thought maybe . . . Well, maybe the cancer . . .' Jo stopped. She couldn't say it; it was too disloyal.

'Lizzie had opened hers,' Jo started again, trying a different tack. 'But her bequest seemed funny – funny ha-ha – by comparison. And then Mona . . . Well, hers is worse. We just didn't know what to do. So we decided not to do anything. We didn't even talk to David to begin with.'

She felt Si pull back, his weight shifting the cushions, rather than saw it. 'You've talked to *David*?'

Oh shit, hadn't she mentioned that?

'We had to . . . I mean, what else were we supposed to do? It's his life, his children, his garden, *him* . . . someone had to.'

'And that someone had to be you?' Si's voice was softer now, resigned.

Jo nodded.

'Hardly surprising. It's always you, isn't it? Always has been. First the bloody business is left entirely on your shoulders with no provision at all for Nicci's replacement, and now this. And what, dare I ask, did you agree with David?'

'Nothing,' Jo whispered. 'Give me some credit, Si. We didn't agree anything. We – Lizzie, Mona and I – just needed to know if he'd had a letter too. If he knew. And he had, he did. Of course. And he felt the same way we did – angry, confused, insulted, obliged. But also scared that she'd – Nicci had – well, lost it.'

'That's it?' Si sounded calmer now, although the fist Jo could see when she risked a glimpse through her fringe was still clenched. 'Nothing else?'

'Nothing else, I promise. We aren't about to have to pay double the maintenance and we won't have two more kids coming to stay every other weekend.' The joke fell flat, as

138

she should have known it would. God, Jo, she thought, dig that grave a little bit deeper, why don't you?

'But you've all known this for months, everyone except me?' Si paused, his voice hurt. Jo knew it was about so much more than Nicci's letter. 'Not . . . please tell me Gerry doesn't know. That would be the final insult.'

'Of course, not.' Jo shook her head. 'Shit, yes, he does, but not everything, not about us and the girls and Mona and David. Lizzie only told him about the garden.'

Si rolled his eyes, before rubbing his hands through his hair. It was a sign Jo recognised. They were through the worst. He was beginning to thaw. The other conversation still needed to be had, but that could wait another day.

'Oh, well, that's something to be grateful for,' he said, taking her hand and squeezing. 'At least bloody Gerry didn't know I now have shares in four kids before I did. He'd kill himself laughing.'

NINETEEN

'How did he take it?' Lizzie looked at Jo anxiously over a corkscrew that protruded from the bottle of something cold and white in Lizzie's hand.

'How d'you think?' Jo said. They were standing in Nicci's kitchen. Again. Jo sounded exhausted, but she looked better, Lizzie thought. Less dishevelled, and her skin, which had been dull for weeks, had regained its healthy glow. And had she had her highlights done?

'Put it this way,' Jo grinned, 'he's just about speaking to me.'

'Really?'

'No, not really,' Jo laughed. 'He's surprisingly OK. I mean, he's not thrilled, but it's not as if he thinks it's my fault or anything. The only thing he's cross about is me not telling him straight off. And he's right: he should have been the first person I told about Nicci's letter, not the last.

'Not for me, thanks,' she added as Lizzie waved the bottle at her. 'I'm drying out.'

'You're what?' Mona turned from where she'd been staring silently out at David's back garden. She'd been so quiet, the other two had almost forgotten she was there.

140

The day was warm – typical early British summer, poured with rain at weekends, tantalisingly hot during the week when everyone was trapped indoors – and the soft evening light emphasised Lizzie's handiwork. Pruned clematis, weed-free flowerbeds, emptied pots lined up along the terrace ready to be planted. The grass could do with cutting, but that wasn't Lizzie's domain.

'Really? First Little Miss Brown Fingers here takes up gardening and manages not to turn it into the killing fields, and now you give up alcohol. What the hell is going on around here?' Mona shrugged. 'I feel like I've woken up on the wrong side of the looking-glass.'

'What happened to live and let live, each to their own and all that?' said Jo, filling the kettle. 'Want one?'

Lizzie, who'd been about to pour herself a glass, put the bottle down. 'OK,' she said. 'Why not?'

'Oh, Lizzie,' Mona rolled her eyes, 'don't be such a drip. Have what you want, for once in your life.'

Lizzie flinched. If she noticed, Mona didn't stop.

'Do you want tea? No. You want wine, so have wine. And pour me one while you're at it.' Mona turned to Jo. 'Why are you drying out anyway? I'm not sure I've seen you without a drink in your hand since 1993.'

'Probably not.' Jo took a peppermint teabag from the kitchen cupboard, found the most hygienic-looking mug in the sink and rinsed it half-heartedly under the hot tap. When she'd finished, the brown ring circling the mug's rim remained. Grimacing, she tossed the teabag in anyway.

'That's the point, really,' Jo said. 'Wine's always been my drug of choice. And since Nicci died I've been drinking more and more. Plus, I'd stopped running and that was my real problem. I don't know what came first, the stopping running or the starting drinking every night. Every time I should have put on my trainers I reached for a bottle instead. It just got to the point last weekend where I kind of came to in front of the fridge. I'd only just got through the door, I still had my coat on, I hadn't even put my bag down and there I was about to pour a drink. To be honest, I scared myself.'

Lizzie glanced at the white-wine waist her baggy sweater was struggling to hide and resisted drawing attention to it by tugging at the waistband of her jeans. Jo wasn't the only one drinking too much lately. Lizzie couldn't remember the last time she'd got in from work and put the kettle on instead of finding a bottle. And it was starting to show. That and the chocolate biscuits that had taken up residence in her freezer. Freezing them was meant to stop her eating them, but it just made them taste better. Not that food was an exercise replacement for her. Lizzie had never been big on fitness. She'd left that to Jo with her running and Mona with all things yoga. Nicci, typically, had been so skinny she didn't bother with it. With Lizzie it was all or nothing. She ate or she didn't, and that was that. Right now, she was eating. And drinking. Jo was right. It was over four months now, nearly five. She had to get a grip. Right after this glass.

It was only their third wardrobe-clearing session but already Jo had established a routine. Once a month they'd go to David's house, and David would go out with some people from work. And then, having put the girls to bed, Jo, Lizzie and Mona would fill another box from Nicci's huge wardrobe.

The last session hadn't yielded much. Vintage Smiths and Stone Roses T-shirts that might have had value to a collector (if David hadn't extracted them from the box and vanished them into his own wardrobe when he got home from the pub) but that was about it. The night's spoils had been divided between Chuck/sell and Charity. And the group had gone home feeling somehow cheated.

'Oh, I forgot,' said Jo, opening the wardrobe doors and

142

reaching up for the next box along. If their guess was accurate and the wardrobe was arranged autobiographically, they should have reached about 1996, when Nicci got her first job as a trainee buyer in a department store.

'Forgot what?'

'I've advertised for a head buyer/stylist for Capsule Wardrobe. Our budget can only stretch to one person who's brilliant at both.' Like Nicci was.

The others looked at her, sympathy in their eyes. 'Oh, Jo!' Lizzie said, making a move towards her friend. 'Are you OK?'

Jo shrugged and made a show of manoeuvring the box through the wardrobe doors. If Lizzie noticed Jo kept her back to her, she didn't say.

'I'm fine,' Jo said. 'Got to be done. You've all been telling me so for months. Well, Si has. It just took me a while to get there in my head. I mean, replacing Nicci . . .'

'Does David know?' Mona asked.

'Of course, he knows,' Jo said, amazed at how quickly her moods could swing from sorrow to irritation. 'He's a partner in the business. He has a right to know. But I don't need his permission.'

Turning with the box in her arms Jo saw their faces. 'Give me a break, guys,' she said lightly. 'You've all been on at me for months to get help. Quite rightly, I might add. Well, now I've done it and you're looking at me like I've exhumed Nicci's grave.'

'She was cremated,' Mona said flatly.

Scowling, Jo dumped the box on the bed and sat beside it.

'We're just surprised you didn't mention it earlier, that's all,' Lizzie said, sitting beside her and handing Jo her glass. 'You always seemed so resistant to the idea whenever anyone tried to raise it.'

Having taken a long gulp from Lizzie's glass, Jo handed it back. 'Enabler,' she smiled. 'I *was* resistant. Then it all came crashing in last weekend: I can't go on like this. I'm not a buyer. I'm not a stylist. I'm an accountant and a bloody good one. The wardrobe streamlining isn't that hard. Anyone can tell a client they don't need ten pairs of black trousers. Then all you have to do is follow Nicci's ten key pieces philosophy: you know, the whole grey sweater, dark skinny jeans, black jacket thing . . . But the creative side's where the profit is – the seasonal top-ups – and that was Nicci's gig. I literally didn't give that a second's thought from one month to the next, other than to tell Nicci when she'd blown the budget. Her team are doing their best, but they're just following Nicci's rules, they don't have the vision to add anything new. So I need to find someone who can.'

'Any interesting applicants?' Mona asked, picking at the parcel tape that sealed the box.

'Yes, that's what I was about to tell you. We're swamped. I started getting CVs the minute the ad went online on Monday. It's only been up four days and I have, I don't know, fifty, maybe sixty? Most are wrong: under-qualified, over-qualified, not qualified at all – you know, people who think that because they love shopping they could be a buyer – and then there are the applicants who spelt my name wrong.' Jo shook her head and mimed ripping the CVs in half. 'But I've already earmarked seven or eight who look worth interviewing.'

'Sounds promising.' Something in Mona's voice implied it was anything but. 'Let's get on with this, shall we?' She turned to Lizzie. 'You know where they keep the scissors around here?'

Opening her mouth to ask what Mona's last slave died of, Lizzie thought better of it. Instead she headed along the corridor, slowing as she passed Charlie and Harrie's room to listen at the crack in their door.

Silence.

It couldn't hurt just to check.

She pushed the door open just enough to slip through. They were in their big girls' beds now, one either side of the small room. A colourful handmade rag rug covered the lime-washed floorboards. And a white-stained chest of drawers sat between their beds. Lizzie vividly remembered Nicci sanding, staining and then painstakingly stencilling the chest. On top an opaque toadstool emitted a pale blue glow that lit two small heads. Lizzie felt her heart contract. Was Mummy with them in their dreams? Did they understand what had turned their lives upside down? And what would happen now Jo had told Si about the letters? Why had Nicci chosen Jo, and not Lizzie, to guard her precious girls? The thought was too painful so Lizzie pushed it away.

Her hand itched to reach down and stroke the downy hair, but Lizzie resisted. They were fast asleep and she knew there was only one person in the room in need of reassurance.

Instead she stood, just for a few seconds, listening to the soft breath of two small slumbering girls. From the other end of the landing, Lizzie could hear the low drone of Mona's voice. *Why is Mona so scratchy tonight?* Lizzie wondered as she tore herself away from the girls' room and headed down to the kitchen in search of something approaching decent scissors.

It wasn't unusual for Mona to be prickly. Prickly was her default state; or had been since she came home from Australia. Lizzie didn't blame her. Mona wasn't the type to let people in, but she'd let Greg get close and look what happened. But that was years ago now. And if you asked Lizzie, which no one did, Mona still didn't seem to be over it.

'Found some!' Lizzie marched back into the room brandishing a pair of scissors. 'Oh . . .'

145

'We got in without them.' Mona hovered over the open cardboard carton, a matt black box with iconic white type in her hands. 'Sorry,' she added, seeing Lizzie's scowl. 'You were gone ages.'

Defeated, Lizzie shrugged and tossed the scissors onto the bedside table. 'What is it anyway?' she asked.

'This,' said Mona with an air of faux ceremony, 'is Chanel.'

'Not just any Chanel,' Jo said, taking the black box from Mona's hands and resting it on her knee so she could coax the lid off. 'If your autobiographical theory is correct, this is *the* Chanel.'

'*The* Chanel?'

'From 1996. The first, and the best. Don't you remember? Nicci was determined to go straight in at the top, so when she got that job as trainee buyer at House of Fraser she bought herself a 2.55.'

'What's a 2.55?'

'Oh, Lizzie,' Jo laughed. 'Nicci would turn in her—' She stopped. '*This* is a 2.55. It's the classic Chanel flap bag.' She wiggled the black lid upwards until finally it came away. Inside, shrouded in white tissue paper, framed by its gold chain, lay the black quilted rectangle for which Nicci had saved so hard and starved so long. Despite using it often, Nicci had obviously lavished attention on the bag. Its leather was smooth and polished, and the gold double-C clasp shone.

'I thought it was frumpy when she got it,' Lizzie said. 'Shows what I know. Not to mention it cost a bloody fortune. David hated it, said his granny had one just like it.'

'Lucky David,' Jo grinned. 'My granny's finest came from C&A.'

'Mine too,' Lizzie and Mona said together.

'And Nicci's, probably,' Jo added. 'That's why she wanted it. I thought it was just a stupidly expensive handbag. Nicci

146

wasn't having it. Claimed it was an investment. Collectable. That it would hold, even increase, its value. Remember?'

Lizzie nodded, but Mona shook her head. 'I don't think I was there, was I?'

'No,' Jo said. 'You'd gone travelling. It was typical Nicci. She was going to build a library of heirlooms, classic pieces that were worth passing on. This was the foundation stone.'

TWENTY

The Chanel 2.55 Bag
Earlsfield, South London, 1996

'How much?!' Jo dropped the cheese salad sandwich she'd just made on getting in from work, too shattered to cook. Its contents splashed across the table and tomato pips splattered the sleeve of her work suit.

'Nic!' Lizzie yelped. 'You're kidding? That's . . . that's telephone numbers.'

'God, listen to you two,' Nicci said. She had one eye on Jo, the other on EastEnders. Someone was getting married, someone was having a baby and someone else had just had a brain haemorrhage. Pretty much an ordinary day in Albert Square.

Lizzie was sitting on a grubby cream sofa they'd given a new lease of life by covering with a pink throw Mona had sent from Kerala. 'If I planned to spend a thousand on a car or put ten times that down on a flat you wouldn't bat an eyelid.'

'That's not the point and you know it,' Jo grumbled, dabbing at the juice and seeds that speckled her sleeve. Damn, now she'd have to get it dry cleaned.

'God,' Nicci rolled her eyes, 'you're such a pair of killjoys.'

'I'm not being a killjoy,' said Jo, 'but that's more than you earn in a month. Before tax. And it's, well, it's three months' rent. And . . .' she took a deep breath, unsure whether to cross the line, 'I thought you were saving for a flat with David.'

Nicci waved her hand airily, as if to say, Oh, that. Over her shoulder Jo saw Lizzie's eyes bulge in warning. Don't go there. But Jo already had. Her accountant's brain had gone into calculator mode.

Jo knew she sounded like Nicci's mother, or like she imagined Nicci's mother would sound if any of them had met her. She certainly sounded like her own mother. But she couldn't help it. It was so much money.

'A thousand pounds,' Lizzie was muttering like a mad woman counting out coppers. 'I mean, a thousand pounds . . .' She didn't say, because she didn't need to: On a handbag.

'God, how did I wind up with you two?' Nicci groaned, dumping her leather jacket on the floor and dropping into an empty seat at the table beside Jo.

She was only half joking.

Having looked at Nicci's skinny black trousers, pointy black flats and white men's shirt buttoned to the neck, Lizzie glanced down at her own Next skirt suit and mid-height heels, and felt envy surge. Just as it had the first day they met. Just as it always would. Nicci's outfit would make anyone else look like a waitress, but not her.

Nicci had it, Lizzie didn't. Lizzie accepted that. It was the way of things. She had other things, after all. Like Gerry, for a start.

Admittedly it was still early days. They'd only been on a couple of dates, but Lizzie had a good feeling about Gerry. A very good feeling. For their third date, last Saturday, he'd taken her to Quaglino's in Mayfair. All men in suits accessorised with expensively made-up blondes. If she was honest, Lizzie had felt totally out of her depth, but she'd been impressed too. And with Gerry by her side she'd felt safe. He was fun, charming, and solicitous. And, so far, he hadn't

149

tried it on. Not yet, anyway. Lizzie hoped that wasn't a bad sign. Because she liked him. He was the first man she'd liked since . . . well, there was no point thinking about that. That one was well and truly taken.

'Show me this bag then,' she said.

'Yes,' said Jo. 'Let's see the masterpiece.'

Reverentially Nicci laid the expensive matt black card bag she was carrying on the living-room table and extracted a matt black box the size of a large packet of cereal. Emblazoned across the top was a bold white logo that would have been familiar to the others, even if they hadn't spent the last five years sharing a variety of flats with a woman who lived and breathed fashion. 'It's not three months' rent, anyway,' Nicci said, her face alive with concentration. 'It's more like two and a bit. And it's worth every penny.'

Excitement made her fingers clumsy as she eased the lid from the box and placed it carefully on the table in front of her.

'This,' she said, lifting a polished rectangle of quilted black leather from its tissue paper shroud, taking care not to let the gold links of its strap clatter on the table, 'is the 2.55 flap bag. A design classic.'

The others stared at the bag and then at Nicci. It was a black quilted rectangle with a gold chain for a handle. That was it. Not rock and roll. Not boho. It wasn't even Prada, Jo thought. It looked like something a particularly grand aunt might carry.

If Nicci had been expecting a celestial fanfare it wasn't forthcoming, but that didn't stop her. 'Gabrielle − Coco − Chanel created the shoulder strap,' she said. 'Slinging a bag over your shoulder? Imagine it! Suddenly women were freed from having to carry a bag in their hands. For the first time they were able to have both hands free. It was radical.'

Jo caught Lizzie's eye and stifled a giggle. But the truth was she was closer to crying. She'd worked twelve hours straight, fourteen yesterday, and had been looking forward to Brookside and an early night before another 6 a.m. start tomorrow.

Fat chance.

'People just don't realise how revolutionary Chanel's designs were,' Nicci continued. 'It wasn't just the 2.55. Your entire wardrobe is down to her.'

Jo opened her mouth to protest that she was pretty sure Chanel would want nothing to do with the meagre contents of her wardrobe, and then decided not to bother.

'Before Chanel designed the little black dress women were restricted by elaborate constructions that required them to be strapped into painful corsets. And trousers! Chanel made it acceptable for women in polite society to wear trousers.

'This . . .' Nicci announced, 'is a radical invention. Hold out your hands,' she told Jo. 'I mean both of them, flat, like that,' she added, when Jo reached out one hand.

When Jo obeyed, she placed the bag in Jo's hands as if it were a baby.

Jo couldn't look at Lizzie. If she did, she knew it was all over. In a way she wished David was here. David never mocked when Nicci got all heavy about the social significance of clothes. She could talk for hours about how, contrary to appearance, fashion wasn't just frocks. Fashion was art. It was history. It was culture. And David never laughed.

To Nicci, clothes were never 'just clothes'. They were as historically significant as architecture or literature. Van Gogh, Charles Rennie Mackintosh, Chanel, Austen – they were all the same to her. She'd even managed to write her English literature dissertation on it.

'In your hands,' Nicci said, 'you are holding a little piece – no, a big piece – of history. That is not just a bag. It is the bag. My pension. Or the first part of it. You should be proud of me, Jo. You're always banging on about how we should get pensions.'

'Erm, Nicci,' Jo said, 'I meant a real pension. If you want one I've already told you I can fix you up with a financial adviser. If you start investing now . . .'

Nicci rolled her eyes and didn't grace the suggestion with a reply. 'For the nine hundredth time, I don't need a financial adviser,' she said. 'But I do need a favour . . .'

'That sounds ominous.' Jo couldn't help wondering if that was why Nicci had asked her to hold the bag. To stop her reacting.

Hefting it, she felt its weight and wondered if she dare threaten to throw it at her friend.

'No, no, not ominous,' Nicci continued. 'But like you said, it's almost three months' rent. Well, two and a half. Two, if I don't bother with food. After all, eating is cheating.'

'Nicci, I thought we agreed . . .'

Jo raised her eyebrows to remind Nicci that Lizzie was huddled behind them on the sofa, her arms covering her body as she stared pointedly at the television. 'Eating is Cheating' had been Nicci's mantra at uni. She'd always passed it off as cover for her student poverty, but privately Jo suspected Nicci had believed it. But they both knew that Lizzie, always battling with her body, had taken the phrase to heart.

'Two months rent,' Nicci repeated. 'That's all. You earn so much more than me at the moment, you could cover it for me. Just for a couple of months. I've saved about half already and I'll pay you back the rest as soon as I get promoted, if not sooner.'

'But, Nicci,' Jo gasped, 'you only started last week! That could take years.'

'A year, tops. They've already said that if I do well I can expect to be promoted to buyer with a several grand pay rise.' She paused. 'But if you don't want to, I can ask David.'

Sighing, Jo looked from Nicci to the bag and back again. She knew she was the boring one, the accountant, the safe pair of hands. The one you could trust with your life's savings. Nicci had the ideas. She had vision and an instinctive eye for what people wanted – this month, this year, even next. And Lizzie . . . well, Lizzie was lovely, but Jo was sure Lizzie was still trying to work out who she was.

Right now, none of that helped.

Jo might be fast-tracking her way up the graduate programme at the big-five accountancy firm she'd signed up with in her final year at university. And if she carried on the way she was going, her mentor kept telling her, she'd make partner by thirty. It sounded so old, such a long way from twenty-four.

It wasn't something she'd shout from the rooftops, it wasn't exactly cool, but Jo loved numbers. She loved what she could do with them, the way they changed in her hands. But there had to be more to life than auditing, killing herself working twelve- to eighteen-hour days to line someone else's pockets. Nicci was right, Jo did earn twice as much. But then she worked absurd hours, sometimes seven days a week to earn it.

Jo looked from Nicci's expectant face – alight with anticipation and the certain knowledge Jo wouldn't refuse her. And if she did? David wouldn't – to the quilted leather rectangle that sat in her hands, its perfect finish putting her ink-stained fingers to shame.

It's not just a bag, *she told herself.*

After all, if it was 'just a bag' she could buy fifty like it for the same price. But without the quality, without the craftsmanship, without the heritage, and without the label . . .

It's a piece of history. It's an investment. It's a legacy.

But try as she might to look at the world through Nicci's eyes, Jo couldn't see the art in her hands. All she could see was the money.

TWENTY-ONE

'I know this is my Saturday on, but I was wondering if I could swap shifts?'

Mona pushed her glasses up into her hair and sighed. If she had a tenner for every time she heard that she could retire and live a life of luxury in . . . well, anywhere, but preferably somewhere fabulous and hot and far away from here.

The boy on the other side of the beaten-up wooden table that passed for her desk was looking at her expectantly, shifting nervously from foot to foot. He wasn't huge, less than six foot, but the office was so small he nearly filled it. And not much older than Daniel. Five years, six at most. Involuntarily, Mona shuddered. When had that happened? How had her boy turned from the tow-headed infant she carried back to England, via a stopover in Hong Kong, with his *Star Wars* rucksack full of matchbox cars, into the gangly almost-man, whose endless dirty laundry now filled their flat?

'Well, can I?' Caleb's voice jolted her back to the crammed storeroom that doubled as the restaurant manager's office.

'I'm sorry, Caleb,' she said. 'I would, but I've just this

minute redone next week's rotas so I know I don't have anyone available to swap with you. Even if you could persuade them to give up their Saturday night, Poppy and Irina have already traded shifts and Lec has asked to do earlies instead of lates. I've got breakfast and lunch covered, but I can't spare anyone on Saturday evening, I'm really sorry.'

This was the problem with running a business on part-time and casual labour. Apart from Mona and the chef, most of her staff were students, travellers or recent immigrants, Australians and Eastern Europeans mostly. Biding their time, finding their feet or just paying their share of the rent, as they were at almost every café and restaurant within the M25. It wasn't that they didn't work hard – they did – just that work wasn't their priority. Mostly, their priority was funding the next leg of their journey (Australians), sending money home (the rest). But then, wasn't funding trips how it had been for Mona in her early twenties? Each job lasting as long as it took to save up for the next plane ticket. Working a beach bar in Koh Pha Ngan, teaching English in Seoul and waitressing in the Tokyo hostess club. Maybe she'd still be travelling if she hadn't stopped off in Sydney.

Even when Mona had wound up at The Green Table, a horrifying nine years ago now, she'd only been looking for casual waitressing to boost her income from yoga teaching. *Nine years . . .* How had that happened?

'Mona,' Caleb said. He was looking at her now with an odd expression on his face, 'I think there might be one person I could swap with. If that person didn't mind me asking and didn't have anything else on. I wouldn't ask, only it's important.'

Mona knew what qualified as important to most of her young staff. Sex, mostly. Love, occasionally. And sport. If she cast her mind back she could remember when at least two of those three things had mattered to her too. Until finding reliable childcare became the single most important thing in her life. The thing that defined whether a day was good or bad. Childcare, and earning enough money to pay for it.

'Cut to the chase,' she said, 'because I've been looking at this rota for the last hour and I can't for the life of me think who can swap with you.'

The boy swallowed, his Adam's apple bobbing beneath the shaving rash on his skinny neck. He was nervous. Oh, bless him, Mona thought. *She* made him nervous. She stifled a laugh. If only he knew her top drawer was full of guide-books and travel brochures to places she'd never go, not in this life, at least.

'Come on,' she said, running her hands through her hair and knocking her reading glasses onto the table. 'Who?'

The boy forced himself to look her in the eye. 'You,' he said. 'You're not working Saturday and I wondered if, just this once, you'd swap with me. I wouldn't ask if it wasn't important. Really important.'

Suddenly Mona knew what it was that put her off him. It was the accent. The way every sentence ended as a question, whether it was a question or not. He sounded like Greg. If he was anything at all like Greg in other ways, she thought, the really important thing he needed tomorrow night off to do involved shagging someone who wasn't his girlfriend.

That's not fair. Mona caught herself. *All Australian men aren't Greg.*

It wasn't fair. But then life wasn't, in Mona's ample experience. And, anyway, she had plans. Plans that would qualify in Caleb's eyes as really important: Sex. Love. Neil.

This was Mona's first full weekend off in a month. Dan's football team were away and he'd be gone from ten till at

156

least seven, maybe later. And Neil's wife was taking the kids to her sister's for the day . . .

A whole Saturday. With Neil. This was a big deal. An apology. Things had been wobbly lately, but this was progress.

She'd hardly dared believe it when he'd called to suggest it. 'It'll be fun,' he said.

Mona had started planning immediately. They'd have lunch at home, just the two of them. A bottle of wine, or two. Talking, lots of talking. They so rarely had time to talk properly. There would be sex, of course, lots of that too. But it could wait. There was no hurry. They had all day.

Rolling the words around in her head, Mona luxuriated in them. *All day.*

She had things to tell Neil. About David for a start. She still hadn't mentioned Nicci's ridiculous letter. And she wanted to. Neil was the only one she *could* talk to. No one else. Not Lizzie and Jo because, as far as they were concerned, Neil was old news. Not just last year's news but the year before's. For the thousandth time Mona wished she hadn't lied to them. But back then she didn't feel she had a choice.

What would they say if they knew? Would things be different? Of course they would. For a start, if they'd known she was still with Neil, Nicci wouldn't have sent that bloody letter. But she did, and they didn't, and Mona couldn't change things now. She was on her own. Just as she'd been on her own, with Dan, ever since Greg left.

Mona eyed the boy on the far side of the table, his eyes bright with hope as he awaited her verdict. No, she could not, would not, swap. But neither could she explain to him why.

Picking up her glasses from the desk she perched them on the end of her nose, fancying they made her look authoritative. 'I'm sorry, Caleb,' she said. 'I would, but I've got plans too.'

* * *

Caleb avoided Mona for the rest of his shift. And she was sure the others were looking at her with something approaching disappointment. Not that Mona had much time to notice. The Green Room was so busy nobody got a lunch break, let alone time to sit and chat. Even Mona, who rarely waited tables these days, was bustling around with the rest of them. Her shift was due to end at six but it was almost eight before she managed to tot up the takings so far, and lock them in the safe.

Grabbing her coat and bag from the back office, she loaded half a leftover quiche from the lunch menu into a brown paper bag for supper and checked her mobile. There were two messages. The first, an hour ago, from Dan: *Ordered pizza. Meat Feast for me, Veg for you. OK?* ☺

No need for that quiche after all.

The second was sent a couple of minutes after six. Just as she would have knocked off, if she ever knocked off on time.

Sorry M, change of plan. T not away after all. Call you Mon. N.

Mona read the text a couple of times. Began to key in a reply and then thought better of it. She wasn't surprised, just let down. Let down and now totally, horribly, at a loose end all weekend. Even Dan was busy.

Dan was always busy these days. His diary put hers to shame. She didn't even have the yoga class she usually taught on her Saturdays off because she'd cleared the decks.

For Neil.

Mona tried never to think of Nicci and Neil in the same thought. Now she couldn't help it. What would Nicci say? 'You mug,' Mona muttered, edging back around the desk, inching open the drawer to pull out a yellow bottle of Rescue Remedy. 'You total mug.'

And then Mona stopped. That wasn't what Nicci would say. It was what Nicci would have said when she was alive.

Mona couldn't help feeling Nicci would say something different now. Nicci would give her a look – knowing and annoying in equal measure – and her expression would say, 'I've got this covered'.

That thought stopped Mona in her tracks. 'Don't be ridiculous,' she told herself. 'Nicci couldn't possibly have known . . . ?'

Shaking away that thought, and all the things she'd like to say to Neil, Mona went in search of Caleb. Maybe there was still time to swap?

TWENTY-TWO

What a mess.

Eyeing the metal filing box crammed with papers, David sighed. He couldn't believe this bloody mess passed for Nicci's personal accounts. No wonder she'd been so dependent on Jo. It was chaos. *Filed* was in no way an accurate description of the random pile of bank statements, letters and receipts he found himself confronted with.

He'd never gone through Nicci's papers before and he didn't want to have to start now. Jo had the business covered. Their domestic finances all went out of a joint account that Nicci let David manage – in fact, begged him to. Maths had never been her speciality, even with a calculator.

To be honest, he'd forgotten this account existed until his solicitor reminded him it needed to be wound up for probate. Then its contents could be transferred to his own account. Or a new account opened for Charlie and Harrie.

He carried the red metal filing box from the spare room into his study and up-ended it onto the rug. There were no files to remove, just paper. Piles and piles of paper: receipts, bank statements and letters going back to the nineties. Some folded, some crumpled, some wedged any old how, into every available space.

It wasn't as if he had anything else to do with his Saturday. No hot dates certainly. David shook himself. He'd never had a hot date in his life until he'd fallen hook, line and sinker for Nicci Gilbert. And he'd never wanted one since. Doubted he ever would. It was just . . . The house was so quiet without the girls in it.

Nicci had been dead for well over four months now, but in reality she'd been gone longer.

'Forget me, David,' she'd said, the day after the consultant told them conclusively that, as he'd warned it might, the treatment had failed.

The date was etched on David's heart: 6 November.

'You're young, you're gorgeous, you're successful.' She held his face in both hands and kissed his wet cheeks. 'You need to move on.'

'What if I don't want to?' he whispered, like a small boy. Stubborn. Petulant. Heartbroken.

'You will,' Nicci promised. 'Once I'm gone. It's human nature. You will. Eventually. I promise.

Two months later she took her final turn for the worse. A month after that . . . David closed his eyes and counted slowly down from ten, twice . . . A month after that, she was gone.

It was the first time he'd been able even to think it with dry eyes.

Pushing the thought to the back of his mind, David rifled through the paper, pulling out Loyds Bank statements and setting them to one side. He had to start somewhere. He might as well start with those.

David had felt sick to his stomach when his mobile rang midweek and it was Jo. He didn't know why, or how, but somehow he just knew what she was going to say, the minute

161

he saw who was calling. He was only surprised it had taken her this long.

'How are the interviews going?' he asked, a lame attempt at heading her off at the pass.

She wasn't having it. 'O . . . K,' she said. Her voice was cautious but heavy with determination. 'Actually, not that OK. Pretty disappointing, if I'm honest. But that's not why I called, David. You see, I've been thinking . . .'

He had to restrain himself, almost literally, from shoving a fist in his mouth to stop himself completing the sentence for her. 'I'd like to spend more time with Charlie and Harrie, if that's all right with you? It's not just the letter – Nicci's letter, I mean – it's that I'm their godmother, so I'd want to anyway. Is that all right?'

She sounded as uncomfortable as he felt.

'You will say, won't you?' Jo said. 'If it isn't?'

And then what? David wanted to ask. *What if I do say, No, it isn't? What happens then?*

Feeling his fingers cramp, David had forced himself to relax his grip on his mobile. He'd been expecting this, but that didn't make it any easier to deal with. 'It's fine,' he said. 'I mean, it's not, fine, exactly. But it's what Nicci wanted.'

'Yes,' Jo said.

And then she said something he didn't hear and David realised she was in traffic. It was almost 9 p.m. Surely she wasn't on her way home from work at this time, again? He owed her. He owed Si. And Si would probably tell him so next time they met. He did so pretty frequently these days, although David knew from Nicci that the business was the least of Jo and Si's problems.

'If it's really all right, would this Saturday suit you? I thought I could pick them up at ten thirty. Take them to soft play, maybe the park if the weather's good. And maybe after that, Pizza Express?'

David laughed. He couldn't help it. 'Say hi to all the every-other-weekend dads while you're there, won't you?'

'Not funny,' Jo said, 'not even slightly.' But she was laughing too.

The doorbell had rung that morning at ten twenty-nine precisely, according to the clock on the DVD player. Charlie and Harrie were ready; Peppa Pig lunchboxes packed with every toy they might need in case of emergency; their parkas on, even though it wasn't cold; bows tied on their matching mini Converse.

They'd been ready long before ten.

By ten fifteen they had taken up their posts on the bottom of the stairs to await what they called 'fun'. It would have been cute if David hadn't felt his heart tearing in two.

'They can't wait to be shot of me,' he said as Jo shepherded them down the path, a hand on each fair head. 'If you were anyone else I'd be offended.'

Over her shoulder, Jo gave him an apologetic grin and then bent to whisper something to his daughters.

'Bye, Daddy!' Charlie called.

'Bye, Daddy!' Harrie echoed.

'Be good,' David called back. He was pretty sure they weren't listening.

When he'd separated all Nicci's bank statements from the detritus he started on her receipts. There were surprisingly few, given all the clothes he knew she'd bought, and all dated back several years and were for significant purchases.

A Chanel receipt, dated 1996. He didn't need to read the details. He knew what it was for and how much that bag cost. At the time it had been the cause of a big, almost fatal, row. Until now, it was the only time he'd felt she'd put herself before them. They'd been saving up the deposit to

163

buy a flat, and she'd blown everything – everything she had and plenty she didn't – on a bloody handbag. To say he'd been hurt was an understatement But then she'd been hurt too, in tears – real tears, not cynical ones – because he didn't get it. In the end he'd backed down. As he often did. Just as he still was, even now she was gone.

Next out of the pile was a hand-written invoice for the £350 Jimmy Choo sandals. So strappy and princessy, so un-Nicci, but beautiful all the same. And another for £200 for a pair of Church's brogues with a lifetime guarantee. She'd bought those for David's first Christmas after they married. He hadn't been convinced then either; thought they looked like something his dad would wear. But Nicci was right about those, too. Over the years he'd taken to buying his own. He'd hardly taken them off since except to sleep and clean them.

After the receipts came the endless, pointless scraps of paper. Letters from charities thanking her for this or that donation. A smear recall she'd had before she got pregnant that, thankfully, came to nothing. An ancient and, looking at it, criminally inaccurate CV. Flipping the pages, he decided you could probably be sued for that these days. It followed the rest of the papers into the pile to be shredded later when the girls were back. They had an unhealthy love of shredding. It qualified as 'fun'.

Glancing at his watch, David discovered two hours had passed.

All these random letters and receipts were getting him nowhere fast. Climbing to his feet to stretch his legs, David wandered to the window overlooking his back garden. The first time he'd looked out and seen Lizzie's head bent over one of the flowerbeds he'd felt intruded upon, uncomfortable in his own house. Wasn't his home his own any more? But today he was surprised to feel a ripple of disappointment that the garden was empty.

Determined to get the sorting over with, he made a fresh pot of coffee and returned his attention to Nicci's bank statements. Even after sixteen years together, it felt wrong to be rifling through her personal things. Like snooping. If she'd wanted him to know she'd have told him. And she wouldn't hide anything important anyway. Would she?

If you'd asked him that last year, David would have said no. He'd have been prepared to swear on his precious babies' lives that he knew Nicci inside out. That she didn't keep secrets. But that was before he picked up the phone to find her mother on the other end of it. Now he wasn't so sure.

Picking up a random selection of bank statements spanning more than a decade he let his eyes skim the information. At first he'd thought it was a savings account, but even a cursory examination showed it wasn't. The credits never amounted to more than a couple of hundred pounds a month. And exactly the same amount went out. Except for the occasional large sum that almost always tallied with his birthday or Christmas, the entries were just a handful of Standing Orders and Direct Debits, set up to go out at various times of the month.

There was £25 to the NSPCC, another £25 each to Oxfam and War Child. And £100 on the fifteenth of each month to something called Safe Shelters. Safe Shelters? David couldn't place it. A homeless charity, presumably. Not one he knew. To judge by Nicci's other choices, David assumed it was for children. But why the larger amount? It wasn't that they couldn't afford the money. It was just it being four times more than the other charities didn't make sense.

Pulling statements from the pile, David tracked back. Her statements came in no particular order: 2000, 2002, 1997, 2003, 2009, 2007.

In 1997 Safe Shelters received £15 a month. This went up to £25 in 2000. Two years later Nicci increased it to £50.

It hadn't reached £100 until 2006, the year Charlie and Harrie were born.

Had she doubled the payment for them?

Suddenly, it came to him. He'd seen that name before and he'd seen it today. In the 'To be shredded' pile, he found it. *Thank you for your continued support.*

It was a standard letter. If not computer-generated, then the kind set up and ready to go. But it was the subheading under the logo that made his heart race.

Protecting families from domestic violence.

Sitting back on his heels, David closed his eyes and concentrated on breathing. *Nicci, Nicci, Nicci*, he thought, *why didn't you tell me?*

A quick Google search confirmed what, somewhere in the back of his mind, David realised he'd known ever since he met Nicci's mother. Safe Shelters was a domestic violence charity based in South London. The one that had helped house Nicci and her mother when they ran away from home. The one that started Nicci on the path to the woman she became.

Nicci might never have spoken to her mother again but she had never forgotten. She'd started repaying the charity that helped them as soon as she could and she continued until the month she died.

The cigarettes he'd restarted buying when Nicci's cancer was diagnosed, but had been trying not to smoke for the last month, were half-heartedly hidden from himself at the back of the junk drawer in the kitchen. Sliding a Marlboro from its packet, David ignited the cooker, waited for it to *pfft* to life and bent towards the flame, watching as the tobacco glowed orange.

Having taken a bottle of Becks from the fridge, he picked up his mobile phone and headed for the garden, glad now

166

that Lizzie wasn't there. His instinct was to go to Nicci's shed, to try to think where she'd thought. But it wasn't Nicci's shed any more. It was Lizzie's. Instead, he sat on the edge of the terrace and dug his heels into the grass. Long overdue for a cut, he thought. He should cut it – would cut it – as soon as it dried. He owed that much to Lizzie. Even when he didn't see her out here he always knew when she'd been. Because slowly, patch by patch, she was stroking Nicci's garden back to life.

Taking a long gulp, David placed the bottle on the slabs beside him and wiped his mouth with his hand before picking up his iPhone and scrolling through dialled numbers. He'd be seeing Jo in a couple of hours but this couldn't wait. He needed the answer now.

She answered on the second ring.

'David,' she said, before he could open his mouth, 'we're fine, the girls are fine. We're on the swings. Don't worry. I promised I'd call if there was a problem.'

He smiled, surprised at himself. It hadn't occurred to him to worry. 'It's not that,' he said. 'I need to ask you something. Something that can't wait.'

He winced at his own words. They sounded so melo-dramatic. It was bound to get her antennae tingling. Too late now. 'You remember the charities Nicci wanted the money from selling her clothes to go to?'

'Uh-huh,' Jo said. In the background David could hear small children squealing. They sounded like they were having the time of their lives. 'What about them?'

'Can you remember which they were? The names, I mean.'

'Um. Think so . . . Macmillan, definitely. A couple of kids ones. NSPCC maybe? I can't remember the others right now. Let me think.'

There was silence while Jo thought and his daughters shrieked with excitement in the background.

'Shelters Something? Domestic Violence, I think. I remember being surprised. I mean, Nicci was never big on that stuff. She never mentioned it to me, anyway. Why?'

'Uh, no reason,' David muttered. He knew it was lame; there was no way Jo would fall for it. 'Just going through her stuff, you know.'

'Jojo higher!' Harrie's voice came over the phone and David grasped his opportunity. 'Sounds like you've got your hands full,' he said. 'I better let you go.'

Ending the call before Jo had a chance to protest, he stared at his iPhone's screen and weighed up his options.

Nicci hadn't forgotten her mother; first the photo, now this. Maybe she hadn't forgiven, but she'd never forgotten. Sadness engulfed him. She had been paying, literally, her whole adult life, every year they'd been together. This had been in her head, in her heart, everyday, and he hadn't known.

Why hadn't she felt able to tell him? He wished he could go back and undo it: that he could do something to change things. Wished he could understand why she hadn't trusted him with it all. But somehow, he supposed, she had. Nicci must have known that, once she was gone, he'd follow the paper trail and find this.

Just as, once his sorrow at being excluded from part of her life had passed, she knew he'd understand why she hadn't told him about her stepfather . . . He had questions, so many questions, tumbling around his mind. The only person who could answer them was the person he'd so skilfully avoided contact with for the last few weeks.

Slowly, David started scrolling through his iPhone's address book. There was nothing there. Nothing under L, nothing under W or C or even G, and nothing under N for Nicci's mother. The Received Calls log was useless; because he'd never given her this number. He hadn't wanted her to be able to call it.

168

The junk drawer in the kitchen yielded nothing. Nor did the drawer beside his bed, his various jacket pockets and the wastepaper bin in his office. Although he wasn't sure why he even bothered looking. He knew there was nothing to find.

David remembered scribbling Lynda's number on a scrap of paper that first night she'd called, saying he'd call back. He recalled shoving it into his pocket so the girls wouldn't find it. And he could picture himself throwing it away in a fury as he strode away from Starbucks all those weeks ago, the balled-up scrap of paper bouncing in the wind behind him.

The same went for the postcards that had arrived, religiously, one a week, since that day. He'd told the woman not to call him – he'd call her, if and when he was ready – and obediently she hadn't. But that didn't mean she was about to let him forget her. He knew where the cards were, but that was no help. Because he'd taken perverse pleasure in watching the seemingly innocuous pieces of card be innocently shredded by the granddaughters Lynda longed to see.

Draining his beer, David sighed. There was nothing to do but wait. And hope: that his mother-in-law hadn't finally decided to do what he'd asked and leave him alone.

TWENTY-THREE

Her small rented terrace was dark when Mona's minicab pulled up outside. For a second panic surged. Where was Dan? It was gone ten. Had something happened on the way back from football? But as soon as she had her key in the lock and pushed open her front door the familiar boom boom boom of Grand Theft Auto and a strip of light under his bedroom door reassured her he was safely in his room.

Far from dreading being home alone, her teenage son seemed to love it. No one to point out that junk food included none of his five a day. No one to tell him he should be doing his homework, not ritually slaughtering his virtual enemies. Once he was glued into that machine the house could collapse around him without Dan noticing, let alone the small matter of darkness falling.

Tapping softly on his door, Mona twisted the knob and pushed it open without waiting for an answer.

Dan was sprawled on his bed, his lanky body almost as long as the bed itself – head and torso dangling off the end, fair head lit by the glow of the TV screen. 'Hey, Mum,' he said without looking up, his fingers dancing furiously on a keypad. 'How you doing?'

'Sorry I'm late. Did you get something to eat?'

'Stopped at Burger King on the way back from the match.'

Mother fail, Mona thought, automatically reaching into her bag, taking five pounds from her purse and dropping it onto the bed beside him. She knew he'd far rather eat burger than whatever macrobiotic leftovers she scavenged from the restaurant, but that wasn't the point.

'How was the game?' she asked, perching on the end of the bed beside him, careful not to tip him off balance.

'Meh. Richards was sent off in the first half. Dick-wad.'

'Dan, don't swear,' Mona said. It was her parent reflex.

'So we had to play the entire second half with ten men,' Dan continued as if she'd never spoken, his thumbs punching furiously at the keypad all the while. 'Lost two-nil. Dropped to fifth in the league. Anderson went f—. Anderson went ballistic.'

'Not surprised,' she said.

Game Over flashed on the screen and Dan tossed his control pad aside, rolling over to face her.

'Sorry,' she said, reaching out to tousle his hair. It was as close as she could get to hugging him these days. She'd tried the 'You're never too big for a cuddle' routine but he'd shaken her off with an, 'Eugh, Mum, don't.' And, fearing rejection, she hadn't tried since.

'Was that my fault, interrupting you?'

'Nah,' he grinned. 'I was crap anyway. They were destroying me.'

Hauling his lanky body, all arms and legs, into a sitting position, Dan adopted a serious face. 'You work too hard, y'know? And when you're tired you're kind of . . .' he paused, 'grumpy. You need to chillax.'

The change of tone took Mona by surprise. 'Sorry, hon,' she said, trying to dismiss it. 'You know how it is. We've

171

been short-staffed so I've had to do a few late shifts the last couple of weeks. I've got a couple of new waiters starting next week, and then we'll be back to normal.' She nudged him. 'Enjoy the junk food while it lasts. You'll be back on tofu before you know it.'

'—s'not that,' Dan said. 'I just think you need a day off. It's late and you're not even supposed to work Saturdays. And since, Nicci, y'know, *died . . .*' his face screwed up when he said the word, like it could be catching, '. . . well, we've only been round to David's a couple of times. I kind of miss him, y'know? And Si. Even Sam and Thomas. A bit,' he added grudgingly.

Guilt surged in Mona. How could she have been so dumb?

She'd been so busy steering clear of David rather than risk any awkwardness that it hadn't occurred to her how that would affect Dan. Apart from teachers, David and Si were the only adult male company Dan had. Role models, even.

She didn't regret removing his father from Dan's life, not for one moment. And it wasn't like Greg had bothered with more than the occasional birthday card in the early days. Now even those had dwindled to nothing – not that Dan ever commented. But David and Si were good influences. They hung out with Dan, played football with him, and she knew that as they kicked balls at each other he talked. And they listened.

Mother fail, she thought again. *Mother fail*.

Braving rejection, Mona pulled her son close and squeezed him tight. She was grateful when he didn't just tolerate it, but hugged her back, his strong arms taking her aback a little. She had to resist the urge to bury her face in his T-shirt to stop the tears.

'I worry about you, y'know, Mum,' he said.

172

Mona bit back tears. This was the wrong way round.

'I'm sorry, kiddo,' she said as she pulled away. Although he was so far from that now it was ridiculous. 'You're right. Let me talk to the guys and fix something. Maybe next weekend, if David's free? Anyway, what are you?' she said, punching his upper arm lightly. 'My mum?'

Dan's face was serious. 'Someone's got to be round here.'

Something has to give, Mona thought, measuring three drops of lavender oil into the hot water drizzling into her bath. And it can't be Dan.

Swiping at the steam that clouded her bathroom mirror, Mona eyed her tired face. What little makeup she'd put on much earlier was long gone. Her shoulder-length dark hair needed a cut. And, if she wasn't mistaken, thin stripes of grey had started to show at the sides where she pulled it into a bun for work. Swiping more condensation away, she looked at herself critically.

If she saw herself on the street, an anonymous woman passing the other way, what would she see? A woman in her mid-to-late thirties with everything still to play for? Someone youngish, fit and – somewhere deep inside – still full of hope, if she could only find it? Or someone approaching middle age, weighed down by responsibility and sore at life's missed opportunities?

Putting down the toilet lid, Mona sat down, swinging her feet up onto the side of the bath as she watched the water creep to the halfway mark. Her nail varnish was chipped but her naturally dark skin still bore the remnants of last summer's tan. When was the last time she'd given herself a pedicure?

She'd spent the whole day working out her pent-up rage at Neil for letting her down. Now, thinking about it made her furious all over again, this time with herself. Mona prided herself on her 'life is what you make it' approach. And yet it had taken her fourteen-year-old son to point out that, if it was her life, only Mona could change it. Even if Dan hadn't actually said so in as many words.

Well, she was the grown-up. The *parent*. It was about time she remembered that. In Mona's experience there were few problems that couldn't be fixed by changing your job, your relationship or your house (in extreme cases, your country). Somehow, though it was tempting, she didn't think Dan would be happy to pack up his PS3 and follow her around the world again. So that left the first two.

Setting her mug of tea on the side of the bath, Mona ticked off the problems on her fingers.

1) Crap job, fallen into nine years ago and never got out of . . . Resolution: retrain funded by teaching yoga? Mona snorted. Hardly. Yoga wouldn't pay the rent, let alone the rest.

2) No money for any fun stuff . . . Resolution: a) work harder, or b) see above.

3) Grumpy (Mona couldn't help smiling. Dan was right). Resolution: she couldn't think of an answer right now. Probably, see above.

4) Toxic relationship (*relationship* being a generous description of what she had with Neil. In the past Mona would have done anything for him. Actually, had done . . . But it was becoming increasingly obvious that was no longer a two-way street. Maybe, not even one-way, any more).

Resolution . . .

Mona watched as cloudy water reached the overflow. The bathroom was heavy with lavender-laden steam but, for the first time in months, her thoughts were clear. There was a resolution to problem four. A resolution that could solve problems one, two and three.

It involved David.

'You could have made a bit more effort.'

The front door was barely shut behind them but Lizzie had been expecting this for the last half-hour. With the atmosphere set to frigid as soon as the Audi's doors were closed, they had completed the ten miles from the house of Gerry's boss (a box-fresh version of their own but with six bedrooms and four bathrooms in best commuter-belt neo-classical style) in silence. No sound but Gerry sucking in his breath every time Lizzie crunched the gears, while Lizzie carefully didn't mention that if he wasn't three, if not four, times over the limit, she wouldn't have had to stop drinking after the first glass so one of them would be in a fit state to drive.

It was one of Gerry's things; he wouldn't argue in the car, never had. Perhaps there was some deep-seated reason but Lizzie didn't intend to ask. Maybe his parents always argued in the car. Or maybe, being his prized possession, the Audi was sacrosanct, like a shrine, or something. The latter seemed more his style.

'Gerry,' Lizzie sighed, 'I knew it was a big deal. Take a look at me. That's why I'm frocked up to the nines with killer heels. I had a blow dry specially. It's also why I spent twenty quid on a bottle of Châteauneuf-du-Pape and a further thirty on a bouquet for our hostess. I call that effort, don't you?'

All right, so she'd bought her frock last summer and it was a bit tight, but that was a minor detail. Although not one Gerry was likely to have missed. And not one that would have by-passed Lianne, his boss's wife.

'You barely said a word the whole evening.'

'They barely said a word to me.'

'I've spent the last bloody ten years hanging out with your friends,' Gerry hissed. 'The least you can do is be civil when you're invited to dinner with mine.'

Civil?

'I *was* civil,' Lizzie said, trying not to let her hurt show. She'd tried really hard tonight. Not naturally sociable, making small talk was her idea of purgatory and she'd spent the last four hours trying to do it. And obviously failing.

Dropping her handbag on the table in the hall, Lizzie hung her wrap on the rack and started off up the stairs. If she was lucky Gerry would head for the kitchen to pour himself a whisky and a confrontation would be averted. By morning it would have blown over, settled with all the other unspoken resentments biding their time.

No such luck. His voice sailed up after her, immediately followed by the sound of his dress shoes on the treads. 'That was an important dinner, Liz. These guys are my colleagues; Michael's my boss, for fuck's sake. Their wives make an effort, why can't you? Don't you want me to get that promotion?'

'Of course I do.' Heading into the bedroom, Lizzie crossed the room to draw the velvet curtains. Gerry flicked the light on behind her.

'So why aren't you more sociable?'

'Those women know each other,' Lizzie said. 'They do coffee mornings and lunches and go shopping. They have things to talk about. I've only met them a couple of times.'

She stopped short of saying they were corporate wives, that was their job, because she knew what his answer would be. But it was too late.

'You could be friends,' said Gerry, taking off his dinner

jacket and flinging it across an armchair, 'if you made an effort. You only have to try a bit harder. They'd welcome you with open arms.'

Lizzie suspected they wouldn't, but stayed silent.

She and those women were just different. They were twenty-first-century women living 1950s lives, with perfect gym-honed bodies, perfect three-times-a-week-cleaner houses and perfect prep-schooled children. They made her look like a bag lady. And they certainly made her feel like one.

'I haven't got time to sit around drinking coffee,' she said, wandering into the en suite and starting to take off her makeup. Within seconds one eye had vanished, leaving her strangely lopsided.

'You could make time.' Gerry had come into the tiny room behind her.

'I work hard at school, I have my own friends and—'

'But you don't *have* to do any of that.' Standing close behind her, Gerry rested his chin on her shoulder and slid his hands around her waist, under the top layer of her wrap dress, his fingers stroking her stomach. Instinctively Lizzie breathed in.

'You don't have to work at all now, babe, not with the money I'm making. There are other things you could do . . .' He kissed her neck.

'What about my job?' Lizzie couldn't believe they were having this conversation. Again. Just as she couldn't believe he'd think she'd want sex with him after this evening.

'It's hardly a "career" is it?' His voice made speech marks around the word.

Hearing his sarcasm, Lizzie started counting down from ten.

In the mirror she could see their faces: his ruddy from an excess of red wine, her own, pale and freckled, one eye on, one eye off, makeup wipe still in her hand. Gerry caught her gaze and held it. She felt him press his hips against her. 'There are other things you could do,' he repeated.

It was the same old story whenever they did anything connected to Gerry's work, Lizzie thought as she lay in the dark, staring at the triangle of light on the bedroom ceiling. Beside her, Gerry's breathing slowed and grew heavier. Were all men so simple? she wondered. Come, roll over, crash out? How was she supposed to know? There had only been one other, and that was so long ago, so mutually inept, she'd wiped him from her mind.

As quietly as possible she shuffled the pillows under her head to get the angle right. She was in for the long haul now. Wide awake and likely to remain so until dawn broke. She might as well be comfortable.

These evenings always started off well, full of expectation and hope. With Lizzie trussed up like she was going to a wedding and Gerry cooing over her, saying how pretty she looked 'when she made an effort', Lizzie ignoring the inference that she didn't usually; look pretty or make an effort.

But by the time four types of wine had done their work on him, and three hours of listening to people she hardly knew talk about private schools and house prices had done their work on her, the row was inevitable.

Deep down Lizzie suspected their rows had little to do with how much effort she made, and everything to do her not being a size eight blonde who'd produced three delightful children and kept a perfect house. Like Lianne, his boss, Michael's, wife.

No, that wasn't fair and she knew it. She knew Gerry didn't want Michael's wife. He wanted Michael's *life*. Preferably with Lizzie in it. But looking and behaving more like Lianne.

And with three perfect children, of course.

Sometimes she thought that Gerry would have been happier if he went to sleep and woke up in an episode of *Mad Men*.

The what-a-rewarding-job-motherhood-is line was a recent development, and one Lizzie would have welcomed not so long ago, when Gerry still lived to work and Lizzie wanted nothing more than to start a family with him. Lizzie had always believed motherhood was rewarding. She could see that in her friends and colleagues. Nicci for one. She'd seen Nicci's face suffused with a love Lizzie couldn't begin to comprehend, just as she'd seen Nicci grey with exhaustion in those first difficult months as she'd realised her life was no longer her own.

Lizzie wanted those feelings for herself.

Then, about the same time Gerry started peppering his conversation with words like 'pension' and 'property', it became clear that, for him, motherhood was Lizzie's new role in the relationship.

Beside her Gerry's breath caught in his throat and a resulting snore half roused him from his slumber. His hand flopped across her belly and pulled her towards him. Inadvertently, she froze. For a minute, maybe more, she lay completely still, keeping her breath regular as she waited for him to settle. Then, when she knew he was asleep, she carefully removed his hand.

Things had started out so well. How had their hopes and dreams grown so far apart? With a start, Lizzie realised she'd never thought about that before. She'd been so flattered when Gerry asked her out that it hadn't occurred to her to say anything other than yes. When he'd told her he loved her, she couldn't believe it. Men like Gerry didn't fall in love with women like her.

It had never occurred to Lizzie to wonder, if she could get inside Gerry's head and peer out at his world, whether she would see the same things she saw through her own eyes. Or whether what he wanted from life, and the future he had planned for them, would look different.

TWENTY-FOUR

Lizzie slept, eventually, just as light began to seep above the horizon and the birds began to stir. A worrisome dream in which she was five, but everyone else was grown up and living in her house. In the dream she tried to explain that she was really thirty-six and needed to go to work, but nobody listened.

When she opened her eyes it was to the hum of Gerry's electric toothbrush, the sound of him peeing, a loo flushing. Multi-tasking for men. Lizzie didn't need to check the alarm clock to know the time. It was Sunday, Gerry was up. Lizzie would put money on it being eight forty-five.

Through half-closed eyes, she watched him creep cartoon-like from the bathroom, scoop up a pair of shoes and head for the door. At the last minute he paused for the briefest of backwards glances, his expression telling her nothing, other than that he had the hangover from hell and today would not be his day at the eighteenth hole. The nineteenth may be a different matter. Then he was gone.

For a while Lizzie lay there, listening to the almost-silence. A baby crying in a nearby house, an occasional grumble of traffic, crows shrieking, a car door slamming. Life happening.

Just as hers should be, if she didn't want to be late.

Rousing herself, she stretched first her right leg, then her left. And zipped up her abdominals as she'd learnt in Pilates, in faint hopes of stretching her stubby spine and adding an inch to her height. Placing her hand flat on her stomach, Lizzie tried to feel her muscles clenching as she knew they must be. Yes, under the recently gained layer of podge she was sure she felt movement. She was getting bigger and she knew why. It wasn't rocket science. Lizzie wasn't one of those people who blamed their metabolism. There was only one thing responsible for the weight gain: food. She had to stop eating. And she had to stop drinking so much. But how?

The question lingered as Lizzie washed, cleaned her teeth, rinsed with mouthwash and tried to put on makeup without looking too closely at herself in the bathroom mirror. She didn't much like how she looked from the neck up. From the neck down was even less palatable, and getting worse every day. She knew enough about herself – like everyone her age she'd read *Fat Is a Feminist Issue* at uni – to know her eating was stress, or depression, or both.

What she didn't know was how to stop it. Glancing around, she flooded with shame. Look at all the things she had. Lovely house, good job, successful husband, two cars. Whatever she wanted, within reason . . . Talk about middle-class problem.

Opening the wardrobe she reached, without really looking, for her 'parents evening' clothes: a well-cut black skirt, grey cashmere sweater, trench coat, sensible mid-height heels. The only items she owned that could possibly make her feel grown up enough for the very grown-up thing today had in store.

* * *

182

Her little Renault seemed to know where it was headed as soon as she turned the key and reversed out of the drive. The first few times she'd visited the care home, Lizzie had got hopelessly lost, not helped by the sat-nav Gerry insisted on having fitted that recommended a winding route through Oxshott, Ewell and Carshalton. Now she didn't even bother to turn it on. She could drive there in her sleep.

Radio Four was her constant companion on these drives. The end of *Broadcasting House* segued into *The Archers*, just at the point she pulled into an M25 service station and bought a grande latte, full fat, as a treat to herself, pre-payment for the challenge ahead.

Around the time *The Archers* bled into *Desert Island Discs* she left the motorway. By the time a business magnate she'd never heard of had chosen his second track and skated over his impoverished Liverpool upbringing, Lizzie was taking a left through the trees lining The Cedars' car park.

It didn't look much like a care home, and Lizzie had seen enough of those when she was trying to find somewhere for Mum to know the many ways care homes disguised themselves. Driving past The Cedars, you'd be more likely to mistake it for a travel lodge built in the eighties by someone who'd taken the lodge bit a touch too literally. The inside was much the same: faded motel décor, magnolia walls, floral furnishings, matching velour cushions and curtains. The front was clad in cedar (or wood stained to look like cedar) with square windows overlooking the grounds, which consisted of big conifer-lined lawns at either side and a car park at the front. Now Lizzie couldn't remember why she'd thought it looked so nice. She could only assume that was relative.

'Come on.' She rested her hands on the steering wheel, counting her breaths in and out again. 'The quicker you get in there . . . the quicker you can get out again.'

Glancing in the rear-view mirror to check her face was

where it should be, she fixed her 'Little Johnny is doing fine' smile in place, grabbed her handbag from the passenger seat, straightened her jumper and opened the door.

A middle-aged woman with short greying hair and glasses looked up from her computer when Lizzie tapped at the screen door.

'Hello, Mrs O'Hara,' the care home manager said. 'We expected you last Sunday.'

'Hello, Janet.' Lizzie smiled and tried to stop her teeth clenching. With that economy of words, the woman could teach a passive-aggression masterclass.

'School's busy at the moment,' she said, trying not to let her irritation show. 'It's not always possible for me to come weekly. I did mention a couple of weeks ago that I might have to miss a visit or two.' Just as she'd mentioned more times than she could remember that while she was a Mrs and she was a O'Hara, she wasn't Mrs O'Hara. How could she be, when her mother was?

'How's Mum?' she asked.

Janet pursed her lips and Lizzie could almost hear the air whistle through her teeth. She was the care home equivalent of a car mechanic, all sucked teeth and 'well we can fix it, but it's going to cost you'.

'Not good, Mrs O'Hara.' Janet paused, frowning at Lizzie over her spectacles. 'As we discussed last time, the signs of aggression your mother started to display a few months ago are becoming more pronounced. She lashed out at the nurses and our rules are strict on that.'

Lizzie nodded slowly. She knew what was coming. She'd read enough books on the subject. Before gardening took over, books on Alzheimer's were all she'd ever borrowed from the library.

'Your mother needs specialist care. Now, as I explained,

184

you can buy that in, which would be better for your mother, less unsettling. Or you can move her to somewhere better suited to her new needs. It is, of course, your decision.'

Lizzie felt the grown-up desert her. No amount of armour could protect her from this. It wasn't a surprise, but she'd been in denial since Mum's mental deterioration was first raised, working Nicci's three-memo rule. The first time someone mentions something, ignore it; the second time, assume it might need some thought; the third time, act on it. This was the third time.

Grabbing the grey plastic chair on her side of the desk, Lizzie dropped into it and fixed her gaze on the framed certificates on the wall behind Janet's head. Health and Safety this, Excellence that. Behind her NHS glasses, Janet's eyes softened.

'What does Dr Clifton advise?' Lizzie asked.

'That's for him to tell you.' Everything about Janet's tone implied it was more than her job was worth. 'Unfortunately, he's not on duty this weekend. Perhaps we could make an appointment for you to come back when he's here? He could see you later this week, if you can be available. Your sister, too?'

Lizzie bit back a bitter laugh. 'Karen is happy for me to make the decisions.' The lie came easily. Karen had made it clear she was anything but. But as far as Lizzie was concerned, unless her elder sister got her arse on a plane and came to see their mother, she could live with whatever decision Lizzie made. Not that Lizzie would say that to Karen's face.

'I'll look at my diary when I get home and give you a ring,' Lizzie said. 'When I've heard Dr Clifton's recommendations I'll talk to Karen.' She took a deep breath. 'To be honest, though, it's unlikely we'd choose to move Mum at this point. So if you could also let me know the probable costs I'd appreciate it.'

185

The manager nodded her approval and pushed back her chair. 'Well,' she said, 'let's go and see if we can find Mrs O'Hara, shall we?'

It was just a nicety, Lizzie knew. Where did she think Lizzie's mother had gone? Popped to the West End for a bit of shopping?

Lizzie's mother was where she always was. In her room, in an armchair, looking out of the window over the empty lawns. Sometimes there was a blackbird or even a woodpecker to keep her entertained. Other times, excitement of excitements, a gardener mowed the grass or rabbits played under the trees that lined the perimeter. Once, Janet claimed, Lizzie's mum had seen a deer. Today, nothing. A low murmur cut through the silence. The first time she'd heard it Lizzie assumed it came from the common room at the end of the corridor. Now she knew better. The murmur was her mother, lips moving in endless barely audible conversation with herself. Sometimes low murmuring, like today; other, more disturbing times, loud and fraught with internal dispute.

'Look who's come to see you, Mrs O'Hara,' Janet said, as if speaking to a child. 'It's your daughter Elizabeth.'

No reaction, just the low murmur.

'Hello, Mum,' Lizzie said. 'It's me.'

Janet and Lizzie exchanged glances. Lizzie knew what Janet was asking and she shook her head. It was bad enough her mother mistaking her for Aunt Kathleen without encouraging her by pretending to be someone who was dead.

Pulling up a padded footstool, Lizzie perched on the edge, inclining her head towards Janet to let her know she could take it from here.

'How are you feeling, Mum?' asked Lizzie conversationally, as Janet pulled the door to but didn't shut it behind

186

her. 'You're looking well. I always did like that dress. Blue suits you.'

For the first time, her mother's eyes flicked towards her, then away again. Her mouth moving all the time, the murmur never abating. Much of the time her mother's gaze was blank, as if the essence of her had shut up shop and left. Right now Lizzie could see she was in there. Or someone was. Then the murmuring stopped and her mother's gaze fixed on her.

Daring to hope that this might be a good sign, that the decline might have been a blip, Lizzie leant forward, took her mother's hand and squeezed it gently. 'It's so good to see you looking a bit better.'

Her mother didn't remove her hand but nor did she return Lizzie's squeeze. Her hand lay limp and cold in Lizzie's, her fingers clammy. When she started to speak, Lizzie had to lean in to hear.

'I'm not surprised you like this dress, Kathleen,' she said. 'You have one just like it, don't you remember? We made it from that pattern Mother bought from the Co-op. Don't tell me you've forgotten?'

Instantly Lizzie knew the dress her mother meant.

There'd been a picture on the sideboard when she was a child. Betty and Kathleen, still teenagers, arms linked as they beamed at the camera. The girls wore identical shirt-waisters, made from the same Vogue pattern; her mother, Betty's, cornflower blue, Kathleen's primrose yellow. Or so Lizzie's mother had told her, many times. The picture was black and white, its monotones fading to grey even when Lizzie was small.

Lizzie's first emotion on leaving The Cedars was always relief. That usually lasted long enough for her to get out of the car park. Increasingly, the second was guilt; closely followed by despair. Sometimes that didn't strike until she'd reached home and poured herself a large alcoholic drink. Today it hit within minutes of putting the conifer-lined grounds of the care home behind her. As she pulled on to a dual carriageway, tears blurred the cars that bore down on her. Without signalling, Lizzie pulled sharply to the left, braked hard and flung the gear into neutral before slumping over the steering wheel.

Once she'd started the sobs came hard and fast; huge gasping breaths bordering on hyperventilation as she fought to compose herself. Crying for Mum, for the girl her mum had once been; the girl in a cornflower-blue shirtwaister, full of hope and the possibility of what she could become. Crying for the tough-disciplining mother she'd turned into; sharply spoken, unforgiving but protective. A woman whose sense of what was proper would have recoiled to see what had become of her.

And then she cried for herself, because however grown up she was meant to be, with her house, her job and her husband, she would never be grown-up enough for this.

TWENTY-FIVE

David nearly didn't bother to answer the phone. He was halfway down the garden, knee-deep in lawnmower angst when it started ringing. Pulling the starter repeatedly and being rewarded with total silence. Out of petrol. Nicci's voice echoed in his head. *It's always out of petrol.* Why they hadn't bought an electric one was beyond him. But Nicci had this theory that oil-driven lawnmowers were more efficient. Even now he couldn't see the logic in that.

Mowing the lawn was right up there on his list of least favourite things. It wreaked of suburban Sundays and middle age. But Lizzie's gardening was putting him to shame. If he didn't cut the grass soon he wouldn't be able to bring himself to look out of the window. Plus he'd been thinking it was time he asked Dan round for a kickabout. He hadn't seen Mona's son since Easter. But asking Dan meant asking Mona . . .

'I was just about to hang up,' said Mona, when he answered. 'Thought you must be out.'

'Nope, just down the garden, trying to do my bit to keep up with Lizzie . . . Good to hear from you,' he added, surprised to find he meant it. 'I was just this second thinking about you.'

189

'Really?' Mona said. 'Spooky.' She laughed, but something in her voice put him on alert.

'Well, I was thinking about Dan really,' David said hastily. 'Wondered if he fancied coming round for football and pizza? I can ask Si too, and Sam and Tom, if you think he'd like that—'

'We'd love to,' Mona cut in.

'Well, um,' David pushed his hand through his hair. Nicci used to call it his anxiety gesture. 'I was thinking boys' night . . . if that's all right?'

'Oh, um, sorry,' Mona gave a nervous laugh. 'Stick, wrong end of. Dan would love that. Let me find out when he's not at football practice and get back to you.'

'Good, great,' David stared at the receiver, bemused. He and Mona hadn't exactly been relaxed around each other since the letter business. But, Christ, this was painful. Like meeting your ex and her new lover in the street and having to engage in small talk until one of you can think of an escape route. Looked like that duty fell to him.

'So, well, good of you to phone. Let me know when Dan's free,' he said, trying to wrap it up gently.

'That's not why I phoned.'

'It isn't?' David had a nasty feeling he knew what was coming.

'I've been thinking,' Mona said. 'You know, about things.'

'Things?'

'Nicci's letter.'

'Ah.'

'Haven't you?'

'Erm, no, not really,' David said. The truth was he'd thought about little else. *Those letters. Nicci's bequests. And Lynda.* That was why he'd bothered to run for the phone. In case it was Lynda.

'Well, I have.' Clearly Mona wasn't to be put off. 'And I

feel, well, we haven't talked about it, have we? You and me. I mean, I know you've talked to Jo about the girls, and Lizzie's working away on the garden, and I thought . . . well, we should . . .'

'There's no need, Mo, really,' said David hastily. *Did she mean what he thought she meant?* 'I appreciate the thought, I do, but it's hardly the same as a bit of hoeing, is it?'

Mona forced a laugh. 'Don't let Lizzie hear you say that. You'd think she was preparing for the Chelsea Flower Show the way she goes on about it, not doing your weeding.'

They both laughed and David forced his clenched fingers to loosen their grip on the receiver. Maybe the moment had passed.

'So . . .' they said simultaneously.

'You go,' Mona said.

'No, you go,' David replied.

She took a deep breath. 'OK, like I was saying, I was thinking about Nicci's letter and I thought well, we should meet, talk about it.' Mona hesitated. 'Go for a drink, out for supper, maybe?'

She heard her voice rise at the end, part remnant of her years in Oz, part question, part pleading. *Don't say no. Not after I've spent a whole night psyching myself up to call you.* But even as her voice hung in the air she could sense his horror in the silence echoing down the line.

'Mo, Mona, I mean, thank you for asking, I appreciate it, really I do.' David was stumbling over his words, like a guy the morning after, frantically trying to climb back into his trousers, find his shoes and get out of the door. Mona knew the routine. She'd seen enough of it in her time. Hell, she'd done it herself as a student: woken up, thought W.T.F. and run for the exit, one shoe on, one shoe off, underwear shoved in her bag on one ignominious occasion.

David was still talking. 'Thank you,' he said. 'But no. To be honest, I don't know what Nicci was thinking about any of this. I mean, I like you – I'm not saying I don't – but it's too soon to think about seeing anyone . . . No, thank you, though, very much, but . . .'

Mona could stand no more. 'It's fine, David,' she said. 'Really, it is. Forget I ever mentioned it.' And she ended the call before he could make her feel any worse.

David stared at the telephone in his hand in disbelief. The plastic was still warm, the vibrations still rippling through his hand, his knuckles still white from where his fist clenched it.

Had that just happened?

He glanced out the window, as if checking. Yes, the sun was still high in a cloudless sky. Charlie and Harrie were still at his parents'. The cricket was still on the radio. The mower lay lifeless on not-quite-dry grass. And yet everything felt different.

Had Mona just done what he thought she'd done? Had she tried to ask him out? Nicci was dead barely six months. What had possessed her?

Tossing the receiver into the cradle, David went to the fridge and pulled out a bottle of Becks, flipped the lid off with the end of a spoon and took a long swig.

Bloody Nicci had possessed her. Who else?

David's road was quiet when Lizzie pulled into it, Sunday lunchtime quiet.

Nicci's restored green Mini was there. Glancing around, Lizzie checked the parked cars for David's people carrier. It wasn't outside the large Victorian semi, nor outside the slightly smaller houses opposite. Just as she'd hoped, he was out.

There was a space, a few doors up from David's house, and Lizzie slid her Renault into it. She didn't want to intrude on his Sunday unannounced. And the truth was she didn't want him to intrude on hers. But if he was out, she could tend his garden in peace, take her frustration out on the enormous – and so far nameless – green shrub blocking the path to the greenhouse. It would not defeat her, even if she killed it in the process. Ugly thing, anyway. She couldn't imagine why Nicci had planted it.

It would be a relief to think of something else. For the entire drive – only stopping at her own house for as long as it took to change into jeans, T-shirt and trainers, and not a second longer – her brain had buzzed with problems: Mum, her job, Gerry, Mum . . .

Nicci's home had been the default setting on Lizzie's inner post-Mum sat-nav for three years now. Immersing herself in the company of friends and whatever bottle of wine was cold and open. So what if Nicci wasn't here to pour a drink, listen to her problems and, nine times out of ten, tell Lizzie exactly what she should be doing? At least if David was out Lizzie could enjoy the quiet of Nicci's garden and lose herself in pruning and weeding, a blissful few hours with an empty head.

Lizzie O'Hara enjoying gardening. Who'd have thought it? Her mother had always said gardening was therapeutic. She'd never believed her. Now, she understood.

Thanks to David doing a little sanding, and warmer weather drying out the wood, the gate was no longer too swollen for its frame. Lizzie had opening it down to an art. A twist of the key, a slight shoulder push at the same time as she lifted the handle and she was in. Shutting the gate behind her, she leant back and closed her eyes. It was even quieter in here. The murmur of a radio, probably from next door, the low thud of a kid a few doors down kicking a

193

ball in the garden, the drone of a mower like a distant mosquito. Feeling her tension ease, just as it always did here, Lizzie dropped her bag and jacket onto the terrace and strode down the garden.

A second later, she stopped.

Concealed by overgrown grass, David's mower lay on its side, its bucket dismembered, an empty petrol can beside it. Turning on the spot, she peered back at the house, listening hard. Still the murmur of a radio, still a kicked football and a mother up the road calling her children in for lunch. Nothing else, and no sign of movement from inside the house. Perhaps David had started to tackle the grass and then lost interest.

'Attention span of a gnat,' Nicci always moaned, 'if it's something he doesn't want to do.' Privately, Lizzie thought it took one to know one, but she'd never said so.

After a second's more staring, she roused herself and, arms swinging, and humming some annoying jingle she'd picked up from the car radio and hadn't been able to shake, she headed for the shed.

He was staring blindly at his sketches for a supermarket that probably didn't need to be built outside a small Wiltshire town that probably didn't want it, and wondering why he bothered, when he heard the click and scratch of metal on wood below.

Let it be next door, he thought.

But wood scraping against wood was followed by the unmistakable click of his own side gate shutting again. Then silence. The silence lasted nine or ten seconds – just long enough for David to get his hopes up that it had been next-door's gate after all – when there was a gentle thud and a head of auburn curls appeared below his office window.

Shit. David closed his eyes and threw himself back on his office chair so he couldn't be seen if Lizzie glanced up. Was a little Sunday peace in his own house too much to ask?

It certainly looked that away. Had been since he married Nicci and her entourage came too. That clearly wasn't about to change now. Nicci had seen to that with her stupid bloody letters. Closing his eyes, David took a deep breath. And another. And another. As darkness spun inside him.

Fucking Nicci. He missed her so much the pain was physical.

Sometimes, when he woke in the morning, he had a blissful split second . . . Then realisation hit that she wasn't there in bed beside him. And grief convulsed his body so violently it shocked him. Most of the time he felt a long dull and lonely ache, so constant he noticed it only in the fleeting moments it left him.

Opening his eyes and seeing sunlight glint against Lizzie's head, briefly igniting her auburn hair, David shut them again.

'Why, Nicci?' he moaned quietly. 'Why?'

'Bloody stupid idea,' his father had said. 'She couldn't have been in her right mind. Just ignore them.' And David had wanted to – how he'd wanted to – but the look on his mother's face had told him something different. That she, too, felt they were all, somehow, emotionally, if not morally, bound by them. So now Jo was doing time-share on his daughters, Lizzie was rocking up in his garden unannounced, and Mona . . .

Groaning aloud, David caught himself. What the hell was he going to do about Mona? It wasn't that he didn't understand where she was coming from. Perversely, he did. After all, he'd had that thought too. Mona had no one. He had no one. They both adored Dan. Relationships had been built on far less. And when he looked around their house – his house – and felt the silence, David couldn't bear the thought of feeling it for ever. Being here alone, watching his girls grow up. Just as he couldn't yet imagine being here with someone else.

David dragged his thoughts back to the woman making herself at home in his garden. He had only himself to blame for that too. He could have said no. No one forced him to do the whole *mi casa es su casa* thing.

Below him, Lizzie examined the mower, peered at it, and then turned to stare at the house. For a second, she seemed to look right into his study window and, thinking she'd seen him, David rolled backwards. Then she shook something away. A fly, or a thought. Her curls bobbing as she did, and she headed down the garden towards Nicci's shed, body swaying in time to some imagined beat as she went.

'Fancy a cup of tea?'

Lizzie jumped and dropped the secateurs on her toe, hopping backwards, too late to avoid them.

'Sorry.' David bent to pick them up. 'I didn't mean to scare you.'

'God, no. I'm sorry. I was miles away. How long have you been here? Sorry, that was rude. It's your house, after all. I meant, I didn't hear you come back.'

David looked sheepish. 'Oh, not long,' he said.

Lizzie wiped her hands on her jeans. Her palms were clammy, sweaty from the work, the heat and something else. Then she shut the secateurs, clicking their safety button. 'I should go,' she said. 'Just let me clear up my –' she paused – 'I mean, Nicci's stuff.'

'Stay,' David said. 'You're fine. You're not disturbing anyone. The girls are at Mum and Dad's. I'm just, you know, hanging around.' He glanced over his shoulder. 'Doing nothing at all, except cutting that bloody grass.'

They grinned at each other.

'You sure?' Lizzie asked. 'I mean, I can go, if you'd like some peace. What with this being your house and all . . .'

David shook his head. 'It's fine. I wasn't doing anything much.'

'I just thought I'd tackle this.' Lizzie pointed needlessly at the enormous bush in front of her, 'before it blocks the path completely.'

'Futile task,' said David. 'Grows like a bastard. And the more you cut it, the more it grows. Fugly thing.'

Lizzie smiled. 'It never used to look ugly. Maybe I just haven't got the knack.'

'Or maybe you never got that close to it before. I was about to put the kettle on. Earl Grey? Or something stronger?'

'Tempting, but I better not, I've got the car. Earl Grey, please. If you're really making.'

'As good as made.'

She watched his back as it receded up the garden.

The more distance David put between them, the more his shoulders sagged. Like the ascent of man in reverse. How much effort did he have to put into appearing bright and happy? It reminded her of Nicci's wake. The night, they'd watched him from the shed, walking from the light thrown by the shed window into darkness and then emerging into the glare of the open kitchen door. His shed no longer his own, taken over by his wife's friends. His kitchen no longer his own, full of relatives and mourners. His wife . . . nowhere to be found. His shoes scuffing in the mud, shoulders slumped, weighed down with responsibility, worry and grief.

*   *   *

'Thanks,' she said, taking the cup and sipping the hot liquid tentatively. 'Don't know why I didn't make one myself.' She jerked her head towards the shed and the kettle inside. 'Think I just wanted to defeat this monster.'

'I've told you,' he grinned, 'you won't beat it. Nicci battled the damn thing for years. Never won. She was on the verge of admitting defeat and digging it up wh—'

His smile slipped. For a second he sat in silence, hugging his mug and trying not to think about the battles Nicci hadn't won. He was surprised to realise the silence wasn't uncomfortable.

'I hope you don't mind me being here?' Lizzie asked him finally. 'I know I should have called. I'm sorry. I just dropped by on the way back. On the off-chance. And when you weren't home, well,' she shrugged apologetically, 'I just let myself in.'

'On the way back from where?'

'Mum's care home. You know . . .' Lizzie's voice trailed away.

'How is she?' Poor Lizzie, he'd forgotten her mum had Alzheimer's. Not that the two of them had ever discussed it. He'd just heard fragments of conversation as he'd lurked tactfully in the background, keeping Gerry well oiled, while Lizzie cried on Nicci's shoulder. But he'd forgotten almost everything in the last few months – everything that didn't revolve around Charlie and Harrie, and their immediate day-to-day existence.

'Not good, to be honest.' Lizzie sipped her tea, holding the mug in front of her face a beat longer than necessary. David had the distinct impression she was hiding behind it.

'In fact . . .' seeming to come to a decision, Lizzie took a deep breath, '. . . she's pretty bad. She just sits there in her own little world, chattering away to herself. She hasn't recognised me in months. If she speaks to me at all it's to call me Kathleen.'

David watched her eyes well up as she stared hard at her cup, as if willing the tears away.

'Who's Kathleen?' he asked.

'My aunt, sort of. Mum's cousin. The sick thing is . . .' Lizzie looked sideways through her hair, forcing the corners of her mouth upwards, but her eyes shone with a more complex emotion, '. . . Mum didn't even *like* Kathleen. When I was growing up she didn't have a good word to say about her. It makes me feel . . . Oh, I don't even know how it makes me feel. Guilty, resentful, sorry for her, sorry for myself, helpless. But more than anything,' Lizzie took a deep breath, 'it makes me want to run away. There are days I just want to get on a train going anywhere as long as it's far, far away from here.'

Shifting uncomfortably, she looked down suddenly finding the freckles on the back of her bare hand engrossing.

'I don't blame you,' David said, when she didn't look up again. 'But you should give yourself a break. I mean, you're doing all you can, aren't you?'

He remembered Nicci railing privately about Lizzie's 'useless bloody sister'. And that was the printable version. He'd always just let Nicci get on with this stuff, the constant ups and downs of her friends' lives washing over him. Now it all seemed more real.

Lizzie made herself look at him. His expression was kind, his tired eyes full of concern.

'Mum is not going to get better.' She paused, listening to her own words as if hearing them for the first time. It was true. Her mother was only going to get worse. Inevitably, inexorably worse.

Turning to David, she said again, 'Mum is not . . . going . . . to . . . get . . . better.'

He looked at her, waiting for what came next.

'It's unavoidable, and it's speeding up, even the doctor says so. It's months since she's been able to dress herself, months more since she's recognised me. And now she's becoming aggressive, lashing out at her nurses. She doesn't remember, of course. And it's hard, you know? I mean, Mum and I had our ups and downs. Who doesn't?'

David's smile was wry, but he didn't interrupt.

'Dad was never around much when I was small. Always at work or on a train, the classic commuting father. Endless years doing a job he hated. Waiting for a promotion that never came. It was just the three of us: me, Mum and Karen. Until Karen left home. Most of the time I felt it was her and Karen against me. The grown-ups against the baby. The wanted child versus the accident. And she could be tough, harsh even. But now Dad's been dead a while and Mum's so helpless, and Karen's three thousand miles away and Mum doesn't even know who I am. Well, it's hard, you know?'

Stopping, Lizzie took a deep breath. Where had all that come from?

She'd known David for years. After Nicci, Jo and Mona, he was her oldest *friend*, she supposed. Although it occurred to her she hardly knew him at all, other than through the filter of Nicci. Certainly not to talk to like this. She didn't even talk to Gerry like this.

'God, David,' she said, handing him her empty mug and looking purposeful. 'I'm so sorry. First I break into your garden and spoil your Sunday. Then I dump all over you.

As if you haven't got enough problems of your own to be getting on with.'

'It's OK.' Reaching up, David gave her hand the briefest of squeezes. 'That's what friends are for.'

TWENTY-SIX

'No Mona tonight?' Lizzie asked.

'Apparently not.' Jo raised her eyebrows and her eyes glinted in a way that instantly raised Lizzie's suspicions.

'What?' Lizzie asked 'What have I missed? Something. I can tell.'

Jo shook her head, but her grin gave it away.

'Nobody tells me anything,' Lizzie grumbled. She sounded petulant. 'Has she got a date? She must have. With Mona, there's always a man involved.'

'Oh, there is and very close to home.' Turning her back on Lizzie's enquiring gaze, Jo started to drag shoe boxes out of the wardrobe. Each one was semi-transparent plastic, with a Polaroid taped to the front. Most of Nicci's shoe boxes were the same. But the plastic of these was yellowing with age, the Sellotape had browned and the Polaroids had begun to curl and fade.

'*Close to home?*' Lizzie slid off the bed and knelt on the floor beside a pile of boxes, hitching up her work skirt to avoid creases. Her eyes widened as realisation dawned. 'Close to *this* home?'

Lips twitching with amusement, Jo nodded.

'*David?*' Lizzie almost shrieked. 'Don't tell me David asked Mona out? Why didn't she tell us?'

'Getting colder.' Jo was enjoying this too much for Lizzie's liking. She'd always been a withholder of information, Nicci's closest confidante at college and beyond. It made Lizzie feel peripheral, as if it didn't matter to the others whether she was there or not. Whereas her world revolved around them, always had.

'Stop pissing about,' she said.

'*Shhh.*' Jo cocked her head towards a half-open bedroom door. But there was no noise coming from the girls' room. 'Keep your hair on. It's not like you to get so riled about a bit of gossip.'

'It's not "a bit of gossip",' Lizzie said defensively. 'This is Mona and David we're talking about. This is A BIG DEAL.'

'Don't be such a drama queen. There is no 'Mona and David.' Jo looked at Lizzie with interest. 'And David didn't ask Mona, Mona asked David.'

'Shit! You're kidding me. When? Why didn't Mona tell us?'

'Ooh, can't imagine,' said Jo. 'But I guess your reaction right now might have something to do with it.'

'How did *you* react then?' Lizzie asked. She knew she sounded huffy; she couldn't help it. *Why didn't Mona tell us she was planning this? Why didn't David? What happens to us if they get together? What about the garden? What about Charlie and Harrie? What about . . . ?*

'Same as you, to be honest.' Jo leant back against the bed, on the other side of the pile of shoes boxes. 'But I waited till I'd put the phone down first. And then I shrieked at Si, but that was no fun because he's a bloke and claimed not to know what all the fuss was about.'

'Men.' Lizzie shook her head. 'You could have called me.'

'True, but Mona only told me this morning when she phoned to bail on tonight. You would already have been on your way to school.'

'I don't see why that means she couldn't come?'

'Obviously because she didn't want to run into David.' Jo rolled her eyes. '*Again*. It's like *Groundhog Day*. I hope this thing isn't going to run and run. If we're lucky David will meet someone else.'

Lizzie gave her a sharp look. 'You don't mean that.'

'No, I don't,' Jo admitted. 'Not yet, anyway. But I wish one of them would, so we can ditch this particular slice of Nicci-induced madness and get on with our lives.'

'But what happened?' Lizzie persisted. 'When Mona asked him, I mean. What on earth made her do it?'

'No idea,' Jo shrugged. 'She didn't go into detail, but in a nutshell? He blew her out.'

'No way!'

'Yes, way. Knocked her straight back. Didn't even say he'd think about it, just to be polite.'

'That doesn't sound like David. It's not like him to be cruel.'

'Oh, I don't think he was. Mona said he was "very David". Which I took to mean lovely, embarrassed, apologetic, audibly squirming. Mo said it was agonising. Which is why she's not here. She can't face seeing him. It is a bit of a pain, but I don't really blame her.'

Nor did Lizzie. She couldn't even begin to imagine how embarrassed she'd be in Mona's shoes. She'd never leave the house again. 'When did this happen?'

'Last Sunday lunchtime, apparently.'

Turning her attention to the shoe boxes, Jo reached for one that had fallen from the pile and pulled it onto her lap.

'What about you?' she asked, turning the box towards Lizzie so the other woman could see the one she'd chosen: Jimmy Choos, their spindly four-inch heels and cubic zirconia-studded straps captured for ever in faded Polaroid. 'It was your weekend for seeing your mum, wasn't it?'

Lizzie nodded – at the Polaroid and the question.

Yes, they were the shoes Jo thought they were, and yes, it was her weekend for seeing her mum. She didn't feel like elaborating on the latter right now.

'How are you? Really?' Jo persisted. 'No point asking if your mum's any better, I suppose?'

Shaking her head, Lizzie reached for her glass on the bedside table. 'Same old, same old,' she said dismissively, taking a sip. But she was thinking, *Sunday lunchtime? I was here Sunday lunchtime, David must have been on the phone when I got here. Why didn't he tell me?*

And then, next thought: *Why should he . . . ?*

TWENTY-SEVEN

The Jimmy Choo Heels
Wimbledon, South London, 1999
*The function room was aglow with fairy lights. It might have been
at the back of a less than salubrious pub in the grotty end of
Wimbledon (the bit that's Wimbledon in postcode only), where they
spent almost every weekend, but Lizzie still thought it was the most
beautiful thing she'd ever seen.*

*With the fairy lights, and the candles, and Radiohead playing
in the background, it didn't matter that this wasn't all for her,
Lizzie still felt transported. As if, in some other, fairy-tale life, it
could be.*

*She turned to Jo. 'One day someone is going to do all this for
me.'*

*Jo wrapped her arm round Lizzie's shoulders and squeezed.
'What? Decorate the back room of a shitty south London pub with
plastic lights and pay for limitless warm white wine out of a box?
Ooh, you old romantic.'*

*'Better a romantic than a cynic,' said a familiar voice. A skinny
bare arm with a fine chain-link tattoo braceleting its bicep encased
Lizzie from the other side and she found herself in the centre of a
three-way hug. 'You realise,' Nicci added, 'that every time you say*

something like that, a fairy dies. Not to mention a bit of your rapidly shrinking soul.'

'I'm not a cynic,' Jo said. 'I'm a realist. One of us has to be.'

The girls laughed. If Mona hadn't been halfway round the world the evening would have been perfect.

'You look fab,' Nicci said with a huge smile, pulling away to take in Lizzie's long charcoal Ghost dress, with a denim jacket thrown over her shoulders.

'Tell it to the stylist,' Lizzie grinned back. The stylist was standing in front of her.

'Someone will do all this for you,' Nicci said, 'one day. But – and I hate to be the one to tell you this, honey—'

'Then don't,' Lizzie said.

Nicci ignored her, instead she leant in and kissed Lizzie's cheek, leaving a red stain where her lips had been. 'That someone isn't going to be Gerry.'

'I like Gerry,' Lizzie protested. She knew she should be angry, but she wasn't, not really. Just disappointed. She just wanted her friends to like Gerry, approve of him at least. Was that too much to ask?

'He's not the one for you, my love,' Nicci was saying, in that way she had of saying things that hurt but making them sound like it was because she loved you. And Lizzie knew it was. 'You don't even look at the world with the same eyes.'

Lizzie gazed around. How did Nicci know what eyes she looked at the world with, anyway?

The room was filling up with old uni friends, and Nicci's new fashion friends, who made Lizzie feel even more uncomfortable than the besuited fast-trackers Gerry hung out with, even if she had been styled to pass for one of them (though most would rather die than leave the house in a size fourteen). Plus a couple of awkward-looking blokes who had to be from David's work.

'I'm serious,' Nicci said.

'I know you are.'

'There are any number of lovely men who'd happily worship at your feet.'

'Huh! That's easy for you to say . . . Look at you.' Lizzie waved a hand at Nicci's beaten-up combat trousers, rolled at the ankle, topped and tailed with a tiny vest that had been showered with sequins, and stratospheric sparkly heels, which made her almost as tall as Jo in bare feet.

The heels were a birthday present from David, under strict instruction from Nicci. Jimmy Choo, apparently. A shoe designer Lizzie and Jo had never heard of. That was enough to make Nicci widen her eyes in horror and declaim loudly that everyone who was anyone was stocking up on him right now, before he went 'really mainstream'.

Nicci had everything.

The looks, the style, the confidence and a lovely man who always looked at her as if, on the eighth day, God had taken time out just to create her. Why couldn't she let Lizzie be happy with the little she did have? Gerry might not be Nicci's type – or Jo's, or Mona's – but Lizzie liked him. She thought she might even love him. And some people thought he was a catch. People like Lizzie's mother. And that was enough for Lizzie, since it was the first time in living memory she'd managed to do anything to impress her.

The tables had been pushed aside and the resulting square in the centre of the room was swarming with bodies when The Chemical Brothers faded out mid-track.

'Oi!' came a voice from the corner.

It was Mad Phil, David's mate from uni, although not so mad now he was a houseman at St Thomas' Hospital. Nicci always said that if she was lying on her deathbed and saw Mad Phil walking towards her brandishing his stethoscope she'd use her dying breath to run for it.

'Shut up, will you! Dave's got something to say.'

There were jeers and muttering but gradually silence fell, and the crowd dropped back to form a horseshoe around David. 'I just want to toast the birthday girl, before we're all too bladdered to remember,' David said, and everyone laughed. 'Plus I splashed out on some champagne—'

'Cava, I bet,' came Nicci's voice from behind him.

'Er, excuse me, vintage champagne,' David repeated. 'And I want us to drink it while we can still taste the difference.'

'How could we taste the difference if we've never tasted it?' Lizzie whispered to Jo.

'We haven't,' Jo grinned. 'But there are people here who have.' She eyed Nicci's workmates gathered in one corner. 'And Nicci's one of them.'

Lizzie felt a nudge from behind and turned just as a glass was thrust into her hands. Jo took one too.

'Everyone got one?' David was asking.

After some muttering and shuffling, everyone had.

'Nicci, Nicci, where's Nicci?'

'Over here,' said another voice, and Nicci was pushed into the centre of the room.

'Oh God,' she said, 'all this fuss, just for a bloody birthday. Who wants to celebrate being old?' But she was loving it. The centre of attention and Nicci had always been friends.

David pushed a glass into her hand. 'To be honest,' he said, quieter, 'it's not "just for a bloody birthday". It's for so much more than that.'

Lizzie felt the hairs on the back of her neck prickle. It wasn't so much the words, as his tone of voice: so much more than that. And it was as if the rest of the room did too because silence descended. Lizzie and Jo exchanged glances. Was this what they thought it was? Was this it?

'Nicci . . .' David's voice cracked.

And then he did it, in front of the entire room.

At least half of them he didn't know, had probably never met before in his life. At least half of them were so cool they could

209

probably freeze their own reflections. But David didn't care about them, what they thought or what they wore. He only cared about one thing and that was the woman standing in front of him.

Oblivious to everyone else, he dropped on to one knee.

'David . . .' Nicci hissed, her skin growing pink, 'what are you—'

'Shhhh,' he said. And everyone did. Even Nicci. 'Nicci, I love you. Will you marry me? Please?'

'Oh . . .' Lizzie muttered, '. . . I think I'm going to cry.'

She clutched Jo's arm, nails digging into bare flesh. 'She will, won't she?' Lizzie said. 'I can't bear it if she doesn't.'

'Of course she will,' Jo said, beaming, putting her arm around her. 'He's the love of her life. And if she doesn't, I bloody will. Or you can. One of us. I'm not bothered either way.'

'I think David would be' Lizzie started to say. But her words, and Nicci's answer, were drowned in the roar of approval that filled the room. Suddenly everyone was hugging and kissing and crying, like love was catching. Or they hoped it might be.

When Lizzie and Jo fought their way through to where they'd last seen David, Nicci was on her knees beside him. Her arms wrapped around him, their faces locked together, champagne, friends and fairy lights long forgotten.

They didn't look as if they'd take too kindly to being disturbed.

TWENTY-EIGHT

'You do realise planting season ended months ago?' The voice of the girl at the garden centre was faint with disbelief. How could the person standing in front of her with a question mark for a face have got to the great age of thirty-whatever-she-was without knowing that?

Lizzie felt herself wilt. She'd never been good at standing up to authority figures and this girl, who couldn't be more than twenty-three – all ruddy cheeks, outdoorsy glow and perky ponytail – was looking at her with the same scorn Mrs Lambert, her maths teacher, had once reserved for Lizzie's homework.

'Seedlings are out of the question as well. My advice would be to go for fully grown plants. They're already potted and hardy enough to plant them straight out.' The girl waved her hand in the general direction of a wall, lined floor to ceiling with racks of plants. Four tiers of tumbling blooms, reds and oranges, pinks and yellows and whites, and every permutation in between. To the right was a label announcing 'BEDDING', to the left, 'HANGING BASKETS & POTS'.

'It's flowering season for most of these now,' the assistant said, lowering her voice. 'If you start earlier next year – much earlier – you'll save yourself a fortune.'

Lizzie didn't know whether to feel patronised or grateful. As it was, the latter won, just.

Gardening was hard work, not to mention complicated. Whilst cutting, pruning and tidying, Lizzie's confidence had begun to grow. How bad could it be if the worst she could do was prune at the wrong time and stop a shrub flowering for another year?

She'd almost started to look forward to the hours she spent lost in her head with only plants for company.

Mona might have said something about the earth's vibrations. If Jo had been there, she'd have laughed and said that was a load of old bollocks. But Nicci had been into gardening so she must have got something out of it; other than a vivid, living watercolour outside her kitchen window.

To Lizzie it was rapidly becoming a form of meditation, time out from the demands of her life. A chance to think about the problems she usually pushed out of her mind: her mother, her job, Gerry . . .

Or a time to not think about them.

Maybe that was why Nicci had become so obsessed with gardening. Not that she'd ever have admitted it. Maybe it was why Lizzie's own mother had. That thought brought Lizzie up short and she pushed it away.

But planting things? Making something live and bloom and grow, nurturing it? That was a whole different ball-game. One someone had forgotten to give her the rulebook to, unless they had once tried to and she hadn't been concentrating.

When she was at junior school, Lizzie's mother had given her her own little patch of soil, a kiddie-sized trowel with a red plastic handle, and a packet of seeds blazing with red and orange flowers, called Na-stur-*shums*. Lizzie had been enthusiastic at first, eager to transform the seeds – which looked more like the dried beans her mother soaked overnight and made into a gluey soup than anything with a life inside – into the riot of reds, oranges and golds the packet promised.

Kneeling beside her mother, Lizzie mimicked her every move, digging little furrows in the soil with the tip of her trowel and placing the seeds one by one in tiny trenches before covering them with soil. 'To keep them warm,' her mother said. 'Like a blanket.'

Lizzie watched and watered, rushing home from school each day to see if any green shoots had poked through in the hours she was away. But as days and then weeks passed, the only shoots that showed were weeds. And Lizzie, learning another little lesson in self-defence, lost interest rather than face the rejection. Adding gardening to her internal list of things she wasn't any good at.

Lizzie is not naturally athletic.

Lizzie tries hard but this is not always reflected in her grades.

Lizzie does not have green fingers.

Now, after hauling her plants and two enormous bags of multipurpose compost onto her trolley, Lizzie waited in the queue to pay and picked up a pot of tiny crystals that claimed to hold water if mixed into compost. Which meant less watering. It sounded too good to be true to Lizzie, but the woman in front bought some, so she did too.

'That'll be £68.39 please.' Lizzie hadn't even noticed the blonde girl was ringing up the shopping until she spoke.

'Sixty-eight . . . ? Are you sure?' Sixty-one pence more and Lizzie could have bought those ankle boots she wanted from Zara.

'Yes, but I can do it again, if you want to check?' The girl smiled and eyed the queue behind Lizzie meaningfully.

213

Glancing over her shoulder, Lizzie took the hint and handed over her card. The boots would have to wait.

Was that right? Lizzie knelt back on her haunches and eyed the first pot critically. It looked blousy, tarty even, to coin her mother's phrase. The reds and crimsons and pinks of the begonias, fuchsias and geraniums were overpowering. Was this what Nicci would have done? In Lizzie's mind's eye, Nicci's pots were a heady mixture of fluorescent pinks and Marlboro-pack reds, but somehow they looked classy, modern. Like a Chanel Barcelona Red pedicure with candy-pink Havaianas. Like Nicci.

Lizzie was afraid her pot was trying too hard. Like someone copying a head-to-toe look they'd seen in a magazine and failing to pull it off. So she tried again, this time mixing the tiny country garden flowers with the geraniums. That looked too prim.

By the time she was four pots down Lizzie had tried every permutation she could think of. Nothing looked right. She longed to ask Nicci where she was going wrong. Just as an hour earlier in the garden centre she'd longed to ask her mother for advice on soil types and compost.

In the distance, through the birdsong and passing traffic, Lizzie could hear the sound of ringing. A phone. Maybe David's, maybe a neighbour's. The ringing stopped and she returned to the pots in front of her. White. That's what was missing. A bit of white to break up the colour. She should have got some white begonias, some paler pink fuchsias. There was still time to go back to the garden centre but Lizzie had been patronised enough for one day. Instead, she upended what remained of the first bag of compost into a marbled green pot that she suspected was meant to look like aged copper, shook in some water-retaining crystals and reached for her old-fashioned plants, filling the pot with every last one and pressing compost down around them.

Leaning back and wiping her muddy hands on her jeans, Lizzie couldn't help smiling. It was so . . . pretty.

'Twee,' said Nicci's voice in her head. 'Ditsy.'

Nicci spoke with the sort of scorn she reserved for Laura Ashley prints and anything that smacked of a tea dress; despite the fact she'd worn both with Doc Martens and her beloved leather jacket when Lizzie first knew her. Lizzie could see Nicci's face, nose wrinkled, tongue out like she'd been forced to eat worms. 'It's not me at all. If I wanted an English country garden I'd have planted one.'

Lizzie shrugged. She'd tried channelling Nicci and it wasn't happening. Sitting among the plants she'd chosen, not because she liked them but because she thought someone else would, Lizzie realised she had no choice but to be herself.

'Hello?'

Lizzie jumped and glanced around. She seemed to be alone, but the voice sounded like it was coming from next-door's garden.

'Hello? Is anybody there?'

From where she was kneeling, Lizzie couldn't see anyone, but she clambered to her feet, went to the wall and peered over. Nothing. Lizzie was about to return to her potting when the voice came again.

'Hello?' This time it was accompanied by knocking.

Now she was on her feet Lizzie could tell it was coming from the far side of David's gate. Instinctively, she froze. She hated unexpected visitors. Even in her own home she would keep cartoon-style quiet and hide at the back of the house in the hope any unwanted visitors would go away.

Lizzie wrestled with herself. Whoever it was wasn't there to see her, anyway. And the person they had come to see was out. But what if they'd come a long way? What if David had been expecting them but forgot?

Not your problem, she told herself.

'Is anyone there?' The voice was female, the age of its owner difficult to place; not young – older than Lizzie – but definitely not as old as her mother. It was also on the cusp of giving up.

'Hang on a sec,' Lizzie called, driven in part by her instinctive good girl, part by idle curiosity. 'I'll be right with you.'

Glancing at her reflection in the kitchen window she tried ineffectually to tame the frizz that haloed her face and then went to open the gate.

The face that greeted her was familiar and yet not. Older than the voice. Cropped grey hair, birdlike features, eyes wide with a surprise that matched her own.

'I'm so sorry to disturb you,' said the small woman carrying a large brown paper carrier bag. 'I must have the address wrong. I thought David Morrison lived here.'

'He does.' Lizzie smiled, but something about the woman was niggling at her. There was something familiar . . . It hung, like a forgotten memory, just out of reach. 'I'm afraid he's out at the moment, though. I'm not sure when he'll be back. I'm just here doing the garden. But I can give him a message?'

'Oh.' The woman sounded bemused. 'You're the gardener?'

Lizzie laughed. 'Hardly! No one in their right mind would pay me to look after their garden. No, I'm a friend, I just . . . It's a long story; I'm just helping out.'

The woman looked past Lizzie into the garden beyond. 'Nice pots,' she said.

'Really? Do you think so? I wasn't sure. I'm what you might call a beginner.'

'Those ones,' the woman said, nodding towards the riot of red and pink. 'They're gorgeous. That nearest one, though,' she pointed at the tiny cottage garden flowers Lizzie had just finished potting, 'well, it's a bit . . . ditsy . . . for my taste.'

'*Ditsy?*'

'I don't mean to be rude.'

'No, it's not that, it's just, *ditsy*, I don't know many people who use that word.'

The woman shrugged. 'Really? I suppose I got it from my mother. Truth be told, I was never much of a one for flowers. In my experience, a man bearing flowers is a man who's been up to no good.' She shifted awkwardly. 'Look, I only came to drop this off for the girls.' She held up the bag, with two sparkly pink parcels poking from the top. 'Do you think I could leave it? I know I've missed their birthday but I still wanted to get them something.'

'Sorry, yes. You must think me so rude.' Lizzie stepped aside to let the woman pass, then something stopped her. 'I'm sorry,' she said, 'but before I let you in I do feel I ought to know who you are.'

'Of course,' the woman said. 'I should have said. My name's Lynda Cummings, Lynda Webster as was. I'm Nicci's mother.'

217

TWENTY-NINE

'Herbal tea or herbal tea?'

They were sitting in the shed – well, Lynda was sitting, in the beaten-up old leather armchair where Nicci had sat so many times before. Lizzie was plugging in the kettle and holding up boxes of herbal tea, mainly for something to do that didn't involve looking at the ghost of memories past.

'Camomile, peppermint, blackcurrant or rosehip?'

'What's blackcurrant like?'

'Hot Ribena.'

'Sounds nasty. What about peppermint?'

'Same principle – warm toothpaste.'

'Peppermint then,' Lynda said, her longing for PG Tips obvious.

Flicking on the kettle, Lizzie dropped a peppermint tea bag into one mug, a blackcurrant one into another.

'I'm sorry,' Lynda said, when Lizzie had poured hot water into the mugs. 'I can see I've given you a bit of a shock.'

Lizzie handed the woman a mug and leant back. 'It's not that so much,' she said, then stopped. What was the point of lying? 'Well, actually, it is. I don't really know how to put this . . .' She searched desperately for some kind words.

'It's all right.' When Lynda's grey eyes paled and her mouth turned down there was no denying her similarity to Nicci. 'You didn't know Nicci had a mother.' Lynda shrugged. 'Why should you?'

'It's not just that,' Lizzie said. 'It's, well, I guess it's none of my business, but if David knows about you, I can't quite get my head around why he didn't tell me. Tell us, I mean.'

'*Us?*'

'David hasn't told you about us then?'

'David hasn't told me anything much. I've done most of the talking so far.'

'Ah . . .' Lizzie swallowed the questions that were bubbling in her head and gave the woman their potted history. The story of well, *them*. Nicci's other − she just stopped herself saying *real* − family. Explained their group, how it worked. How Mona and Jo and she and Nicci became friends at university and stuck together, more or less, since then.

How David joined them just before they left university. And, became one of them. An honorary girl. Only allowed to be with Nicci with their approval. Although Lizzie knew that wasn't strictly true. That Nicci, if it had come down to it, would have gone to the wall for David. If they'd forced her to choose, which they wouldn't, since all three of them loved him as much as Nicci did. Like a brother, in their own ways.

'So, I've known − knew − Nicci,' Lizzie swallowed. She still couldn't get used to talking about her best friend in the past tense. 'We've been friends seventeen years. And I've known David fifteen. I'm so sorry, but Nicci never mentioned you. I don't remember it, but Jo says she once said her dad left when she was tiny and you and she fell out in her teens.'

Nicci's mother nodded grimly. 'Both absolutely true.'

'It was only the once. We'd had a bit to drink and she

219

never referred to it again. Subject closed. With the benefit of hindsight I realise Nicci went out of her way to steer clear of childhood stuff. We've talked about it since she died, tried to pool all our memories to discover if we'd missed something significant. A clue, if you like. In the end we reached the only conclusion we could: Nicci never told us about you, her father, her childhood, any of it, because, well, she didn't want to.'

'And you just went along with it?'

Lizzie bristled. 'She's my best friend,' she said, aware her voice was sharp but past caring. 'Family, even. Nicci didn't want to talk about it, I didn't want to make her unhappy. When you love people – in my experience – you make allowances for them.'

The woman coloured, whether with shame or hurt Lizzie didn't know, but she was on a roll now and not about to start worrying if she hurt some total stranger's feelings.

'And now you're sitting here, in her shed, her private place, telling me you've spoken to – had coffee with – David. Surely you're not surprised I'm struggling with that. The idea David spoke to you, saw you and never told us something so significant?'

The other possibility – that David might have told the others, Mona and Jo, but not her – was too awful to contemplate.

Lynda was watching her calmly as if waiting for her to finish.

'Your turn,' Lizzie said, as forcefully as she could manage. 'Now it's your turn. I want to know *everything*. What happened. Why you fell out with Nicci. Why you never bothered to come looking for her – your own daughter. How you found David. Why you're sitting here now.' Lizzie's voice was rising. She forced her anger back down again. 'Make me understand.'

The woman nodded. 'I'll tell you. But because I want to.

Not because I owe you anything. I don't owe anyone anything.' She paused, stared hard at her tea. The lime scale from the kettle had formed a film on top of the liquid. 'Except Nicci. And it's too late for that. It's because I can't make it up to Nicci that I want to make it up to the people I can. My granddaughters.'

'*Lizzie!* Where are you? Are you still here?'

David was halfway down the garden before she realised he was back. Lizzie had been so engrossed she hadn't heard him open the back door, or seen him through the shed window. Exchanging glances with Lynda, she opened the shed door and waved.

'In here,' she called. 'We're in the shed.'

A grin lit David's face. 'The pots look fantastic, thank you. Not that I'm any—' In the doorway he stopped, taking in the two women as his brain caught up with her words. 'We? Ahh.'

'You have a visitor,' Lizzie said.

'So I see.'

'I suppose I should make myself scarce.'

'No need,' said David. He reached out to stop her and her arm goose-pimpled under his fingers. 'What's the point? There are no secrets around here. Not any more.'

'I'm sorry to force your hand like this . . .' Sitting at the kitchen table, Nicci's mother looked suddenly nervous.

Lizzie knew she should tear herself away and leave.

'But what else could I do?'

She should leave Nicci's husband, and the mother-in-law no one knew existed, to do whatever it was they had to do. Say whatever needed saying. But Lizzie couldn't. She had to know how this played out, to know what there was to know about Nicci's past. To own the little part of Nicci that had always been denied her.

221

'You gave me no choice,' Lynda was saying. 'You said you'd call me and you didn't.'

'I needed time to digest everything.'

'I played by your rules. I sent you cards in case you'd lost my number. Still you didn't call. The woman's small mouth was a thin line across her face. So like Nicci when her patience was wearing thin. 'I gave you time. Months. Now here I am. Can you blame me?'

Her expression was defiant.

David shrugged. 'I threw them away,' he said flatly. 'Really, what did you expect me to do?'

The air in the kitchen was frigid with tension. Suddenly Lizzie wanted to be anywhere but in the middle of a battle between Nicci's mother and Nicci's husband.

Taking a deep breath, David opened his mouth to say something cutting, then seemed to change his mind. 'Until a few days ago,' he said, 'if you'd turned up like this I'd have told you to leave. And if you'd refused to move I'd have called the police. And if they refused to deal with it I'd have thrown you out myself. Until recently, I had absolutely no intention of letting you anywhere near my children. Since you were obviously incapable of looking after your own.'

The woman looked like he'd slapped her.

His gaze was firm and he obviously meant it. 'Because I thought that was what Nicci would have wanted. But something's changed. And . . .' David shook his head, 'as it happens, I *did* try to call you.'

'You did?' Lizzie and Lynda spoke in unison.

'Sorry.' Lizzie mimed zipping her lips.

'Well, not exactly. But I looked for your number and I'd have called if I'd been able to find it. The point is, I *wanted* to call you. I need to speak to you. I have stuff to say.'

'I can . . . you know . . .' Lizzie forced herself to do the right thing, though she didn't want to. 'I know you said no secrets. But if you want some privacy?'

'You know,' David said. 'If it's really all right with you, I might take you up on that.'

Trying not to let her disappointment show, Lizzie pushed herself off the worktop, tipped her still-warm coffee down the sink and padded across the kitchen. As she passed David, he reached out and pulled her in for a brief hug, as he'd done a hundred times before. But this time Nicci's mother was sitting in Nicci's chair, her pale eyes sharp with interest.

Embarrassed, Lizzie pulled away.

'I'll call you later,' David said. 'I'll tell you everything. I promise, no more secrets.'

'Nicci did leave you something,' David said when Lizzie had slipped on her muddy Converse, grabbed her bag and vanished through the front door. He knew she hadn't wanted to go, but he had to do this on his own.

'She did?' Lynda sat up, her face alive with hope.

'Hang on, hang on.'

Shit, he wasn't playing this right. He'd got her mother's hopes up with clumsy wording and now he had to dash them. 'I don't mean literally.' As he'd expected, her excitement waned, leaving Lynda looking old and tired.

'Wait here a minute.'

Taking the stairs two at a time, David shot into his study and scooped the pile of Nicci's papers from his desk. Within seconds he was back.

'Here,' he said, dumping them on the table. 'These are Nicci's personal bank statements. Look at them.'

Lynda picked up one, then another and then another. The confusion on her face didn't clear. 'What am I meant to be looking for?' she said eventually. 'They're just bank statements.'

David pointed to a payment on 15 February 1997. 'That was the first.'

'I don't –'

'And this was the last.' He passed her a statement for the month of Nicci's death. The payment to Safe Shelters had been made the day before she died. 'She's been giving money to a domestic violence charity every month for years. Almost as long as I've known her. Certainly since she started earning any real money. Nicci didn't tell me. She just did it; month after month, year after year. And she's left them money in her will. Not a huge amount but enough to make a difference to someone's life. That's what I wanted to tell you. Whatever Nicci said, or didn't say, she may not have forgiven you, but she never forgot.'

'Safe Shelters?' Lynda looked at him, recognition fighting the tears in her eyes. Too late it occurred to David that being remembered like this might be worse than not being remembered at all.

'I know it's not you personally,' David said hastily. 'I mean, I know she didn't leave a clause saying "I leave money to Safe Shelters on behalf of my mother, Lynda Webster, Cummings, whatever your name is now". But she might as well have done, don't you think?'

He couldn't translate the expression on the woman's face. Not guilt, exactly . . .

'You need to give me time to take this on board,' she said at last. 'You've had time to think about this. Well, I need time too. I'm not sure how I'm supposed to feel about my daughter paying them back all this time, the people who helped us get away. They gave us a roof and helped us build a new life. Without them . . .' Lynda waved her hands at the kitchen. 'Who knows if all this would even have been possible? And, obviously, Nicci never forgot that. What does it say about me that she found a way to repay them, and

I . . .' Lynda paused. Tears burst through and strangled her words. 'I threw it all back in their faces . . .'

She looked David in the eye, as if hoping to find solace there. When none was forthcoming, she looked away. 'You know I went back to him. Not once, but twice. The second time was just after Nicci's A levels. She told me that if I went she'd never speak to me again. She meant it. Nicci always kept her promises. She said someone around here had to.'

THIRTY

The tick of the new kitchen clock was so loud it surprised him. He was struck by the contrast to the riot of noise he'd lived with just a few months earlier; until Jo had walked him around the house, forcing him, one by one, to turn things off. The television, the radio, the iPod: the cricket, the news, Blur's greatest hits. And then she left, making him swear not to turn them all straight back on again.

Back then, silence had made his brain scream. But in the weeks that had passed, he'd learnt to still the constant snarl of his own thoughts. Not like them, exactly, but they'd reached an accommodation. He'd bought the clock to keep him company. It was a replica of an old station clock. By luck more than judgement its wood frame matched the units he'd had made from old railway sleepers, making the clock look as if it had always been there. Maybe even come from the same country station.

Now, he found its solid tick, tick, tick comforting. Just as the snuffles through the baby monitor nursed his 3 a.m. thoughts. He'd have preferred to be left alone with those thoughts and the clock right now, if he was honest.

But he didn't have that choice. Nicci had seen to that. As always.

When did Nicci buy that? Jo wondered. She wasn't sure she'd ever noticed the clock before. Maybe David bought it. No. She dismissed the idea. For a start, it *went*; which Jo was sure it wouldn't have done if David had chosen it.

He was great on the big stuff; his buildings got shortlisted for awards. The other partners in his practice more or less admitted they couldn't afford to lose him. But David did big picture. Nicci did detail.

'I don't know what to say,' Jo said pointlessly, when it became clear David, Lizzie and Mona weren't planning to speak.

Reaching for the bottle of rosé that stood in a puddle of condensation in the middle of the table, Mona emptied it into her glass. It amounted to half a glass and a few drips. 'Sorry,' she shrugged, seeing Lizzie's face. 'I wasn't thinking . . .'

'. . . I was just drinking,' Lizzie and Jo finished simultaneously.

'Not a problem.' David pushed back his chair and headed for the fridge. 'Plenty more where that came from.'

'I feel so gullible,' Jo said, to no one in particular. 'I mean, seventeen years we were friends. *Seventeen* I thought we knew everything there was to know about each other.'

'Did you?' Mona said, her tone matter-of-fact. 'Because I didn't. Not for one minute did I think I knew everything there was to know about Nicci . . . Oh,' she added, 'I know you two were closer to Nicci than I was, even before I went to Australia—'

'That's not—' Lizzie interrupted.

'You don't have to protect my feelings. You know it's true. It's always been you three.' Mona threw a smile at David,

227

their recent embarrassment temporarily forgotten. 'With me on the outside.'

'But that's not what we're here to talk about, is it?' Jo reminded them.

The women fell silent as David unscrewed the bottle and filled Lizzie's glass, then Jo's, before seeing to his own.

'I just mean,' Mona said, 'that I never thought I knew everything there was to know about Nicci. Remember at the funeral? When we were down in Nicci's shed reading the letters . . .' She threw David an apologetic look, but he just shrugged, and took a swig from his glass, as if to say it was par for the course. 'Jo said Nicci always played her cards close to her chest.'

'I think it was you who said that.'

'Whoever said it was right,' David interrupted. 'I mean, let's be honest here. We all knew that asking Nicci about her family was likely to get us iced out for weeks. Yes,' he said, seeing the shock in their expressions, 'even me. I made that mistake once, and once was enough. We all could have pushed it and none of us did. And now we'll never know what might have happened if we had. We could have got to the bottom of this, but we did what we always did.'

He looked around the table. Only Lizzie wouldn't meet his eye.

'We did what Nicci wanted us to do. Because we were afraid of losing her when maybe, just maybe, if we'd stood up to her we would have found her.'

A murmur came from the baby monitor in the corner of the kitchen. Four heads instinctively flicked in its direction. The murmur turned to a mumble, swiftly followed by a wail. 'Be right back,' David said.

'He's a good dad, isn't he?' said Mona, as the sound of his footsteps on the stairs faded and the wails were quickly replaced by the practised murmurings of a parent. Lizzie and Jo locked eyes and smirked, looking away before Mona could catch them.

'Very,' Lizzie said. 'A good husband, too.'

'And friend,' Jo added. 'A really good friend. It's funny, really. I never thought of David like that, before . . . but now I see it. He isn't just Nicci's husband, he's one of us. Who's making him sit here with us? No one. Nicci's not here to make him do it any more.'

By unspoken agreement, the three women raised their glasses to their absent friend.

'He doesn't have to do it,' Jo said. 'He chooses to. David could have told us to bugger off and mind our own business, but he didn't. Plenty of men would.'

The murmuring from the monitor ended and bare feet padded back down the wooden stairs.

'What I keep coming back to,' David started speaking almost before he entered the room, 'is this. Even if I didn't know – scratch that, let's be honest here, even if I put my head firmly in the sand – somewhere, at the back of your minds, one of you must have had a sneaking suspicion. You knew Nicci for years before I came along.'

'Two and a half,' Jo said.

Lizzie sighed.

'It must have been recent. Still hurting,' David said. 'I mean, the whole gap between A levels and university is hazy. Her mum doesn't know where Nicci went when she stormed off. And you didn't meet her till the end of September. Where did she live? How did she support herself? There must have been something. A slip in her mask, surely?'

As the women searched their memories, David searched their faces, looking for a hint of conspiracy, a sign that they were colluding in burying things, not digging them up. He found none.

'I don't remember anything, do you?' Lizzie asked Jo. 'From whisky night? I certainly don't remember that, since I was mostly unconscious or vomiting. But you said Nicci told you her dad left when she was little and she'd had a big row with her mum the previous year. That all she said?'

'Don't look at me,' Mona shrugged. 'If you don't know, I'm not going to. Jo, are you sure there's nothing?'

Jo sipped her wine and thought hard. 'I've been racking my brains since David told me,' she said. 'But all I know for sure is it was just easier not to ask.'

Jo looked at her hands. *Easier not to ask.* Easier to let it be. Easier to give Nicci her way. How often had the four of them done that over the years?

'There was that Violence against Women march,' Lizzie said thoughtfully. 'But that was a one-off.'

The others turned to her. 'Violence against Women?' David asked.

'In the second year Nicci got involved with the union women's group for a bit, didn't she? And then fell out with them badly. Or am I imagining it?'

'I'd forgotten about that.' Reaching out, Jo took a handful of cashews from a bowl David had put on the table, and chewed thoughtfully. 'She came back from the march really angry and with a bottle of gin.'

'And hated gin ever after,' Mona cried. 'It's one of the few times I've seen her out-of-control drunk. She kept ranting about actions speaking louder than words, and the organisers being their own worst enemies or something. You know that white-lipped angry she got occasionally.'

'I know that kind of angry,' David said, his voice wry. 'I used to try to avoid it.'

'Didn't we all?' Lizzie said with a smile.

'And then there was Donna Brooks.' Jo's voice was quiet,

but something in her tone cut into the conversation. The moment of brief levity was gone.

'Donna Brooks?' asked Mona.

'Who's Donna Brooks?' David said.

'Oh God,' Lizzie said. 'I can't believe we forgot that. I just didn't see the significance until now.'

'*Who* was Donna Brooks?' David repeated testily.

'Ask Lizzie,' Jo said. 'She knew her better than we did.'

'I didn't exactly *know* her,' Lizzie said. She looked at David, her face apologetic. 'No one did. She was on our English course. It was this compulsory module on Jacobean tragedy, second year I think . . . We were studying *The Duchess of Malfi*. Nicci had no time for that stuff so her attendance record wasn't exactly pristine.'

Out of the corner of her eye Lizzie saw Jo rolling her hand. *Cut to the chase*, it said. Lizzie ignored her.

'It was an open secret that Donna Brooks had this thing going with the lecturer, Call-me-Martin something or other. God knows how his wife hadn't heard. Unless she just turned a blind eye.'

'Maybe,' said David. 'There was a Donna Brooks in every year.'

Lizzie shrugged. 'Quite possibly. Right from the start Nicci took against him. Not only was he married, but he was much older than us. Paunchy, balding. Nicci said it was all about power. Got that from some book she'd been reading. Donna thought shagging the lecturer gave her some. And being able to pull an attractive, young student gave him some. But Donna told everyone who'd listen that Martin was in love with her.'

'And what did Nicci think about that?' David asked.

'You know Nicci,' Jo said. 'Zero tolerance.'

'Whatever she thought,' Mona said, 'I doubt she drew the line at just thinking it.'

Jo and Lizzie exchanged looks. They both knew she was thinking about Neil.

'Anyway,' Lizzie said. Unused to being the source of coveted information, she was surprised to find she quite enjoyed holding court. 'One evening, after lectures were finished for the day, I saw them arguing in a corridor. He had her wrists gripped really tight. It must have hurt. Nicci wanted to wade in, but I dragged her away. Nicci was really angry; more with me for stopping her than with him. She didn't speak to me for the rest of the night. Shut herself in her room and turned the Manics up really loud. To be honest, I thought it was a fuss about nothing. She didn't even like Donna. It wasn't as if she was one of us.

'Next day Donna was in tears in the refectory and someone said it was because she'd split up with her boyfriend. I don't know if she had bruises. She was wearing a jumper so we couldn't see.'

Jo and Mona nodded.

'Because of what I'd seen – the row in the corridor – I just assumed she'd dumped him. A few days later someone said they were back together. Nicci was raging, but that was nothing compared to the following week when . . . Oh Christ, I can't believe I forgot this.'

'Well, you've remembered now,' David said impatiently. 'Spit it out. What happened?'

Lizzie looked abashed. 'As far as I was concerned, nothing,' she said. 'Not really. A week after they got back together Donna came to class wearing dark glasses but they didn't even begin to cover the bruising around her cheek-bone. She said she'd fallen over drunk and I believed her. I'd done it myself, after all. But Nicci didn't. Nicci was so furious – irrationally, I thought, at the time – that she packed up her bags and stormed out of the seminar with the lecturer yelling at her to come back. Come to think of it, she never did. Go back, I mean. She wrote the essays and sat the exam, but she never sat in the same room as him – or Donna Brooks – again. She used to copy my notes when I got home.'

David began pacing the kitchen. 'What did she say?'

'Who? Donna?'

'No! Nicci. What did *Nicci* say when you asked her why she stormed out?'

Sheepishly, Lizzie looked at the table. 'I'm not sure I did. I just thought Nicci was over-reacting. She did, often. But that's the point, isn't it? They're connected.'

David slumped back in his seat as if someone had pulled a plug on him. 'Yes,' he said. 'I think you can safely say they're connected.'

'I need a cigarette,' David said eventually, when Lizzie's hurt silence became too much for him.

'Thought you'd stopped,' she said.

'I started again.'

'Anyone care to join me?' He flipped open a crumpled pack of Marlboro extracted from his jacket pocket and offered them round. Only Mona took one.

'Mo . . . ?'

'Special ocasion,' she said, propping it between her lips and inhaling deeply when the match David struck ignited the tobacco. The moment was so curiously intimate he almost wished he hadn't.

'I suppose the real question is, what do we do?' Jo asked.

'Nothing. What *can* we do?' David turned away to look out over his twilit garden. 'It's over. It happened. Nicci's dead. Unless you're thinking Ouija board?' He was trying for humour, but it fell flat. 'Joke?' he said sadly. Only Lizzie smiled weakly back.

'Look, I guess, we have to get used to the idea she died

233

without us knowing significant things about her. And that was the way she wanted it.'

'I didn't mean that.' The bench scraped on slate tiles as Jo pushed it back, walked around the table and leant against the worktop next to him, looking into the room as he looked out. In silhouette David's face was tired, the roundness that once gave him a boyish air developing the slightest hint of jowls. 'I meant Lynda,' she said.

'What about her?' David took a drag, held the nicotine in his lungs as he counted down from ten and then breathed out. Jo tried not to flinch as the smoke crowded her before drifting through the open window.

'What are we going to do about her?' she said.

'We?' The speed with which David turned on her took even him aback. Somewhere in the back of his head a voice was ordering him to remain calm. *She means well*, it insisted. *You know she means well.* He tried to steady his voice, until it came out, not exactly reasonable, but not utterly aggressive. '*We* aren't going to do anything,' he said. '*I* am going to sleep on it.'

Across the room, Lizzie saw Jo's face tighten. Lizzie hated confrontation, always had. Would leave the room, even the house, to avoid it, given the slightest chance. But right now, no chance presented itself.

'David,' Lizzie said carefully, 'this isn't an "I" situation. Nicci . . . She left the care, some of it at least, of Harrie and Charlie to Jo. I know they're your children, but Jo owes it to Nicci to do what she asked . . . And Nicci didn't want her mother around her children. If she had, she'd have let her into their lives while she was alive.'

'Lizzie . . .'

'We're their godparents,' Lizzie said. She sounded stubborn.

234

The kitchen was silent. Just the clock ticking and the girls snuffling over their monitor, and David and Mona inhaling and exhaling nicotine in tandem. Catching Lizzie's eye as she puffed smoke towards the ceiling. Mona inclined her head as if to say, 'Should we get out of here?'

Barely perceptibly, Lizzie shook her head. A large part of her wanted to grab her bag and go, but a smaller, stronger part was determined to stay. What happened now affected all of them, none more so than the two small girls asleep upstairs. The girls in whom – despite Nicci's letter 'bequeathing' them to Jo – they all had a stake. As she said, David was their father, but they – she, Jo and Mona – were their godmothers.

The seconds it took David to take one last drag of his cigarette and run it under the kitchen tap felt like hours.

'I'm sorry, Jo,' he said, finally. 'All of you. Really, I am. Don't think I don't appreciate all you've done. You're a big part of Charlie and Harrie's lives. They love you and I want it to stay that way. But it's my choice. Nicci made her choices, but she's not here now. I wish she was – nobody wishes that more than me – but Nicci's gone and I have to get on with my life. The girls have two grannies. That's one more than they're aware of. Think about it for a moment. Try to forget Nicci and imagine how they'd feel . . . I mean, what if they grew up to find out I'd kept it from them? I think – no, I know – that they deserve to know her. To build a relationship with the only bit of their mother that remains.'

He ran his hands through his hair, leaving a tuft at the front sticking up at an angle, then looked at each in turn, half questioning, anticipating objections. When none came, his shoulders untensed and Lizzie risked a small smile.

She could have sworn she saw the flicker of one in reply.

'And Lynda . . .' David shrugged. 'She made a terrible, life-shattering mistake and no one regrets it more than her. I genuinely believe that. And I genuinely believe she deserves a second chance. I'm just sad Nicci never had time to see that.'

Unless she did, Lizzie thought.

THIRTY-ONE

It was surprisingly hard to get a parking space. Who knew so many people did their shopping at noon on Wednesday? Not David. He couldn't remember the last time he'd set foot in a supermarket. Why bother when everyone delivered?

With the engine ticking over, his people carrier idled behind a Barbour-clad woman unloading her trolley into the back of a mud-splashed Land Rover, waiting for her to vacate the space.

It had taken him less than an hour to track Lynda down. He had her phone number now, she'd made sure of that, standing over him as he keyed it into his iPhone before she left. But he wanted to see her in person; wanted, for once, to have the upper hand. The back foot had become his default position where Nicci's mother was concerned and he'd had enough. He wanted to take her by surprise, say what he had to say, and then . . . well, then, they'd see.

The woman in the Land Rover eventually reversed out of the space and he pulled in behind her.

There's still time to change your mind, he told himself. You don't have to do this. You can call her. Tell her no. Tell her to leave you alone. But he did. He'd decided. There was no going back now. Somehow, after several long dark nights, he just knew this was right thing to do.

Despite the crowds of shoppers – women with small children mostly – the electronic whirr of tills and clatter of trolleys, the constant volley of announcements over the tannoy, and the unfamiliar uniform, he spotted her instantly. It was the similarity to Nicci, he supposed. The curve of her head, maybe? Or maybe he'd just struck lucky. Instead of heading straight for her checkout, he prowled the aisles, picking up milk he didn't need, bread and a box of Weetabix, ditto. On the spur of the moment he grabbed a ready-made trifle, luminous with forbidden E numbers. Charlie and Harrie would love it.

Nicci, on the other hand, would have been furious. But what the hell? As acts of marital betrayal went, it was the tip of the iceberg compared to what he was about to do.

Her queue was not the shortest but he stood in it anyway, watching from behind two fully laden trolleys as her small strong hands scanned groceries and punched numbers, her voice polite but distant. A million miles from the easy familiarity of the woman on the next till, who chattered constantly about her children and the weather and summer holidays, although David was pretty sure she didn't know the person she was serving.

'Would you like a carrier bag, sir?' Lynda had started on his shopping without even glancing up.

'No thank you, Lynda,' David said. 'I would like a chat, though.'

The plastic milk carton slipped through her fingers and bounced off the glass surface of the scanner.

'How did you . . . I didn't . . . Not here,' she said finally.

As usual he couldn't read her expression. Shock, joy, foreboding – all flashed across her face and then were gone.

238

The result of years spent hiding your feelings beneath a smooth surface, he supposed.

'That's fine,' David said. He smiled, but he could see it didn't reassure her. It wasn't really meant to. 'I can wait.' Flicking his wrist, he looked at his Omega. A last birthday gift from Nicci. 'But not for very long.'

'It won't take very long,' Lynda said, glancing at her own watch in turn. 'I'm due my lunch break in twenty minutes. I'll see you outside by the trolley bay.'

'Why didn't you just phone?' she asked. With her beige mac over her cashier's uniform, Lynda looked more like herself.

Shrugging, David ground his half-smoked Marlboro under his brogue. 'Let's talk in the car.'

'I wanted to see you,' he said by way of meagre explanation when they were sitting side by side, windows half wound down. He was trying not to be weirded out by this older not-quite Nicci sitting where Nicci had sat so many times before. Leaning against the passenger window, head propped on her hand in just the same way. It would have been far easier to go for a coffee somewhere neutral. But he had to do it this way. After all, if he really was going ahead with this, neutrality would no longer be an option.

'Ah,' she nodded, clearly understanding what he wasn't saying: *I wanted to take you unawares.* 'How did you know I'd be here, then?'

'It wasn't hard. Not really. You told me you moved back down to Margate when you went back, that second time, and had lived round here ever since. You mentioned you worked in a big supermarket. There are only so many to choose from. Then I rang around and lied through my teeth. If anyone asks, you left your reading glasses at my house, OK?'

239

For the first time, her lips curved in a smile. 'I wondered where they'd got to,' she said.

Lynda watched the man sitting beside her, fighting the urge to tell him to stop biting the skin around his thumbnail. He wasn't man really. Oh, he was, in age and responsibility, but there was something youthful about him, something gentle. His eyes were full of pain, but anyone could see that until he lost his young wife his life had not been hard. It was no surprise that Nicci had loved him, but still Lynda felt a swell of pride in the core of her belly. Pride that, in spite of all she had done wrong as a parent, she had, somehow, produced a woman who could be loved by a man like this.

A good man.

David caught her eye and she turned away, bracing herself for what might come next.

'I've got some stuff I need to say,' he said. 'But first I have a question for you.'

'OK,' Lynda said. 'Ask away.'

'Why now?' David said. 'You've had years and years to contact Nicci and, to my knowledge – which we both know is limited – you haven't even tried, not once. Why now?'

Lynda closed her eyes and took a deep breath. *If she could turn the clock back* . . . How many times had she thought that useless thought in the last twenty years? In the last six months?

'Firstly, I did. Right at the beginning. I sent her three letters. The first two I assume she ignored, but the third she replied to with a very short, not especially sweet, note that told me what she thought of me, in no uncertain terms. She said that while I was with him she wanted nothing more to do with me.'

'And even then you stayed with him?'

Lynda didn't look at him. She didn't need to. She knew

what he was thinking. She was thinking it too. 'You know I did,' she said. She hoped the rest of that sentence, *end of conversation*, was apparent to him.

'Brian died three years ago,' she continued. 'He had cancer too, as it happens. Lung cancer.' She stared pointedly at the pocket-worn pack of Marlboro David had dumped on the dashboard. 'Once I got myself together I wrote to her, via the refuge, but they said they didn't have a recent address for her.'

'How can that be true?' David's knuckles were white against the steering wheel. 'She was giving them money every month, for Christ's sake!'

'I know,' Lynda said gently. 'I've been thinking that too. Wondering if she told them she didn't want to hear from me. But, in my experience, life is rarely as complicated as we make it. I think they just didn't make the connection between Nicola Webster and Nicci Morrison. Why would they? It was twenty years ago. They have more than enough on their plate with people who are suffering right now.'

There was an alternative answer, Lynda knew: that the refuge had made the connection but that Nicci had told them to unmake it. Or worse, that they had forwarded her letters to Nicci and she'd disposed of them . . . Unable to bear that thought, she pushed it away.

The car was silent for several long seconds, just the sound of David's fingers drumming the steering wheel. Once or twice they reached instinctively for the cigarette packet before he caught himself and pulled them away. Lynda stared at her own hands. The age spots creeping across the papery skin, the grooves etching her knuckles.

And she waited.

'OK,' he said. 'You can meet the girls. But –' he held up a hand to stop her interrupting – 'I want you to know some things first. One, this is my decision. No one else's. Two, I don't think it's what Nicci would have wanted. Although how can I possibly know? I can live with that. I'll have to. Three, her friends think I'm doing the wrong thing and they're not happy, but that's tough. I can live with that too.'

He paused. There was no going back. The only way now was forwards, forwards into his life without Nicci.

'I have to put the girls first,' David said. 'I've looked at it from every angle and all I can see is that if they grew up and found out – when they were twenty, or thirty or forty – that they'd had a granny all along and I'd kept her from them, that there'd been a part of their mother they were never allowed to know . . . well, I'm not sure they would ever forgive me. And if Nicci was afraid of history repeating itself, then so am I.'

His body slumped with the enormity of what he'd just done and relief that the decision was made. Whether it was the right decision, only time would tell.

THIRTY-TWO

'It's not a problem, Miss Clarke. Not at all.'

Ms, thought Jo, as she did every time she met Gabriel Monihan. *Ms*. But she had long since stopped wasting precious breath correcting him.

'Capsule Wardrobe is a very healthy business,' Monihan continued. 'And considering the current climate we've been more than satisfied with our returns to date. If the healthy retail side of the business continues as projected we could be looking at growth of fifteen to twenty per cent by the second quarter of next year. But . . .'

Here it comes, Jo thought, mentally smoothing the skirt of her Armani suit and daring her recently highlighted fringe to fall into her eyes one more time.

'You must understand that we're concerned about the personnel situation. Growth aspirations of this level require a cast-iron management structure. It's now, what, seven months, since the death of your business partner? And you don't appear to have made much headway in replacing her.'

Jo gave him her best air hostess smile and focused on the view from the fifteenth-floor window behind his head.

On a clear day she would have a panoramic of the City, with the gherkin in a starring role. Today London was overcast and muggy. Low-hanging clouds threatened rain, just as they had the first time she and Nicci visited Gambit Capital's office to pitch Capsule Wardrobe. It was the fifth of five pitches to assorted venture capitalists and they could almost do it with their eyes shut.

Gabriel Monihan had brought out the worst in Nicci from the start. Then, almost four years ago, Jo had to be the sensible one. The practical one. The one who made Nicci see sense. Jo Clarke and Nicci Morrison weren't good cop/bad cop, they were sense and sensibility; practicality and creativity; hard commonsense and intuition. That was why they worked. Like a good marriage, together they were far greater than the sum of their parts.

'Gambit Capital are good backers,' Jo had told Nicci all the way from Guildford to EC1 by train and tube, and all the way back. She'd said it so many times she'd bored herself. That they couldn't expand the internet side of the business in the way they needed without capital was obvious.

Even Nicci knew that.

Two weeks later, as they sat in Nicci's kitchen with Gambit Capital's offer of £2 million liquid capital, and a credit line to another £2 million, in their hands, Jo was still saying it. Spreadsheets covering every inch of the table, her fingers punched calculator buttons as she scoured GC's terms and conditions for loopholes – after ten years at one of London's big-five accountancy firms she certainly knew where to look – and found none.

'We won't do better,' she'd said propping her head against the wall. 'I'm certain of it. With this much capital we can get capsulewardrobe.com up and running, recruit more merchandisers and open another boutique. We could even relook at that Wimbledon site, if you still think that's the best spot for our first London opening.'

Nicci shrugged as she poured over Style.com on her laptop, checking the cruise collections online for any gems she might have missed. 'Gabriel Monihan's still an arsehole,' she said. 'But this is your area, I wouldn't expect you to tell me whether to buy Isabel Marant or Vanessa Bruno, so just say the word and he can be our arsehole.'

Jo grinned at her business partner, her best friend for her entire adult life, and nodded. 'He's our arsehole,' she said.

Now, as she looked at 'her arsehole' across his freakily tidy glass and steel desk and watched his mouth move, she found him every bit as irritating as Nicci had. Possibly more. Those small, expensive, wire-framed glasses Nicci bet he only wore so he could peer over them condescendingly. His ostentatiously expensive suit; he was a Dolce man, according to Nicci. His still thick, too perfectly dyed hair. His manicured nails. It was the last detail that bugged Jo most. *Manicured nails?* What kind of man has manicures?

Jo tucked her hands behind her to avoid looking at them and then, feeling too much like a schoolgirl in the head master's office, put them back in her lap.

She had dressed carefully that morning, wearing the Armani suit Nicci had all but forced her to invest in. And invest was the word. Even thinking about the price brought tears to Jo's eyes. (She could have bought granite worktops with that money, for the as yet unstarted kitchen extension.)

But her nails looked as if they belonged to a neurotic teenager, all bitten to the quick. Nicci would never have let that happen, even if it had meant a detour to Nails Inc on the way. Given the choice between groomed and on time, Jo knew which Nicci would have chosen. That she chose the opposite tended to confirm Gabriel Monihan's words, whether she liked it or not.

'I have been searching for the right candidate for some time,' Jo said, the tone of her voice adding, *not that it's any concern of yours how I run my business as long as you get your returns.* 'But so far the search hasn't turned up anyone of the calibre we need. Not at the right price, anyway. Few companies at our level are as lean as Capsule Wardrobe. Other companies would kill to have our overheads. Most have several people doing the buying part of Nicci's role alone. In short, Nicci's combination of skills is proving hard to replicate in one person. I've appointed a well-regarded head-hunter, and we're looking at replacing her with two department heads at a non-board level. One to head up buying, one to focus on styling and wardrobe management. The online business is covered, and the boutiques already have managers who can handle the personal shopping as long as they have a clear brief.'

The words were so fluent they sounded credible even to her. They were even true. Almost. What she omitted to say was that time had run away with her and it was now urgent. It hadn't been when she'd reluctantly started looking. Back then she'd hoped to avoid the unnecessary expense of a head-hunter, just stick an ad on Fashion Monitor and let the internet do the rest. Now summer was nearly over, in a matter of days the fashion industry would be back from its annual August break and the spring/summer buying season would begin in earnest. And Capsule Wardrobe wouldn't have a Head of Buying in place.

'What do your partners think of that plan?'

'They're fully behind it.' More lies. She worried herself sometimes.

The fact was, Jo hadn't mentioned this latest development to David, beyond a passing comment. Si knew, but he always went with Jo's recommendations. Discussing it with him was more for moral support than anything else.

The new succession plans had been on her To Do list to discuss with David for weeks, but the time had never been right. There had always been something else in the way. Try as she might to put business before emotion, Nicci's letters made that impossible. And since the row about Nicci's mother they'd hardly spoken. She couldn't exactly drop him a friendly email, 'Subject: Replacing Nicci', now could she?

But it looked like she was going to have to. After all, it wasn't just Nicci's job, it was her legacy. And that was very much David's business.

Concentration was out of the question. Jo had been sitting in Caffè Nero, staring at spreadsheets on her laptop for an hour, since just after the meeting at GC's offices ended and the rain began. Huge great gobs of warm water that drenched her in the time it took her to find a coffee shop.

The numbers in themselves were fine. They did all the things they were meant to do: lined up in rows, added up to a nice round black number with a double-digit black percentage (no brackets) in the next column. In Jo's hands, numbers always added up, but when numbers were dependent on words and pictures she stumbled. And these numbers needed more than just maths, they needed vision to keep them multiplying. If Jo didn't find a replacement for Nicci soon no amount of clever accounting would make this bottom line do her bidding.

The trouble was, it felt wrong. Capsule Wardrobe was her business, hers and Nicci's, no one else's. It sounded melodramatic but bringing in someone new felt like a betrayal. And not the first. Last week she'd stood back as David declared his intent to bring Nicci's estranged mother into his daughters' lives, and now Jo was committing herself to replacing Nicci in their business. Call her superstitious, but it felt like a third betrayal couldn't be far behind.

A tear leaked from Jo's eye and slid down her nose. She batted it away and closed her eyes. How could Nicci do this to her? How could Nicci leave her holding all her babies?

It was time she pulled herself together and went home. They weren't expecting her back at the office, but there was plenty to do at the kitchen table. Plus she'd texted Si and asked him to call David and invite him round this evening to talk business.

He'd wasted no time in telling Jo what she already knew – she was pure chicken – but he'd done it anyway. The meeting was set for 7 p.m.

Jo glanced out of the café's window. It was still raining, a lukewarm, lazy August downpour that was wetter than it looked. One more coffee, she told herself, then I'll go. Rain or no rain.

Keeping one eye on her laptop, Jo rejoined the queue. As it crawled forward, she stared idly around. The tables were full of city types: men and women (mainly men) in suits, consulting BlackBerries, pecking at iPhones, talking telephone numbers and drinking skinny lattes. The type she'd been before Nicci persuaded her to leave the city behind and throw herself into Capsule Wardrobe. Nicci had shown Jo a different way to use her skills and she'd loved it, even on the days she could have happily broken Nicci's neck. And there had been enough of those.

'What can I get you?'

'A grande Earl Grey, please, with skimmed milk, and a lemon and poppy seed muffin,' Jo answered, changing her mind at the last minute. She'd skipped lunch, and she doubted much food would be consumed tonight, so she could get away with it.

As Jo looked away, one of the suits – grey with a fine blue stripe, expensive but not in Gabriel Monihan's league – headed towards her, his arm around a much younger woman in navy blue, her skirt slightly too tight, the lace of a camisole poking above the top of her jacket.

At first glance he looked like every other fortysomething man in the room. Thinning sandy hair streaked with grey. Good-looking, despite a slightly recessive chin, if you liked the type. And to judge by the way the young blonde clung to his arm, there were those who did. There was something vaguely familiar about him, Jo thought, as she handed over a twenty. Had they worked together at the firm she'd joined from college and only left under Nicci's urging?

No, he was too old. Older than Jo by ten years. And you could add another ten to the age gap between him and his companion, Jo thought uncharitably.

As the man drew alongside their eyes met and she was sure there was a glimmer of recognition in his too. Then he put his head down and steered his companion out of the door. Jo could have sworn he sped up.

The suit from the coffee shop bugged her all the way back to Surrey. She knew him. She was sure of it. Not well. But sometime, in the past, maybe just once or twice, she felt sure she'd met him before. And he'd known her too. Enough to hope she couldn't place him.

By the time the train finally pulled in, she'd run through everyone she'd ever worked with, every banker she'd pitched to and every lawyer she'd ever met. Still she couldn't place him. The more she thought about it, the more she decided he didn't look like a city type after all. He looked more like an upmarket estate agent. Perhaps, when she and Si were first house hunting . . . ?

And then she got it. Jo didn't know him at all. She'd only seen him once, not even met him properly. But she *had* seen him, and she was one hundred per cent sure she'd seen him with Mona.

THIRTY-THREE

'You remember that guy?' Jo shouted above the shower thundering down on her.

'What guy?' Si yelled back. 'There are so many guys.'

She leant round the glass divide and flicked water at his face. '*Mona's* guy,' she said. 'The married one. The one Nicci hated.'

'Can't say I *remember* him,' Si said. 'It was ages ago, wasn't it? And I never even met him.'

Jo turned the water off and reached for a towel. As she did, Si reached for her. 'Stop. It,' she said, batting away his hand just as it landed on her nipple. 'David will be here in less than half an hour.'

Si grinned. 'It won't take half an hour.'

Jo returned his smile. 'It will if you do it properly,' she said, pressing her wet body against his dry chest and jeans.

'How about a quickie to be going on with then?'

'Chancer.' Jo tucked her towel around her. 'As I was saying . . . The guy, the married one Mona had a thing with a few years ago. Affair, relationship, fling, I'm not sure which. Anyway, I think I saw him today. With a twenty-something blonde wrapped round him. He's obviously up to his old tricks.'

'Lucky bugger. What's he got that I haven't?'

'A bald patch, for a start.' Jo stuck out her tongue and punched Si, making sure her knuckles hit the muscle in his upper arm.

'Ow, that hurt.'

'It was meant to. For the record, the correct response would have been, "Mona's well shot of him."'

'Mona's well shot of him,' Si repeated, rubbing his arm.

'I don't know what she saw in him anyway,' said Jo, turning on the hairdryer and using it to clear condensation from the bathroom mirror. 'Mona's a babe, she could have anyone.'

In the mirror, she caught Si's eye. 'Well . . . maybe not *anyone.*'

'Not that again,' he said. 'Honestly Joey, what was Nicci thinking?'

Jo shrugged and turned to plant a kiss on his punched arm. 'She must have been thinking something. This is Nicci we're talking about here. She was never knowingly unthinking.'

David was ten minutes late. Jo had expected that. David was always ten minutes late. Compared to Nicci, he was punctual. Nicci thought punctuality was bourgeois. Jo thought it was just polite.

Not that Jo minded. It gave her time to arrange the canapés she'd picked up in M&S on the way home from the station, open a cold bottle of Chablis and drink half a glass to fortify herself for the conversation to come. It also gave her time to clean up after Si got his way after all.

Silence or music?

Music definitely.

Putting the iPod on shuffle she sat down. Abba came on. She got up and turned it off again. Maybe silence would be better.

Sitting at the head of the small glass table, she upended her pile of papers against the glass to straighten them and put them down again, precisely parallel to the edge of the table. She didn't need the papers. It was all in her head, but the sight of the numbers reassured her. If all else failed, she knew she could blind David with figures, just as she'd always been able to blind Nicci. Not that this was about the numbers. This was about people.

'Sorry I'm late.' Following Si into the kitchen, David shucked off his jacket and hooked it over the kitchen door where it began to drip rhythmically onto the floor. Then he dropped into one of the black Eames chairs Si had bought in anticipation of their new kitchen. 'The babysitter was late.'

'Childminder?'

'No, Auntie Lizzie stepped into the breech. The girls are thrilled. She lets them get away with murder.'

'Vino?' Si asked.

'Thanks, mate,' David took the glass from Si's hand and took a sip. 'Wow, this is good. Special occasion?'

Jo shook her head. 'Special offer. Three for two, and another five per cent off if you bought six.'

'You didn't tell me you bought six?' Si said.

Jo stuck her tongue out at him. 'Because I bought three.'

'How did it go with our arsehole?' David's voice cut in.

'You remembered!' Jo was impressed. If he was hacked off with her about last week it didn't show. Visibly, she relaxed.

'We-ell . . .' David threw a glance in Si's direction. He'd always been a terrible liar. 'Not exactly remembered. Si reminded me. I mean, I knew it was soonish. Late August/ early September is always second-quarter-budget reporting and year ahead strategy. But there's no way I would have remembered it was today.'

'That's OK,' Jo said. 'You have other things to think about. He was fine. Arsehole-like, same as usual . . .'

'But?'

'But nothing.'

Raising one eyebrow, David said, 'Jo, don't mollycoddle me, I know a "but" when I hear one.'

Talking of bad liars . . . 'Well, not exactly a "but". Things are good. Capsule Wardrobe is where it needs to be, even better. Second quarter was on budget and up on last year. Which, you know, considering the circumstances . . .'

'That's great, Jo, honestly.' David reached across and squeezed her hand. 'Don't think I don't appreciate everything you're doing with the business. I do. I know I've been worse than useless where Capsule Wardrobe's concerned . . .'

Jo smiled and squeezed back, relieving him of the obligation to mention the elephant in the room. There would be plenty of time for that. 'Just doing my job,' she said. Her heart was racing. She had to do it and do it now. 'The thing is, it's not *my* job that's the problem going forward . . .' She caught herself. 'Sorry, been hanging around too many arseholes today. If you catch me using "blue-sky thinking", "out of the box" or "walk up to the problem" feel free to slap me.'

'Ah,' David said, his face serious. 'To be honest I've been wondering what you were planning to do about Nicci's job.'

'You have?' Jo was taken aback.

'Of course I have, Jo. You told me you were looking for someone and then . . . nothing. I run a business too, you know. All businesses are only as good as their people. One of Capsule Wardrobe's key skill sets has . . .' he paused, dropping his eyes to the table. Si and Jo waited in silence as he composed himself.

When David looked up his eyes were bright. 'Gone.'

Si caught Jo's eye. Told you so, his look said. He's widowed, he's hurting, he's lonely, but he's not an idiot.

'We need to replace her properly,' Jo said. The words rang around the small kitchen. The echo was all in her imagination. So was the little voice in her head screaming, "Traitor".

David understands, she told herself. *Nicci, of all people, would understand.*

'Si told me you'd engaged head-hunters.'

Si told . . . ?

Her husband slid his arm around her. 'Joey, as sleeping partner in this business, I've been keeping the other partner in the picture while you threw your energies into keeping our business afloat. That's OK, isn't it?'

She nodded, too stunned to speak.

'David and I might be blokes, but we do talk occasionally. And sometimes we even talk about you.'

Colouring, Jo felt the tears come. 'I—Yes, I just . . . Thank you. I . . . sorry. I've been so focused on getting from day to day, I didn't think.'

'Yes, you did,' David said. 'You've been thinking and managing everyone's expectations and keeping Capsule Wardrobe going. Frankly, I'm in awe. But you need support, proper support, not another junior. Have you found someone yet?'

'Sort of. She's not ideal. She's half ideal. That's what I wanted to talk about. I know they say no one's irreplaceable, but I've scoured the industry and Nicci's specific skills are pretty hard to come by. So we – I – have to stop looking for Nicci and find someone else. We need two replacements.'

Pulling a sheet from the pile in front of her, Jo pushed it across the table. It was a planogram of her proposed staff structure. Where once Nicci and Jo had sat alongside each other, with Jo heading up operations and Nicci heading up creative, there was just Jo, as Chief Executive. In a line below her were a retail director, a head of buying and a head stylist. All three reported into Jo.

'The buying and styling positions are new,' she said. 'Nicci's old job splits in half, each appointment taking in the extra work that comes with our internet expansion plans. Both report to me, and the shop managers now report to the retail director, which is a new role but not a new member of staff. I'm thinking of promoting Yvonne, so it shouldn't be *too* expensive. She's managed the flagship for three years now and has on-the-road sales experience. So that's three new roles, but two new people. Because if I'm running the business single-handed, I won't be able to micro-manage the retail and internet operations. Obviously, the staff bills will be higher, because Nicci and I took salaries only when Capsule Wardrobe could afford it. But I can't see any other way. I've thought and thought about it—'

'Yeah,' Si interrupted. 'Mainly at three a.m.'

Jo turned to him horrified. 'Did I wake you?'

Si laughed. '*Did you wake me?* Oh, my love, only every single night. Don't worry about it. It's in the job description.'

'Who do you have in mind?' David asked, not particularly subtly dragging the conversation back to the point.

'For the buying half of the role? Nadine Cameron. She's junior but she's keen. Trained at Selfridges, worked on their online set-up, good contacts. I think she'll tune into the Capsule Wardrobe customer easily, and she'll be good for us. The stylist . . . well, hear me out, I'm thinking of going for a magazine person, someone with experience of styling and celebrity dressing, rather than buying, as such.'

She was interrupted by the front doorbell.

'Who's that?' she said. 'No one ever rings the bell.'

'Jehovah's Witnesses probably. Or a chugger,' Si said. 'I'll get rid of them.'

'Sounds good to me,' David said, as Si vanished into the hall. 'I mean, I trust you, and if you think this is the way forward then do it. How soon can this Nadine start?'

'That's the drawback. She's on three months' notice. Everyone remotely good is these days. But she doesn't think they'll hold her to it. Worst case, two months, she thinks, because she's owed three weeks' holiday. It's a risk, but—'

'Ah shit, sorry, Jo, am I interrupting?'

Behind Mona, Jo could see Si making his best 'I'm sorry, but what could I do?' face. Mona was already removing her jacket and shaking droplets onto the tiles. 'I've said it before,' she said. 'But, Christ, I don't call this summer.'

'You spent too long in Australia,' David said. 'Summer's always looked like this from where I'm standing. Here, take my seat for a sec, I'm going to call Lizzie, check the girls went down OK.'

Mona dropped into his chair and looked pointedly at the Chablis. 'My favourite. Any left for me?' she asked. Si got her a glass and emptied what remained of the bottle into it.

'Are you OK?' Jo asked. 'You seem a bit . . . hyper?'

'Not hyper. I just had an idea and I wanted to see what you thought. Although, in the time it's taken me to get here I've gone off it a bit. I'm starting to think it was a moment of madness. Maybe I'll just have a drink and then go.'

Si rolled his eyes and Jo bulged hers back at him.

'You could have called,' Jo said, eyeing her mobile. 'It would have been drier.'

'I did,' Mona shrugged. 'Your mobile was switched off. Your house phone didn't even ring. Just went straight to that non-answerphone message of yours.' Her fingers made speechmarks in the air. 'We're not here. Don't bother leaving a message, just call our mobiles.'

Si laughed. He knew exactly what they'd been doing.

'Well,' said Mona, 'I'm here now, so I'm going to say it. You know I've been thinking I need a change? I'm going slowly mad at the restaurant. Plus I'm sick of working all hours to line someone else's pockets. Sometimes I feel like chief bottle-washer and waitress, as well as manager and cashier. I wouldn't mind if it was my own business, but it's not. Which got me thinking . . .'

Mona was gabbling now. Jo couldn't remember when she'd last seen her so nervous. 'I know you've been looking for a replacement for Nicci.'

Jo raised her eyebrows at Si. He shook his head. *Don't look at me.*

'You said so, remember? Anyway, I'm not saying I'd know where to start with Nicci's job, but I thought maybe I could help out. With the shops, maybe? Build up to overseeing them? I've got tons of retail experience. I know about niche marketing.'

One look at Jo's face and Mona stopped. 'I knew it. Crap idea, right?'

Jo smiled. 'Not crap, exactly. But, Mo, you hate fashion! And your retail experience is in restaurants and organic food.'

'Retail is retail. Customers are customers,' Mona offered, but Jo could see she'd given up.

'I'm glad you're here, though,' Jo said. 'I was just telling David and Si that I've found someone to do the buying.'

'Great.' Mona took a large swig of her wine and held her glass there, obviously trying to hide her embarrassment. 'That's great news. Really. I feel a total idiot now. So let's forget I mentioned it, shall we? What else is new?'

'Oh God, I almost forgot,' Jo cried. 'Guess who I saw today. A total blast from the past. You'll never guess.'

'Give me a clue then.'

'A guy.'

258

'Young, old, fit, ugly? I need more to go on. Do I know him?'

'Obviously! Well, you did. And quite well . . .' Jo grinned and nodded at Si to fetch another bottle. 'Not young, not old, late forties, fit, I guess, if you like the type. Come on, you're not trying. The clue was in "blast from the past".'

'Nope, not a clue.' Mona didn't even pretend to think.

'*That* guy! You know the one . . . what was his name . . . ? Neil, that's it! It's been bugging me all day.'

'Neil?' Mona frowned. 'You saw Neil? Where? I thought you were in the city today?'

'I was. That's the weirdest thing. I know we never met properly. Because . . . well, you know. But I'm sure it was him. I was having a coffee after my meeting and he was in Caffè Nero, in Newgate Street. With this girl. Woman, I mean. But young, twenty-something. Skin-tight suit, all tits and hair up to here, your basic nightmare. I don't know if he's split from his wife, but something about it made me think he's up to his old tricks.' Jo grinned, their previous awkwardness entirely forgotten. 'Mo, you are so well out of that one.'

David didn't even see Mona coming until he took the corner at the bottom of the stairs and she nearly knocked him flying. It was only then he heard Jo's voice calling after her from the kitchen.

'Mo? What's up? Are you OK?'

'Sorry, I've got to go,' she mumbled, fumbling ineffectually with the front door lock. 'I forgot . . . Dan . . . I need to . . .'

'Here, let me get that for you.'

Extracting her fingers from the Yale, David twisted it and turned the door handle below it. 'One of those doors where you need two hands,' he said.

'Th-thanks.' Mona's words were muffled, her face obscured by hair that had fought its way out of the knot at the back of her head.

'Mona?' Jo was standing in the kitchen doorway. 'What's up? What did I say?'

'Nothing,' Mo almost yelled. 'I'm fine, all right? I just forgot something. I have to go home.'

David threw Jo a look over his shoulder – *I'll handle this* – and Jo retreated into the kitchen, confusion etched across her face.

'I'll walk you,' David said. 'It's not far and the rain's stopped now.'

'No need, honestly,' Mona said. 'I'm fine.'

He wasn't sure, but it sounded like she was crying. What the hell had he missed in there? He'd only been gone five minutes.

Jogging to the gate, he held it open for her. When she didn't protest he fell into step beside her.

Truth was, David felt terrible about the whole thing with Mona: guilty, ashamed, awkward in her company. It made life difficult for everyone. He felt he'd behaved badly and he tried never to behave badly. He just wasn't that kind of guy. He had plenty of mates who were – especially where women were concerned – and it didn't seem to do them any harm, it just wasn't him. Even as a student when everyone was shagging anything with a pulse if they were drunk enough not to care, he preferred to be able to look himself in the mirror in the morning.

Of all Nicci's letters, Mona's had proved the most difficult.

To begin with, he'd thought it was ridiculous – some sick joke – and assumed Mona would take that line too. To his shame, David had even wondered just how badly the cancer had been affecting Nicci's judgement at the end. Not that he'd dare say that to the others, and not that he'd dream of using that as an excuse to dismiss Nicci's last wishes, however deranged they might seem.

David had examined Nicci's motives from every angle during the nights he'd lain awake listening to Charlie and Harrie's breathing. Or sitting at the end of their beds in the antique rocking chair Nicci used for feeding, watching them sleep. He'd reached the conclusion she just desperately wanted her friends to stay together. To make sure they supported him in the difficult months that would follow her death.

Not literally for him and Mona to get into bed together.

No more than she'd intended Jo to be the literal day-to-day dressing, feeding, schooling guardian of her daughters. Nicci just wanted him to have a fallback and Charlie and Harrie to have a mother figure, a woman they could turn to when they needed someone to talk sense about 'girl stuff'. Jo was the perfect choice for that.

And Lizzie . . . She'd taken to gardening in a way he'd never have predicted. Clever Nicci. He was surprised to realise he didn't mind Lizzie turning up, increasingly unannounced. In fact, he found the sight of her bent over the flowerbeds strangely comforting.

But Mona . . . he felt sick about that. Sick about the way he'd panicked and rejected her friendship out of hand, when she'd asked him out for dinner. He should have counter-offered, invited her round for a drink and talked it through. She was only trying to do what she thought Nicci wanted, after all. Nothing more. And he understood that. He was trying to do what Nicci wanted too.

As they walked, lost in their own thoughts, the silence wasn't uncomfortable. Almost companionable. And why shouldn't it be? They'd known each other for years. Every so often, David tried to get a look at Mona's face, to gauge what she was thinking, but she kept her head down, eyes fixed on the pavement.

'Mona,' he said, slowing as they approached her street. 'I know it's been difficult since, you know . . . Nicci's letter and everything.'

'It's not that,' Mona said.

She glanced across at him. He was right, she'd been crying. Her eyes were red and still bright with tears. That wasn't his fault, was it? Surely it had to do with whatever had happened in Jo's kitchen?

'I mean, that was, you know, like you say, tricky. But it's not that.'

'Really?' said David. 'Because I know you've been avoiding me as much as you can. And you didn't look too pleased to see me just now.'

'No. That wasn't you. I just didn't know I'd be interrupting a business meeting. I had an idea – a mad idea, I don't know what possessed me – and I wanted to run it past Jo, but it doesn't matter.'

David wanted to take it at face value, but something told him she wasn't being strictly honest. Then, with Mona, who knew?

'Are you sure? Because you know, we shouldn't let Nicci's letter get in the way of all those years of friendship and I was thinking we should talk about it. Maybe go out for dinner?'

Shit. The words were out before he could stop them. That wasn't what he'd been meaning to say. *Come round for a coffee. Let's go for a drink.* Not dinner. Dinner was *loaded.*

On the pavement beside him, Mona stopped and turned. 'Really?' she said. For the first time in weeks, she looked him straight in the eye.

David hoped the doubts that had surfaced the second the words were out of his mouth weren't visible.

'Are you serious?'

David swallowed. He'd started now; he had to finish. Nice guys don't take the piss. 'Absolutely,' he said. 'I think we should go for dinner. Talk about it. Properly.' He hoped his grin looked more natural than it felt. 'Without the entire committee present.'

Mona's face broke into a smile. Her hard features softened and for a moment she looked less worn down. 'It is a bit like that, isn't it? Every decision has to be scrutinised, everything signed in triplicate. It must do your head in. It's certainly never done mine any favours.'

I know, thought David. *Enough to run to the other side of the world to get away from it.* Only what she'd found there had made her run back again.

'Well, let's rebel then,' he said. 'Just the two of us. Let's make a bilateral decision to go for a curry.'

THIRTY-FOUR

'Why am I the designated babysitter?'

Jo held the phone away from her ear, quacked her hand at Si and mouthed *Lizzie*. Snorting, he wandered into the sitting room, and seconds later she heard Jon Snow's voice echoing along the hall.

'Because you're good at it and the girls love you and you're their godmother.'

'*You're* their godmother too.' Lizzie sounded outraged. 'Plus you're *the* godmother, their guardian. The chosen one.' Her tone was mocking, but not bitter.

'Yes, great. Lucky me,' Jo said. 'But *I'm* interviewing all hours for these new positions. I've literally just walked through the door.' It was true. Her coat was still half on, her hand holding the mobile. 'And anyway, it's not my fault. David asked you. I'm hardly going to call him up and say, "David, I'm the chosen one, I should babysit."'

'Well, I'm busy too,' Lizzie grumbled, trying not to laugh. 'I've got marking, and I need to plan tomorrow's lessons. And cook Gerry's supper. And then there's my mother.'

Jo almost didn't bother to answer. 'You can do the marking when the girls have gone down, like you usually do. And you

weren't planning on seeing your mother tonight, were you?'
That was a bit mean, but truthfully Lizzie was getting on Jo's
nerves. What had got into her? She was usually delighted to
have Charlie and Harrie all to herself.

'Honestly, Lizzie,' she said, swapping her mobile to the
other hand and shaking her trench coat off onto a chair. 'I
don't know why you're making such a fuss. I'm not free,
Mona's going out for dinner with David. If you don't want
to do it, why don't you just say so?'

Silence.

'I know you're not big on *no* but this is David we're talking
about. Just say the word and he'll pay a babysitter.'

'That's what Gerry said,' Lizzie said reluctantly.

'Bull's-eye!' Jo mentally punched the air. 'I knew it! The
dulcet tones and generous human spirit of Gerry.'

'Why do you always have to say that? Anyway, I agree
with him. Gerry simply pointed out that I spend more time
round David's gardening and babysitting than I do in my
own house.'

And does Gerry really notice? Jo wondered. These days
he seemed to spend most of his spare time propping up the
nineteenth hole. Come to that, did David realise how much
Lizzie was doing for him? Jo shook the thought from her
head. Instead she said, 'You always did, Lizzie. You just used
to do more eating and less gardening.'

Lizzie's mood wasn't much better when she knocked on
David's door two days later.

'Thank you,' he cried, opening the door and drawing her
into a hug. 'You're a total star for doing this. I owe you.'
He grinned warmly. 'No change there, then. The girls are
bathed and in bed. Not that I expect them to stay there once
they find out you're here. Everything's in the usual place.
Wine in the fridge, also food if you haven't eaten . . .'

Seeming to realise she hadn't yet spoken, he stepped back. 'You OK, Lizzie? You seem quiet.'

Lizzie dropped her bag of textbooks on the hall floor and dumped her cardigan on top. 'Yes, of course, I'm fine. Don't I seem it? Sorry, it's school . . . One week into the new term and already I'm knackered.'

'Are you? I'm sorry,' David looked concerned. 'You should have said.'

It was becoming a bit of a theme. Gerry, Jo and now David . . . *You should have said*. But said what, exactly?

'You look smart,' Lizzie took in his midnight-blue suit and open-neck white shirt. Bar the funeral, which didn't count, she couldn't remember the last time she'd seen David in a suit. 'Going somewhere nice?'

She could have sworn he coloured.

'No, had to put a jacket on to cover the beans Charlie splashed on my shirt. Just the Gandhi for a quick curry. Best jalfrezi south of Watford.' His index fingers made inverted commas in the air.

'Jalfrezi? You two-chilli lightweight,' Lizzie said, shooing him out of the door. 'When you've progressed to Naga, we'll talk.'

He'd been relieved when Mona rejected his offer of a lift to the restaurant. It was too date-y, though he'd felt obliged to offer.

Even now, as he pushed his way through the couples by the bar waiting for a table, he was still trying to kid himself that wasn't what this was. Not a date, with everything that implied, just two old friends having dinner, straightening out a misunderstanding. But when he saw Mona, sitting on a red velvet banquette in a booth towards the back, toying with a glass of tap water, he was in no doubt that, in her mind at least, a date was precisely what this was.

Her dark wavy hair, usually tossed into a bun, was down and blow-dried smooth, and she was wearing a sequin-spattered strappy top that revealed tawny yoga-toned arms. For one awful minute David thought she was wearing a dress (Mona, in a dress?) but when he got up close he could see a long denimed leg sprawling from the booth, on her feet the ever-present FitFlops. Even so, for the first time he realised what other men saw when they looked at Mona, men who weren't looking through the prism of Nicci. A tall, striking woman in incredible shape. Why wasn't she beating them off with a stick? Unless she was and just kept her own counsel. Who could blame her; given the epic bust-up she'd had with Nicci over that married guy? Even David thought Nicci over-stepped the mark that time. But, like all the rows the women had, it had blown over.

'Wow,' he said when he was closer. 'You look incredible. You didn't have to go to such an effort. It's only me.'

'Effort?' Mona smiled. 'Hardly. Washing your hair does wonders for a girl's appearance. Ditto eyeshadow.' Smiling, she pushed her mobile towards him. 'Ask Dan, if you don't believe me. It comes to something when your teenage son tells you your hair is "rank".'

'Not necessary.' David nudged the phone back and slipped in opposite her. 'And you do, you look amazing. I love that top.' *Cringe*, he thought. He'd forgotten how to do this. Not that he'd ever been any good at it. Compliments had always seemed cheesy, like you were after something. And he categorically wasn't.

'This old thing?' Mona waved at the pale pink silk dismiss-ively. 'It just doesn't get out much. Like its owner. You look good yourself,' she said, and they caught each other's eye and burst out laughing.

'God, listen to us,' she said. 'It's like a school disco or something.'

'God forbid,' David shuddered. 'Looks like there's a rush on. Shall we get ordering out of the way? Then we can talk properly.'

'I've never been here before.' Mona opened the menu and scanned it half-heartedly. 'What's good?'

'Best Jalfrezi south of Watford,' he repeated. 'If they do say so themselves. But I can vouch for it.'

'Oh, no, not for me, thanks,' she said. 'Too spicy.' She glanced at the waiter, who'd materialised beside them. 'I'll have two sides please. Chana saag and bindi bhaji, and a roti.'

'Poppadoms and pickles to start?' the waiter asked.

'Yes, please,' David said.

'Not for me,' Mona said.

'Scratch that,' David told the waiter.

'No, don't. Go ahead and have some.'

'It's fine. I won't if you won't,' David smiled. 'You haven't given up drinking, I assume?'

'You won't believe this,' Mona said, and David felt himself freeze. Christ, surely she didn't expect him to do this stone-cold sober.

'Gotcha!' she laughed. 'I have been trying to cut back. But don't worry, the day I give up drinking altogether is the day hell freezes over.'

She'd eat offal before she'd admit it, but Mona *had* made an effort. Partly it was Dan's fault, that much was true. Who wouldn't be spurred into action by her teenage son glancing up from Grand Theft Auto IV just long enough to say, 'Mum, tell me you're going to do something with your hair. It's rank.'

And partly, she'd wanted to make the effort.

She'd done her roots with one of those DIY retouching kits, and blown fifty quid she couldn't spare on the beaded camisole from a boutique she passed everyday on the way to work, and had almost – almost – worn a skirt. At the last minute, she decided that would look too try-hard, and flung on her best jeans instead.

Good call, she thought when David instantly spotted the new top. Some effort was good. Too much was desperate.

Admittedly, Mona didn't get out much these days. What thirty-eight-year-old single mother did? And as for dates . . . The last one had been with Neil, at least a year earlier. When they'd still bothered with dinner, drinks, coffee . . .

Until Greg, Mona had never had the slightest trouble attracting men. As he once decorously put it, 'They clustered round you like flies round shit.' She toyed with them and then passed them on. Not in a heartless way; she'd always been straight about it. She wasn't after anything serious.

The trouble was, serious found her. It found her, picked her up, screwed with her head and tossed her away. And when she managed to pull herself together, for Dan's sake if not her own, she made the mistake of thinking Neil would be the same as all the others. Easy come – easy go. But it seemed she'd left that gene on the other side of the world, along with the debris of her marriage. Like Greg before him, Neil crept under her defences. There was a theory that if you were 'taken' your hormones gave off a 'not available' signal. The theory didn't tell her what to do when your hormones said you were taken but the person doing the taking didn't seem to want you any more.

It was like an out-of-body experience. Even now Mona could hear Jo's words. *What was his name? Neil, that's it! It's been bugging me all day . . . This girl . . . young, twenty-something. Skin-tight suit, all tits and hair up to here . . . You are so well out of that one.*

If only she was.

The storm in her head had taken hours to subside. Instantly she'd known in her heart it was true. She could have kidded herself it was a case of mistaken identity, but the words came out of Jo's mouth and everything about the last few months slotted into place. It wasn't as if Neil had ever been easily accessible; but lately he'd been positively elusive. Even the booty calls had become less frequent. Every Wednesday lunchtime had become every other. Increasingly, not even that. When he did grace her with his company he was distracted. And she was becoming needy.

Mona hated needy women. She hated that she could be one of them. Hated how her voice sounded when she asked Neil where he'd been or when she'd see him again. She'd told herself she could cope with being the other woman. Neil was married. He'd never pretended otherwise. But this was different. Neil was cheating on her.

And then there was David. So not her type, if Mona was honest. Not chiselled and built like a rugby player like Greg. Not sexy in a slightly sinister way like Neil, who not only looked like he might have handcuffs in his briefcase but had also produced them on many occasions.

Picking at the label on her Kingfisher bottle, Mona watched the waiter hovering and David pretend to be engrossed in a menu she was sure he knew by heart. He was kind. He was attractive enough, in that soft-faced tousled English way. He'd noticed she'd made an effort and, if she wasn't mistaken, had made one himself. Both more than Neil had done lately. Maybe, Mona thought, Nicci had been on to something after all.

'You don't really like curry, do you?' David, said after he'd watched her push the chana saag around her plate for as long as he could stand it.

'I do,' Mona protested. 'I'm just not a big fan of chillis.

And, you know, once a vegetarian, in spirit always a vegetarian.'

'But I've seen you eat meat.'

Mona smiled. 'David, I don't think you have.'

'I have, a hundred times. All those Sunday lunches, Easter, Christmas, you name it . . . I know you don't eat lamb or beef, but you've eaten turkey.'

Mona smiled and put her hand on top of his. He tried not to tense, but he could tell she noticed by the tactful speed with which she took her hand away. 'David, I never ate the turkey. I ate the vegetables.'

'Oh, sorry.' He glanced at his own half-eaten curry and pushed the plate away. It didn't taste like the best jalfrezi south of Watford tonight.

'And all the takeaways we've had?'

Mona shrugged and tipped the remains of the Kingfisher bottle into her glass. 'Vegetable biryani, usually.'

'Biryani!' David scoffed.

'OK, Mr Curry Snob,' Mona laughed. 'Point taken.'

'You should have said. We could have gone for Italian or Chinese, or Southern Indian – that's vegetarian, isn't it? Anything you wanted.'

'This is fine, honestly.' She took a deep breath. 'It's just nice, you know, like you said the other night, not to have supper by committee.'

'Not to do anything by committee is nice.' It was David's turn to take a deep breath. 'About that—'

'It's OK,' Mona said. 'We don't have to . . .'

'To . . . ?'

'Discuss anything.'

David swallowed hard and stopped fiddling with his napkin. 'I think we do,' he said. 'We need to talk about it, clear the air. I mean, we're going to go on being friends. At least I hope we are. For Charlie and Harrie's sake. For Dan's.

271

But much as . . . much as I want to be true to Nicci's memory . . .'

'Are you trying to tell me you don't fancy me, David?'

Kingfisher sprayed across the white tablecloth. 'I don't . . .' David blustered. 'I mean, it's not that.'

'Oh, David, don't be so English,' Mona laughed. It seemed Nicci wasn't on to anything, after all. 'Panic's written all over your face. You're a good man, put in an impossible position by your bloody wife. You don't mind if I call her that?'

David shook his head. Mona imagined he could think of plenty of words he'd like to call her right now.

'David,' she said, 'I'm not a fool. I know you're still in love with Nicci. What sort of man would you be if you weren't? You were together fifteen years. A bit of you will always be in love with her. I know that's why you're here now. Because you love her. It's why we're both here. But even Nicci – with her strong will – can't make a man want a woman he doesn't want.'

He made to interrupt but Mona shook her head. 'One more thing. I hope you don't mind me saying. I like you. I like you a lot. As one of my best friends' husbands. But do I want to go to bed with you?'

Tipping her head to one side, Mona pondered the question.

'Nah, I don't. Even if we weren't in this bloody weird situation, where we're trying to do the right thing by someone we both loved, you and I have zero – and I mean zilch, nothing, nada, niet – chemistry.'

For two people who'd known each other so long, David thought, they'd had surprisingly little to say to each other once the serious discussion was over. The remainder of the evening had been full of small talk. How are your children/how's work/

272

repeat to fade. Except they couldn't even do that in any meaningful way, because they both already knew the answers to all those questions.

Maybe his nerves were to blame. Maybe the forcedness of their situation. Or maybe the fact that, if not for Nicci, David and Mona's paths would never have crossed. They would never have been friends. They didn't like the same music (he was sure he'd once heard her sing along to Sheryl Crow), they didn't have the same interests (she loved yoga, he was all about books, films and music), they didn't even like the same food (how could he be with someone who didn't like curry?).

They could both tell a good Pinot from a bad one and talk about their children until the cows came home, but that was it. So why on earth did Nicci think they should be lovers?

He remembered Nicci saying Mona was 'good in bed', whatever that meant. Somehow David just knew that no matter how technically expert and uninhibited Mona might be, he wouldn't be 'good in bed' with her.

When she'd taken control of the situation like that, though, he'd been grateful. It was only now, as he turned off the engine and listened for a second as it ticked down, that it occurred to him how kind she'd been. It wasn't that he'd ever thought Mona was desperate to rip his clothes off. Just that given the irrefutable evidence that he didn't want to rip off hers, she'd decided to put them both out of their misery.

The sound of his key in the lock triggered a chain reaction on the other side of the door. Lights came on in the hall and Lizzie appeared in the kitchen doorway, a pile of school-books held against her chest with one arm, the other already shrugging herself into her jacket.

'You're back early,' she said, hefting her bag onto her shoulder. 'I wasn't expecting you for another hour or so.' But she was still ready to go, as if she was in class waiting to be excused.

'Gone ten on a school night,' David said lightly. 'Work tomorrow.'

'Daddeeeee,' came a wail from above.

'God, sorry,' Lizzie said. 'I thought they were asleep. They've both been a bit antsy tonight. When one settled the other wouldn't, and that woke the first one and so on. I thought they'd gone down. I guess you're used to that, though.'

'Not really,' David said. 'I mean they were, a bit, when Nicci first . . . But not lately. They're usually pretty good. Especially with you. Wonder what's got into them.'

'*Daddeeee!*'

Hooking his jacket over the banisters, David took the stairs two at a time. When he glanced back, Lizzie was heading down the hall. 'Do you have to go so soon?' he called over his shoulder. 'Stay for a drink. It won't take me a sec to sort this out. And I don't know about you but I could do with a brandy.'

'Thanks, but I can't,' Lizzie called back. 'Like you said, school night. Nothing worse than the Egyptians with a hangover.'

'Doesn't usually stop you,' David joked. But when he peered back over the banisters, the front door was already ajar, darkness spilling in from the night outside.

'Night, David,' her voice drifted up.

'Night, Lizzie,' he called. He doubted she heard him through the closing inches of night between door and frame.

'Bye then,' he said softly, surprised at the disappointment he felt. He hadn't known it until he got home, but after the tension of sitting across a table from Mona for two hours

274

he'd been looking forward to a drink and a chat in Lizzie's easy company.

As Lizzie had warned, Charlie and Harrie were doing their best impressions of the two dwarfs Grumpy and Grizzly when he reached their room, their covers kicked away as evidence of their bad tempers.

'What's got into you two, hey?' he said as he sat on Charlie's bed, one sleepy daughter plus assorted teddies on each knee. 'Have you been driving Auntie Lizzie mad this evening?'

'Auntie Lizzie gone,' Charlie repeated sleepily.

'It's late now,' he soothed, laying the child on her bed, before slipping her sister plus bear back under her own duvet. 'Got to go night night.' On cue, she slid her thumb into her mouth and closed her eyes.

'Daddy,' murmured Charlie from the bed behind him. 'Cuddle.'

'I'm here,' he said, turning back to her. But he could tell from her voice she was already drifting off.

Padding downstairs, he poured himself a cognac and crept back up again, slumping in Nicci's rocker and watching as their tiny chests rose and fell.

Twins. So easy, so tidy, so perfect – when there'd been two of them, him and Nicci. Mini-Niccis with just a hint of David to soften their mother's sharp features. He'd been shocked at first, when the doctor told them, and then showed them two tiny but distinct heartbeats on an ultrasound. Neither had twins in their family – well, not so far as they knew. Although as David was rapidly discovering, he knew little enough about Nicci's family.

Back then it had seemed perfect. Get it all over with in one go. The agony, the maternity leave, the sleepless nights, the nappies. It had been perfect. Too perfect, as it turned out.

The rich, dark Courvoisier slid down his throat, a velvet burning, and he leant back in the rocker and closed his eyes. When Nicci died he'd felt outnumbered, but thanks to Jo, Lizzie, and his mother there was always someone willing to help. And gradually, with their help, he'd regained control.

Usually Lizzie was so good with them, flinging one under each arm, unfazed by their dual demands. So unlike her to let them get the better of her. Unlike her to be tired and short-tempered. But everyone had their off days; maybe he just wasn't used to seeing Lizzie on hers.

David had wanted a drink and a chat.

It was a while since they'd caught up, and he'd wanted to get her take on the evening. Although now he thought about it, maybe that would have been disloyal. He wouldn't want to put Lizzie in a difficult position. After all, of all of them it was Lizzie who had most closely followed Nicci's wishes. Although, admittedly, doing some gardening was hardly the same as going to bed with someone on demand.

Which brought him back to what had been bugging him since he opened Nicci's letter on that bleak February morning seven months ago. Why Mona? Of all of them, if Nicci wanted to *keep it in the family*, why had she chosen Mona? She wasn't his type. David certainly wasn't hers.

Whichever way he looked at it, it made no sense at all.

THIRTY-FIVE

'Wow,' Mona said. 'Just wow. It's stunning.'

The polythene came away in Jo's hand and a billow of taupe silk and lace, and beads cascaded to the floor.

'I had no idea how beautiful it was.'

'I forgot,' Jo said. 'You've never seen it before, have you?'

Shaking her head, Mona turned away. Nicci and David's wedding was just one of the many supposedly shared memories sucked into the cultural and emotional black hole that was her six years in Australia.

'Pretty!' Charlie cried.

'Princess!'

'Do you want to touch Mummy's dress?' Lizzie said. 'Then show me your hands.'

Two small pairs of hands were held out.

'Aaaagh!' Mona cried. 'Chocolate! Let's wash that off first.' A chorus of chocklick followed her down the landing.

'No question what we do with this,' Lizzie said. 'Cherish.'

'Yes, but is cherishing it enough?' said Jo. 'I mean, isn't it McQueen? I almost feel it should be given to the V&A. Or at least put in controlled temperature storage to protect the fabric for posterity.'

'Jo,' Lizzie cried, 'you can't give Nicci's wedding dress to a museum!'

'You reckon?' Jo shrugged. 'Fashion is like any other art form, you know how big Nicci was on that. Just because the Picasso's on your wall, doesn't make it yours. This dress is a one-off. We have a duty to look after it properly.'

Lizzie looked doubtful. 'It's her wedding dress, she wore it on the day she married the love of her life. It doesn't belong in a museum or a deep freeze, it belongs to her daughters.'

Jo smiled indulgently. 'Ah, Lizzie, always the romantic.'

Lizzie poked out her tongue. 'It's true.'

'How did Nicci afford it?' Mona asked, coming back into the room followed by the twins, with squeals and giggles, parading clean hands and rushing up to their mother's beautiful dress, only to stop and gently stroke the fabric, their little faces lit with awe.

'How did she afford anything?' shrugged Jo. 'She got discounts, called in favours, had friends in all the right places. Plus, I seem to remember she spent every last penny she and David had on it.'

THIRTY-SIX

The McQueen Dress
David and Nicci's wedding, 2000

'Well, what do you think?' Nicci stood in the centre of the small room. Sketches were pinned on a mood board covering one wall, cardboard boxes piled high along another. Next to her, reflecting her back view at them was an old-school full-length wood-framed mirror like the one that used to be in Jo's granny's bedroom. A young Korean girl sat at Nicci's feet with a mouthful of pins, adjusting the length.

'Walk around the room for me again,' she said. 'I just want to check the flow.'

Nicci did as she was asked.

'Are you thinking floor sweeping or ankle?' the girl asked.

'Floor, definitely,' Nicci said. 'Problem is, I haven't chosen my shoes yet.'

'That is a problem,' the girl said. 'It's three weeks, isn't it? But we still have time as long as you're not going bespoke.'

Jo snorted, earning herself a scowl from Nicci. Jo couldn't help it. This was Nicci they were talking about. Of course she was going bespoke.

'I'm not actually,' Nicci said huffily, surprising them all. 'I'll

279

probably buy something off the shelf.' She added, 'And have them dip-dyed to match. It depends how long the dying takes. I have three choices. I've seen a beautiful satin Jimmy Choo court, with a three and a half-inch heel, but that feels a bit safe. Or there's a vintage twenties mary-jane, or I could go completely flat.'

'Flat?' the girl said. 'Ballet shoe flat?'

Are you serious? Her tone implied. Jo could see why. Nicci was scraping five feet in her socks. She wanted to look gamine, not like she'd raided someone's dressing up box.

'You're right,' Nicci said decisively. 'Assume heels and I'll come back to you when I've decided which.'

'Well, make it quick,' the girl said. 'A two-inch difference in length is a big deal. It affects the drop, everything. We'll need to relook at the skirt if you go flat.'

Rolling her eyes, Nicci turned to Jo, who was sat on the floor behind her, getting dust on the skirt of her dark grey work suit. 'Well, what d'you think?'

'What do I think? What difference does that make? I know nothing about clothes. Or so you're always telling me.'

'Tell me what you think anyway.'

Jo stared at her friend. 'I think you look incredible. But I'm not the words person around here. If I could describe you in numbers it'd be no problem. You should have brought Lizzie.'

'Ah, Lizzie's no use,' Nicci said. 'She's such a softie she'll just say something like, "Oh, Nicci, you look like a princess," which is no use to anyone. I need a good solid objective opinion. That's why I brought an accountant.'

'Well, you do, I guess, look like a princess. But a 1920s princess. Very above stairs. Which I assume is the intention?'

Turning slowly, Nicci scrutinised her skinny body in the mirror. There was no point going for push-up bodices and crinolines à la Westwood, or classic strapless Wasp-style Wang, with her frame. She'd learnt to play to her strengths a long time ago, and the narrow Edwardian-style column, with intricate layers of beaded and pleated lace, which hung straight down from her small bust, made the most of what little she didn't have.

She was only going to do this once.

Nicci had decided that long ago, lying on a camp bed in the room she'd shared with her mother at a South London refuge. And she was going to do it right. There was no room for error. She'd seen that at close quarters. If every family had nine lives, her family's had been used up long ago. You only got one shot at it, Nicci had come to believe that. She was going to get this right, dress included. Especially the dress. Even if it was going to cost the best part of six months' salary. And that was including all the favours she'd called in to do it. People had been so kind.

'What does David think? Jo was looking over Nicci's shoulder in the mirror.

'David? He hasn't seen it!' Nicci said emphatically. 'And he's not going to. It's bad luck. I don't want anything to jinx this.'

Who knew she'd turn out to be such a Bridezilla? Everyone, Nicci guessed. It couldn't have been a shock; given she did everything she gave a toss about with military precision. And if she didn't give a toss? Well, mostly, she didn't do it at all. But there were elements of planning the wedding that threatened to defeat even her. Things like the guest list and the seating plan.

David had one of those extended families that went on for ever. Even though he claimed not to know any of them, his parents had invited every Morrison in the Western Hemisphere. While her side of the church would be conspicuously empty.

Groaning audibly, Nicci rubbed her eyes with the heels of her hands until bright lights flashed inside her lids. The postage-stamp table wedged into the tiny kitchen of their flat was no longer visible beneath the discarded sheets of A4 paper. Most with just one name on. Some with half-scribbled sentences, started and then crossed out. The most recent, with just two words.

'Dear Mum . . .'

'What's up, love?' David asked, coming up behind her and kneading her shoulders. If he noticed her ball up the most recent sheet in her fist, he didn't say. 'Anything I can do to help?'

Just exist, *Nicci thought.* Your very existence helps more than you can know. *But she didn't say it. Instead she shrugged,* 'Not a thing, babe. It's all done. As good as.'

Apart from the guest list, every last detail was slotted into place. Every flower and canapé and champagne flute was just so, generously more than co-funded by David's parents. Nicci knew how much she and David owed them, and not just financially. She wasn't used to being in debt — certainly not emotionally — and she didn't much like it. But needs must. And now there was just this one last thing out of kilter.

'I'm worried about the church,' she admitted. 'Your parents' church, it's so . . . traditional. They're bound to want to do that "bride or groom" thing.'

'So?'

'Well . . .' Nicci swallowed, wishing she hadn't started this, 'the bride's side will be a bit empty.'

Laughing, David kissed her head tenderly. 'Of course it won't be. There's Jo and — what's this one's name, Alan? — and Lizzie and Gerry, and nearly all of our friends are your friends. They just put up with me because they love you.'

Nicci wasn't appeased.

'Don't worry about it,' David said. 'I'll brief Mad Phil to spread everyone out, if you're really worried.'

'And that's the other thing,' Nicci pushed him. 'About the best man called Mad Phil . . . I'm not sure it's the best omen.'

'Uh-uh,' David's mouth set in a stubborn line that made Nicci's heart melt. She loved him when he made that face. It was like a glimpse of the five-year-old he'd once been, refusing to eat cabbage. She'd never admit it out loud — it didn't fit with her image, but then nor did marrying your university boyfriend at twenty-six — but sometimes, when she couldn't sleep, she'd lie in bed *fantasising about the children they'd have. The little Nicci and little David, a small boy who made a face like that, set his feet solidly on either side and said, 'Don't do cabbage.'*

'I'm not compromising on Mad Phil,' David said. 'Love me, love Mad Phil, you know that.'

'Oh, I do,' Nicci said, although she didn't. Love Mad Phil, that is. Far from it. Truth was she barely tolerated him, but because he was now a registrar in Newcastle she rarely had to see him.

'There's one other problem,' she admitted.

'Which is?' Unfolding a second pine chair that leant against the wall, David squeezed it into the remaining floor space and sat beside her, his hand warm on her bare, brown knee.

It was his 'settling in for the duration' pose.

Nicci took a deep breath. 'I don't want to have to give myself away.'

There, she'd said it. If only they'd eloped, run away to Paris or New York, or even Finsbury Park, they'd have had none of this family stuff. Wouldn't have had to keep rattling the can, but she hadn't wanted a register office and two strangers dragged off the street. She wanted to do this properly.

To give this marriage – her marriage, her only marriage, she recited as a mantra in her head – the best chance of success. Superstitiously, she'd decided luck would come from a country church, a traditional reception in a marquee at David's family home, David's sisters' children as bridesmaids, peonies for her bouquet (in fact, peonies everywhere: Jo said Nicci chose August simply because she wanted peonies), a beautiful McQueen frock and hand-dyed Choos. (She'd opted for heels in the end.)

But no amount of obsession with detail could change the fact that she didn't have a father to give her away. Nor a mother to bury her face in a handkerchief and sniffle. She had no one. David was her everything.

'Nic.' David touched her chin and gently lifted it so she couldn't avoid his gaze as she usually did whenever the F-word came up. 'There is a solution—' he started.

283

'Not your dad, David,' she interrupted. 'It's a kind thought, and I do appreciate it—'

'Let me finish, will you? I wasn't going to suggest my father, I was going to suggest your girls.'

'My girls?' Nicci stared at him dumbly.

'Duh, Jo and Lizzie,' said David. 'You always said they were your real family — your fr-amily? Well, if they're your family, they can give you away.'

On her breast was a white metal broach shaped like a filigree star. Anyone looking would have thought it was silver. Only Nicci knew it was platinum, a wedding present to herself.

They'd gone traditional with the music in the end. She'd been tempted to choose something with emotional resonance, but there was plenty of time for that at the reception. There would be first dances and last dances, and all the dances in between to indulge her embarrassing passion for Van Morrison and Fleetwood Mac. But now, here, as she was about to walk up the aisle, Nicci hadn't wanted to take any risks. There was already one, unavoidable, break with tradition. That was enough.

'Ready?'

Nicci held out her arms and turned first to one side then the other.

On her right stood Jo, her hair loosely piled on top of her head, the colour of sun-drenched holidays. Jo crooked her elbow and Nicci slid her hand through it, resting her fingers on the mocha satin of the fifties-style bridesmaid dress she'd had made by a little tailor off South Molton Street.

On her left, Lizzie — auburn curls tumbling over creamy décolletage — squeezed her arm, so Nicci could keep hold of her posy of peonies. She was tearing up, already. Trust Lizzie.

'When you say giving you away,' Lizzie smiled through wet eyes, 'David does realise it's only lendsies, doesn't he?'

From inside the church Nicci could hear the Bridal March playing. Cheesy as hell but, right now, she wouldn't have it any other way.

'Of course.' She smiled. 'But very, very long lendsies.'

Nicci needn't have worried. Her side of the church was crammed.

So what if it wasn't with Websters, or Gilberts, or any other permutation of Nicci's flesh-and-blood family? Nicci's self-made urban family was out in force: bosses and colleagues, old friends from uni, next-door neighbours, even old landladies. The people who made up an emotional life if you didn't have a life ready made for you. Row by row they turned as she drew level, their faces wreathed in smiles of encouragement, admiration, love.

Only Mona was missing. But Mona was in Australia, with a husband and child – a child! – and unable to afford the flight home for Nicci's wedding.

Below the steps to the altar, surrounded by a riot of pinks and creams and every shade of blush between – Nicci having bought up every peony in the country – stood David and Mad Phil. David's purple Mohican and leather jacket were long gone, replaced by carefully tousled brown hair and an immaculate Paul Smith suit; styled, of course, by you know who. And not for the first time, Nicci couldn't believe this man had found her, how after all the things that had gone wrong in her life, this one thing had gone so very right.

As they reached the altar steps, Nicci turned to kiss first Lizzie, then Jo, and then, with one last squeeze, they set her adrift and David took her hand.

That such a big, life-changing thing could be done in such a short time startled Nicci. All the loving and honouring and till death us do parting over in a matter of minutes, a short sermon and a couple of hymns.

'Will you have this man to your wedded husband . . . ?'

'I will' Nicci replied. 'I will,' she repeated, as if she wanted to

285

make sure he knew. 'I will.' And though her voice was low and quiet, there was a peal of familiar laughter from Jo in the front pew and Nicci felt herself flush.

Beside her, David squeezed her hand. 'So will I,' he whispered as he slid the slim gold band onto her finger and she slid a signet ring on to his little finger. 'Oh, so will I.'

'You may kiss the bride.'

And then David's hands were in her hair and she wrapped her arms around his neck. 'I love you,' she whispered into his hair, although she was almost sure he didn't hear her. And then they were kissing and kissing and kissing, and in the distance, outside their bubble, Nicci heard Mad Phil yell, 'Oi, you two, get a room.' And everyone was laughing and somehow tradition was broken and it really didn't matter at all.

As they broke apart and turned into the applause, faces flushed with happiness and passion, all Nicci could see was a confetti of faces: David's parents, his sister and her children, a hundred people she'd never met in her life, and David swore he hadn't seen since his christening, all their mutual friends. When, after the signing of the register, the organ struck up again, Nicci walked slowly down the aisle, feeling, not seeing, the bridesmaids and David's immediate family fall into place behind them.

Since she'd woken at six o'clock that morning Nicci had promised herself she wouldn't do it, wouldn't force her hand into the flame. But her eyes betrayed her, instinctively scanning each pew as they passed. Face after smiling face, a kaleidoscope of noses and eyes and teeth and hair, young and old, black and white, blonde, redhead and brunette. She knew she shouldn't, but she couldn't help herself.

Like picking at a wound that wouldn't heal, she did it anyway. Within seconds she'd stopped pretending and started searching the rows that glowed with life and happiness, that mouthed wishes of love and affection as, arms wrapped around each other, she and David drifted past. Under hats, above cravats and ties, up-dos and long

286

loose-flowing hair, even flowers, she searched, but the face she hoped to find wasn't there.

It wasn't reasonable to expect it would be, Nicci knew that. It was the longest of shots that Nicci's letter had even reached her. The liaison at Safe Shelters had warned Nicci of that when Nicci called to ask her to act as go-between. She would, she said, but only if she could.

Nicci was given a phone number.

The first woman she spoke to hadn't been volunteering long and didn't remember Nicci or her mother, but the woman who called back did. She was, she said, so happy to hear from her. 'A success story' she called Nicci.

It depends, Nicci had thought, on your definition of success.

But still they couldn't really help her. Lynda Webster's last known address was nearly ten years old. They hadn't seen her or heard from her since then.

'We don't know for sure where your mother is, or even where she went,' the woman, Sheila, said kindly. 'We have no way of knowing . . .'

The words hung in the ether; Nicci finished for her. 'You mean, if she's alive or not?'

But despite common sense telling her otherwise — somewhere in the gap between naïvety and sheer force of will — Nicci had still hoped there would be one Webster at least on the bride's side of the church. The child inside her, who dressed Barbie in a riot of home-made colour-clashing outfits, and lived in the place where mums were infallible beings who loved you and looked after you and never let you down, that Nicci had believed she would come, if only Nicci did everything right and followed the rules.

Nicci's letter would reach her or she would see the notice David's parents had put in The Times *and the* Telegraph *(not that Nicci recalled her mother reading anything other than the* News of the World*). Failing that, she would know by some kind of mystical motherly osmosis that her only daughter was getting married, and find her.*

But she hadn't.

Not in the church, hidden out of sight in a back pew.

Not lingering outside, behind a bush or yew tree in the overgrown cemetery that made up the church's grounds.

Nicci had believed she could summon her mother through sheer force of will. For the first time since the bad times, the strength of Nicci's will had let her down. Not for the first time, but for the last, she believed against all evidence her mother would come through for her.

Well, no more, *Nicci thought as the congregation began emerging into the late afternoon sunlight.* It ends here.

The day Nicci's mother left the refuge and returned to her stepfather for the last time, Nicci had erased her from her life, reverting to her father's surname that afternoon. Today Nicci Gilbert was gone too, leaving Nicci Morrison in her place and the past firmly behind her.

'Happy?' said David, his breath warm against her neck, his arm squeezing her tight.

Only dimly aware of the photographer corralling people around them, steering Nicci and David around the gravestones towards the side of the fourteenth-century church, Nicci grasped the rejection that threatened her day and pushed it away.

Backlight from the sun threw David's face into shadow, but Nicci knew every millimetre of his face as if it were her own. Better. She'd looked at it everyday, and planned to do so for the rest of her life. Reaching up, she placed her fingers against his lips and hoped he would assume her eyes were glistening with joy. Because they were.

'Very,' she said, standing on tiptoe to kiss him. 'I love you so much. You're all the family I need.'

This, here, now, with him, was home.

THIRTY-SEVEN

It's just a wedding, Mona thought, distractedly flicking through a magazine left over from the Sunday papers. And a nine-year-old wedding at that.

She couldn't work out why having missed it bothered her so much now, when it hadn't for the past decade.

But then, everything was bothering her right now, every shared experience she hadn't been part of; the wedge she'd driven between the four of them – five, if you counted David in his own right, which Mona had begun to – by going away. The further wedge she'd hammered home by lying to them about Neil.

It was Mona's first day off in a fortnight. She was meant to get two days in seven but, as ever, short-staffing meant compulsory (not to mention unpaid) overtime. Dan was at school. Year ten now, GCSEs soon and then what? Mona tried not to worry about that.

So far today she'd taught a couple of yoga classes at the local sports centre (one Ashtanga, one beginners) from eight until ten thirty. She could be doing anything now. Instead she was sitting indoors, staring at a wall that was long overdue a coat of paint, and waiting for Neil to turn up.

He'd sounded annoyed, then surprised, then pleased when she called him. Her calling him wasn't the way things worked between them. He did the calling; the shots were all his, particularly since they got back together. But from Neil's voice she could tell the break with the norm had got to him. She could almost hear him get turned on over the phone. For a few seconds, it was like the old days. Even now, with him seven minutes late, it crossed Mona's mind that maybe they should have sex first, fight afterwards. Make-up sex had always been good for them, but who knew if there would be any? Maybe this time she would do what she'd known she should do for months.

The tinny buzzing of the doorbell made her jump.

For a second Mona stopped on the stairs, looking down at his profile through the frosted glass of the front door; the strong nose and slightly weak chin. Anticipating the glance he flicked over his shoulder as she opened the door and he slid inside; past Mona and up the stairs to her flat.

'To what do I owe this honour?' he smiled, and dropped onto her settee, his jacket already discarded on a mismatched armchair. Even as she let herself be pulled down onto him, Mona imagined she could see the calculation in his eyes. Ten minutes' chat, thirty minutes' sex, another ten minutes to get back to the office. She saw it, just as she'd always seen it, and almost ignored it as she felt his mouth on her throat and his fingers tug at her shirt buttons.

'In a second,' she gasped, easing herself back on the sofa. Her body had other ideas but for once her brain was in charge. 'Coffee?'

Neil was thrown. 'Er, OK, yes.' Mona could see him try not to glance at his watch. 'Yes, coffee, if you think we have time . . .'

'I do.' Tugging her shirt back down over her jeans, Mona headed for the tiny kitchen.

'Latte, is it?' she threw back over her shoulder. 'I bet the blonde takes hers skinny, doesn't she?' Mona knew it was childish. She would have preferred a more adult opening gambit, but she couldn't help herself.

The only noise in the flat was the sound of water thundering against the stainless-steel base of the kettle.

'What did you say?' Neil's voice was so close behind her she almost jumped.

'I said,' Mona swallowed and turned to confront him. 'I bet the blonde's drug of choice is skinny latte.'

'What blonde?'

For a second Mona faltered, he looked genuinely confused.

'Mona, what blonde?' he repeated.

Don't lie, she thought, taking two mugs and a jar of instant from the cupboard. *Whatever you do, please don't lie. Treat me with the contempt I've earned. But don't lie.*

'The blonde,' she said, forcing herself to look Neil in the eyes. 'Twenty-something, skin-tight suit, all big hair and tits up to here. The one wrapped around you last week in Caffè Nero.'

The emotions that crossed Neil's face in the next few seconds were almost like watching Voldemort change. Confusion, panic, alarm as he visibly pondered the wisdom of lying to her. Or, Mona thought, maybe he was just deciding whether he cared enough to make the effort to lie convincingly.

'Don't bother to lie,' she said, ostentatiously spooning granules into the mugs. 'You were seen.'

'Where and by whom?' he said. His face had settled now. He looked calm. Not like a man who'd been caught red-handed. But also, she reassured herself, not like a man who didn't care if he had.

'By Jo in Caffè Nero in The City. Newgate Street'

Hang on, why was he the one asking the questions? Why was she even bothering to answer?

'Jo? Your friend Jo? I've never met her,' Neil said entirely truthfully. 'Whoever she thought she saw, it wasn't me. Haven't been anywhere near Caffè Nero, let alone one in Newgate Street. Haven't even been up to London for weeks. There must be plenty of blokes who look a bit like me in the city. Could have been anyone. Mo,' he slid his arm around her, 'I can't believe you think I'd cheat on you.'

'Other than with your wife, you mean?' Mona said. But her heart wasn't in it.

'Obviously,' said Neil. 'But I hardly think that qualifies as cheating, do you? You always knew the score. You said you were OK with it. That it suited you. Mona?' He lifted her chin up so she couldn't avoid his gaze. His eyes didn't look like those of a liar. Well, no more than usual. 'What's changed?'

Where to start? Mona shrugged.

Her stomach was churning with uncertainty. Neil had a point. Jo said herself she'd only seen him once. She just *thought* it was him. And what *would* Neil be doing in the city when he lived and worked in Guildford?

'Mona, seriously,' he said, pulling her closer. 'Mona, love. I mean, really. What do you take me for?'

'She was sure it was you.' Doubt had set in. Mona knew she'd lost this round before the end of the sentence was out of her mouth. 'She said you recognised her.' Her voice was a whisper.

Neil kissed Mona's forehead, then her nose, then her lips. The gesture was so affectionate, so unlike him, that she almost took a step back.

'How could I recognise her?' he asked reasonably. 'Even if I was there, which I wasn't. I've never even met the woman.'

'You have,' Mona said. 'Once, definitely. Seen,' she corrected herself, but not loudly.

292

'Well, if I did it was years ago,' Neil said, stroking her hair. 'And I don't remember. I certainly wouldn't recognise her across a crowded café. Honestly, Mona, give me some credit. Mind you,' he smiled, 'I'm flattered you think I have it in me. Between you and Tracy and working all the hours God sends, trust me, even if I wanted to, I don't know where I'd find the energy.'

Mona smiled despite herself.

Of course, she was being ridiculous. Jo was mistaken. Why had she been so quick to doubt him? 'I don't know what I was thinking. I just hadn't seen you for a while, and . . . Oh, I don't know, things haven't been great between us lately. It's nearly a month since we last saw each other and . . .' She slid her arms around him and under his shirt.

'I know, babe, and I'm sorry. Things have been crazy at work. The market had this freak boom early summer. You remember? Especially at the top end. Any property over £750,000. Things have been so bad for the last couple of years, we had to make hay while we could. I've been working all hours. And then there were the school holidays . . . You know how hard it is during the holidays. For both of us . . .'

His hand was on the small of her back, sliding up to where her bra would have been, had she been wearing one.

They'd had sex. Why wouldn't they? It was what they were there for, after all. But it had been quicker and more perfunctory than usual, and neither of their hearts had been in it.

We don't even care enough to make up properly, Mona thought, as she prowled her flat, picking things up and putting them down again once he'd gone. The *we* came as a shock. Not *he* – Mona was beginning, too late, to realise he didn't care – but that *she* didn't care . . . That was new.

Mona felt cranky and aimless. She wanted to eat but she couldn't find anything she was interested in cooking. She wasn't in the mood to do yoga, plus Dan would be home soon and there wasn't room for yoga, chanting and Dan in their tiny flat. If she'd been a reader she could have lost herself in a novel, found solace in someone else's problems. But she wasn't. And, as ever, there was nothing on TV. Even her precious travel brochures held no attraction.

He's cheating on me, he's lying to me and, worse, I let him.

Yes, Mona thought sadly, she knew the score. And this wasn't it. Being Neil's other woman – well, Nicci might not have approved, but it was the deal Mona had made and, until now, she'd been content to live with it, more or less. But being a bit on the side of another bit on the side? That was a different thing entirely. Mona didn't know why he hadn't just dumped her there and then. Put them both out of their misery.

Why didn't you just dump him? Nicci's voice said in her head. It was a good question. One Mona didn't have an answer to.

She had to get out, get some air. Talk to someone. Tearing a page from one of Dan's exercise books, Mona scribbled a note and stuck it to the fridge door with a Simpsons magnet.

Danny,

Gone to Lizzie's. Do your homework. I'll be back to make supper at seven. Don't be gone out and don't order pizza, or else.

Love Mum x

THIRTY-EIGHT

It was two bus rides or forty minutes' walk to Lizzie's house, so Mona walked. Walking always cleared her head anyway. But she also knew Lizzie wouldn't be back from school until four o'clock at the earliest. Mona didn't know what she was going to say, but she knew she was going to say something. She dreaded to think how Lizzie would react, but this *was* Lizzie, not Nicci or even Jo. Lizzie wouldn't sit in judgement. Lizzie would listen.

Only Lizzie wasn't there.

After twenty minutes sitting on a garden wall, waiting for Lizzie's Renault to pull into her cul-de-sac, Mona stood up again. The street was almost completely silent. Nobody came, nobody went. It was a Stepford street: no one to talk to, nothing much to look at; each of the executive homes identical but for detailing to the brick, presumably intended to add a smidgeon of individuality. There were few homely touches at Lizzie's house. Not so much as a pot by the front door. No sign of the girl Lizzie had been when Mona first met her. She couldn't imagine how Lizzie stood it.

Reaching for her mobile, Mona punched in a text: *At yours. Where you? Mx* There was no answer. Unable to sit there for ever, and reluctant to go home, Mona ran through the places Lizzie might be. Then it struck her. Where was she always these days? In David's garden. Even David called it Lizzie's garden now. Everyone did, except Gerry.

Mona grinned at the thought. Could be worse, could be married to Gerry. Not that she'd dream of saying as much to Lizzie.

Nicci had, of course. Before the wedding.

It nearly led to the kind of falling out Nicci and Mona had later. And much as Lizzie didn't want to fall out with Nicci, it turned out Nicci didn't want to fall out with Lizzie either.

But she was happy to fall out with me. The bitter thought popped into her head. Mona pushed it away and turned her back on Lizzie's house. She'd liked Nicci far more than Nicci liked her, she was sure of that. Thinking about it didn't help. That way madness lay.

She could do without seeing David. They'd become adept at avoiding each other, David managing to leave the house before she arrived for wardrobe clearing. Mona was pretty sure he wouldn't be home from his office until six, and it wasn't yet half-four. This way she could talk to Lizzie in peace and wangle a lift home. At worst, it would just be the childminder and Mona would have a wasted trip. But least she'd get some exercise; a chance to stomp the bad mood out of her system.

For someone who wasn't a sharer, Mona felt strangely light at the prospect of telling Lizzie about Neil. Speaking the name of the thing aloud can loosen its power. As Mona turned the corner into David's street she almost skipped. Why hadn't she thought of this sooner? Lizzie would understand. Lizzie was different. Lizzie would know what to do.

Stamping her feet on the doormat, Mona leant on David's bell, ringing it once, twice, three times, before remembering that, if Lizzie was here at all, she wouldn't be indoors. Trotting to the sidegate, Mona knocked hard on the weather-faded wood and shouted, 'Lizzie? Are you there? It's me, Mona!'

'Lizzie's not here, I'm afraid. Can I help you?'

The unfamiliar voice behind her made Mona jump. 'God,' she said turning to look at the woman behind her. Shorter than Mona by nearly a foot, slim, birdlike even, with short hair and what Nicci always called 'nan jeans'.

She was, Mona realised, her heart pounding, very nearly Nicci.

'I . . . you're . . . You are . . . *aren't you?*'

The woman weighed Mona up, her grey eyes taking her in. Self-consciously, Mona patted the halo of frizz she knew had escaped from her bun as she walked.

'Nicci's mother?' the woman said. 'Yes. I didn't know whether to answer the door or not. But when I heard you calling Lizzie I thought I should. I hope David won't mind me letting you in.'

Wiping her hand on her jeans she held it out. 'I'm Lynda and you must be Mona, the missing friend?' She waited until Mona had shaken her hand, then turned and headed for the open front door. 'Do you want to come in?' Lynda said. 'I don't know if Lizzie's supposed to be here. David didn't mention it. But I'm sure you're welcome to come in and wait?'

Shrugging, Mona followed her into the house. 'I'll text her again,' she said, and frantically punched in a message: *Now at David's looking for you. You're not here but Nicci's mother is!!!! Where are you?! Mx*

'I'm sure David won't mind if I suggest a coffee.'

Oh, I wouldn't bank on it, Mona thought. She hadn't seen David since the date that wasn't, and she still didn't feel ready to. He was right, she didn't know what Nicci had been thinking either. But still, it hurt to have someone so obviously not want you. Especially when they had 'decent bloke' written through them like a stick of rock.

'Herbal tea, please.'

When the woman looked confused, she added. 'It's in that cupboard there. Above the sink.'

'I can't see the attraction, I have to say,' Lynda said, dropping a fennel teabag into a mug on Mona's instruction. 'Just funny-tasting hot water, if you ask me.'

Mona laughed. 'It's good for you,' she said. 'Or so I tell myself. It offsets the alcohol consumption.'

'David does know I'm here, you know.' Lynda said, pushing across a steaming mug of funny-flavoured water. 'I'm not single white female. I do know when I'm not wanted.'

Mona shrugged. 'I'm sure you do. After all, I've never met you before and I knew Nicci for sixteen years, give or take the years I was away.'

'So it follows that I'm not wanted?'

'I didn't say that,' Mona blew on her tea. 'It follows you *weren't* wanted, and you knew it. At least not by Nicci.' She glanced up as if suddenly realising something was missing. 'Where are . . . ?'

'My granddaughters?' The woman paused, obviously adjusting to the way the words felt on her lips. Mona could almost see her rolling them around her mouth. *My granddaughters*. Mona knew Nicci hated the woman sat opposite her. At least, Mona thought she must have done. What did she really know? But she couldn't help feeling sorry for her. That was then, after all. People make mistakes. People change. Not everyone, but some.

'At ballet, I think? Are they old enough to do ballet?'

Mona shrugged. 'Probably,' she grinned. 'Knowing Nicci, those two do a bit of everything.'

'David's gone to pick them up.' Lynda took a deep breath. 'I've come for tea.'

'Is this the first time?'

'First time I've met them? No. We went to the park. Well, David and the girls did. I just *happened to be passing*. Do you think kids fall for that?'

Mona shrugged. 'Probably. At that age, anyway.'

'It's the first time I've been here with them. Or it will be. It feels . . .'

'Weird?' Mona said.

The woman's laugh was hollow. 'I was going to say nice, but yes, weird too. Weird for you, I'm sure, seeing me here.'

Mona shrugged and blew on her tea. 'Not my business.'

She meant it. Live and let live. Nicci could have been better at that, in Mona's opinion.

'I know the others don't feel the same. Well, Jo certainly doesn't. She thinks that if Nicci didn't want you in her daughters' lives, David shouldn't let you in now she's gone.'

Hurt flashed across the older woman's face.

'I'm sorry,' Mona said, 'but that can't come as a surprise.'

'It doesn't.'

'If it's any comfort, I'm not sure about Lizzie. I wanted to talk to her about it, actually. For what my opinion's worth – and you should know that's not much around here – I think it's David's call. I don't know what happened between you and Nicci. Well, I know some of it. The rest is between you and her. She chose not to tell us. So I don't see that you should have to.'

Truth was, Mona was dying to ask.

'Thank you,' Lynda said after a while. 'I know David isn't so sure either. Oh, he's coming round, obviously, or I wouldn't be here. But he thinks I need to earn my place in his family. And I happen to agree with him. But you know all there is to know, I believe.'

Mona tried not to look freaked when Nicci's mother dropped, without thinking, without knowing, into Nicci's chair and propped her little pointed chin in both hands. Just like Nicci.

Except the hands weren't Nicci's. The nails weren't neatly manicured, they were bitten and ragged. The woman's hands aged her. If Lynda was in her sixties, which Mona guessed she must be, her hands looked far older.

'I don't make excuses for myself,' Lynda said. 'If Nicci hated me – and everyone tells me she did – she had every right. She was my daughter. *Is* my daughter.' Lynda's small bright eyes filled with tears. 'I should have gone to my grave trying to make it up to her. Instead . . .'

Her head dropped and for several moments she stared at the film forming on the surface of her strong milky tea. 'What about you?' she asked suddenly.

Mona jumped. Nicci's mother had been silent so long. 'Me?'

'Well, you said your thoughts weren't worth much around here. That doesn't sound like good friends to me.'

'Oh, I didn't mean that.' Mona tried to dismiss it. 'That was just a throwaway comment. What I meant was I went away for a few years, travelling. Lived in Australia for a while.' She was deliberately vague. 'I was away when Nicci and David got married. Other things happened that I missed. Inevitably, it left a hole in our friendship. Maybe not a hole, more like a gap. But that's all.'

'That's all?'

'What I'm trying to say is, I don't have first dibs on Nicci's memory, much as I loved her. David is mourner-in-chief and then Jo, I suppose, because Jo and Nicci met first. And then, as you know, Jo and Nicci were in business together. Then Lizzie . . . Well, everyone loves Lizzie.'

Nicci's mother nodded. 'So I see.'

Mona frowned. What did that mean? This woman hardly knew them. When Lynda didn't elaborate, Mona continued.

'Lizzie's lovely, she's a great listener, a good friend to everyone, except herself. She's having a hideous time with her mother – Alzheimer's; to be honest, I don't think her mum will be around much longer – and her sister lives in America and is worse than useless. She's only been over once. Just issues transatlantic orders. Plus Lizzie's got this *awful* husband.' Mona caught herself. 'Actually, that's not fair. Gerry's not awful, he's just, you know, wrong for her.'

'Sometimes people can be bad together,' Lynda said thoughtfully.

Mona looked puzzled.

'Bad for each other. Make things worse.'

'Then one of them should leave,' Mona said firmly. 'Why would anyone want to be with someone who makes them miserable?' Even as Mona said it she knew how absurd her certainty sounded. Who was she to say that? Nobody knew what really went on in other people's relationships.

And why was she having this conversation with a total stranger? Because Lynda wasn't a stranger, not really. The woman nursing a cup of tea on the far side of the table was utterly unknown and yet eerily familiar.

'What's so wrong about him?' Lynda said. 'Does he hit her?'

The way she said it made Mona start. Like that had to be the problem. Of course it did. In Lynda Webster's life, being married to a man who'd turned into a corporate bore somewhere between twenty-eight and thirty-two wasn't a problem; abuse was a problem.

'Of course not. At least, I don't think so. We'd know, wouldn't we?' Then Mona stopped as doubt body-slammed her. Why would she know? She didn't know Nicci had a mother. Nicci hadn't known Mona still had a married lover. Her stomach roiled. What else didn't they know, these women who claimed to know everything about each other?

'That's why I'm here really,' Mona said. Diversion seemed

the best tactic. 'To talk to Lizzie. But she's not here and I don't want to get in the way of your tea party, so I should go.'

'No need,' Lynda glanced at the clock. 'I mean, not if you don't want to. David won't be back till about five thirty. At least finish your tea.'

Partly, Mona felt sorry for the woman, alone in her estranged – her dead – daughter's house. *Her dead daughter.* How must that feel? Mona's body went cold at the mere thought of anything happening to Dan. How must it feel to be Lynda? She wasn't saying Lynda hadn't deserved to be iced out. Little as she knew, Mona was sure she had. But Mona had first-hand experience of life on the sharp end of Nicci's disapproval.

A vibration interrupted Mona's thoughts. *Lynda!!! No way!!! Damn I knew I should have gone gardening, but Mum's worse. At Cedars. ☹ Tell all later. Lx*

'Lizzie,' she said, seeing Lynda's enquiring expression. 'She was planning to come here but she had to go and see her mother.'

'Bad?'

Mona nodded. 'Worse every day.'

'More tea?'

Mona glanced at the clock. There was still half an hour before David would be back and she was surprised how easy Lynda was to talk to. 'Why not?'

Why not? she thought, as she watched Nicci's mother learning her way around the kitchen, looking for things where she thought they should be, not where Nicci had kept them, throwing snippets of chatter over her shoulder about how beautiful the girls were.

Like Nicci but not. Nicci with thirty years of regrets.

Why not? Mona thought again. She needed to talk. Needed some unbiased advice. Who better to give it than this woman Mona felt she knew, but who really didn't know her at all?

'I fell out with Nicci,' she heard herself say. 'Terribly. About three years ago. Over a man.'

'Usually is,' Lynda said reasonably. 'But surely not . . . I mean, Nicci and David, they seem so—'

'Oh God, no!' Mona spluttered. 'Definitely not. Nicci would never, and David . . . No! I was – still am, in fact – seeing a married man.' There, she'd said it. And the sky hadn't fallen in. 'I wanted my friends to accept him, accept me, my life, for what it was. It wasn't how they chose to live their lives but it was mine and it suited me. It was what I needed, at the time. Good sex with a man who made no demands on me, emotionally. But they wouldn't. Nicci wouldn't. And because Nicci wouldn't, the others wouldn't.'

'And did Nicci say why?'

'Only that he was using me. That he'd never leave her. She only cared about me, didn't want to see me hurt, the usual.'

'All true?'

'Possibly. But it seemed more personal than that. Nicci wouldn't let it drop. Demanded I show female solidarity. Claimed it was as low as you can get. Kept demanding I end it.'

Lynda looked resigned. 'It never occurred to you there might *be* something more personal behind it?'

'Like what?'

'Like maybe her father had an affair and left me?'

Mona opened her mouth and shut it again. How could she have been so blinkered? 'Nicci never said.' How lame did that sound?

'Nicci never said very much, by the sound of it.' For a second Lynda's eyes were sharp and Mona could feel her disapproval. But her own irritation was rising. Why did everything always have to come back to Nicci?

'Look,' said Lynda. 'It doesn't matter. I'm not making

excuses for Nicci. But life made her harsh. People disappointed her, let her down. Me, her stepfather. Before either of us, her father.'

'I should have realised.'

'No, you shouldn't. Friends should stick together. Yours didn't. So what happened?'

'I told Nicci, Jo and Lizzie I'd dumped him. We did break up, but it was Neil who dumped me. I said I'd done it. They were so happy they cracked open the champagne. Started fixing me up on dates with "nice men" – David's partners from work, teachers from Lizzie and Si's schools, even an accountant from Jo's old firm. And when Neil came back with flowers and chocolates and lacy underwear and apologies I took him back. And I never told them.'

Lynda's face was sombre. 'Must have been hard, lying to your best friends for all those years.'

'*Ouch*, put like that . . .'

You *are* like Nicci, Mona thought. Or Nicci was like you. More than you realise.

'I just mean, you must be lonely.'

Mona felt her eyes prick. 'Very,' she whispered to the table.

'And now?'

'I don't know.'

Mona told Lynda how Jo had seen Neil with someone else, how despite his denials, she knew he was lying to her and how she had no one to talk to about it. She couldn't talk to Jo, Lizzie or David. She wouldn't dream of talking to Dan. She couldn't even have a sensible conversation with herself.

'You can talk to me,' Nicci's mother said matter-of-factly. 'I won't tell anyone unless you want me to.'

Mona shook her head and sniffed. 'Sorry,' she said, wiping her nose on the back of her hand. 'Gross.'

Lynda slid back Nicci's old chair and crossed the room to

pick up a kitchen roll. 'Are you sure Nicci didn't know?' she said gently, handing it to Mona.

'Yes,' Mona said. 'Quite. Why do you ask?'

'Well, she left you David, didn't she?' Her tone was kind.

'How do you know that?'

'Something David said. Other stuff I just picked up. Lizzie got the garden, Jo got the girls . . . Why do you think Nicci did that?'

'Because she thought I was a single mum and needed a nice man. Because there's no man on the planet more loyal and decent than David. Because Nicci said I'd never gone to bed with anyone I liked. Which isn't true, because I liked Greg – my ex-husband. I loved Greg.' Mona paused, swiping her hand across her eyes. 'Because she wanted us all to stay together.'

Lynda looked at Mona and her eyes shone. 'She didn't have to leave him to anyone.'

'The others aren't single.'

Lynda shrugged. 'Have it your way,' she said. 'But this is Nicci. For what it's worth, I think maybe she was trying to tell you something. All of you.'

THIRTY-NINE

'Let me guess: you're going to David Morrison's again.'

Lizzie took a handful of clean plates from the dishwasher and piled them methodically in the cupboard. Then she reached back for the cutlery.

'Let me guess,' she said lightly. 'You're going to golf again.'

'It's hardly the same,' Gerry said, leaning against the door jamb. 'Golf is my down time.'

'Gardening's mine.'

'Christ's sake, Liz, I know when Nicci said jump you always asked how high, but seriously, listen to yourself. Gardening? You? The woman who can't keep a house plant alive long enough to get it through the front door.'

'I can,' Lizzie said, feeling her back stiffen. Unwise words jostled at the base of her neck. 'I've got that garden in great shape.'

'I'll take your word for it.'

'You could do more than that.' Lizzie tried to sound conciliatory. 'You could come round after golf and see it. It's the other side of town, not the other side of the country.'

Without needing to look, she knew Gerry was rolling his eyes. He'd wasted no time in using Nicci's death as an excuse to 'draw a line under' their Sunday lunches. Lizzie could count on one finger the number he'd been to this year. Not that there'd been many to miss. Sunday lunches had been too sad to be regular, too fraught with the tensions caused by Nicci's letters. Now no one could face them unless there was a special occasion.

'He's taking the piss, Liz,' Gerry said. Out of the corner of her eye, Lizzie saw him take a step towards her and felt herself tense. As if he'd felt it too, he stopped where he was, and when he spoke again, his tone had hardened. 'If you want to be a mug, go ahead and be one. But, if you ask me, if the guy wants a gardener he should pay one. For that matter, if you love gardening so much you could do something with ours.'

Pointedly he glanced at the plant-free square of unloved, unswept slabs beyond the French doors. The only green either of them could see came in the form of weeds that crept through the cracks.

'Look,' Gerry said. 'I've been thinking we should move house again soon. This one is a bit ordinary. When I get that promotion we can trade up, get a bigger garden, flowerbeds, if that's what you fancy. Double garage, more outside space.'

It's not like that, Lizzie wanted to say. *I do enjoy the gardening, but I like being there. I like seeing David and the girls. And Jo and Si and the boys, and Dan and Mona, when she's there. I like feeling close to Nicci. I like the tradition.* But she didn't. He wouldn't get it.

'Come to the clubhouse for lunch,' Gerry said suddenly, crossing the kitchen in two strides and putting his hands on her shoulders.

Taken by surprise, Lizzie jumped.

'I mean it,' he said. 'Forget Nicci's lot. Come and have Sunday roast with my friends, for a change. See you at the nineteenth hole. One thirty sharp. Try not to be late. And, Liz,' Gerry leant round and kissed the side of her face, just missing her mouth, 'get changed first. That gear might be all right for gardening, but the clubhouse has a dress code.'

Mona was there, sitting outside at the metal table in jeans and a body-hugging T-shirt, despite the chill in the air, drinking coffee and nattering nineteen to the dozen with Nicci's mother. There was no sign of Dan, but he was probably at football, maybe with Si and his boys. If it was the latter, Jo couldn't be far behind. Lizzie felt a twinge as she realised they were all going to be there, and no one had thought to tell her. Except, as Gerry said, she was always there, kneeling in a flowerbed, humming to herself. Doing her thing, turning up unannounced. They didn't need to call her because they'd just assume she'd come. So had she until an hour ago.

'Coffee?'

'No, thanks,' Lizzie called when David waved a cafetiere at her. 'Had one before I left home.

'Hello, Lynda,' she said uncertainly. She'd met Nicci's mother a few times now and still found her presence in Nicci's garden uncomfortable. It wasn't anything Lynda did. It just felt wrong.

'Day off, Mo?' she said lightly as she passed. 'Again? What gives?'

'I've put my foot down,' Mona said, her voice full of pride. 'I told them that if they want to keep me I need at least one day off a week, every week. No more unpaid overtime. No more days in lieu that never arrive.'

'Wow. New leaf.'

'Yep,' Mona smiled. 'First of many.'

Lizzie headed down the garden, but not before she caught the conspiratorial glance Mona threw in Lynda's direction.

What was that about? It wasn't the first time she'd turned up to find Mona and Lynda drinking coffee on the terrace, with Charlie and Harrie and a host of dolls at their feet, David reading papers inside. It was . . . cosy.

Surreptitiously, Lizzie glanced back up the garden. Mona and Lynda were locked in conversation, David appeared with a fresh jug of coffee. For the first time it occurred to Lizzie that maybe she was interrupting something, and despite her best intentions, what little remained of her good mood slipped away.

'What I'd really like,' Mona said, nursing her mug in both hands. 'Is to be my own boss. I'm fed up of working all hours for someone else.'

'Know the feeling,' Lynda replied, visibly dragging her attention away from her granddaughters' game. Baby Alives and bears and assorted other dolls were arranged in a circle at their feet, each with a cup and plate in front of them. Some things never changed. 'I've worked full time my whole life and I have literally nothing to show for it.' Her voice wasn't sad or resentful, just matter of fact.

'Well, I don't want that to be me.' Mona stopped, suddenly realising how that sounded. 'No offence—'

'None taken,' Lynda smiled. She looked younger then, Mona thought. Just as she did when she looked at Charlie and Harrie, and her face suffused with love. 'It's just a fact.'

It still unsettled Mona, the way she found herself confiding in this woman she hadn't even known existed a few months ago. It was like their . . . friendship – she supposed that was what it was – had gone from 0–60 in a few short weeks. One minute Lynda was a complete stranger, the next Mona was telling her things she hadn't even shared with her best, her oldest friends. About Neil. And Greg. And her quiet dreams of opening her own restaurant.

The age difference was immaterial. She barely noticed that Lynda was over twenty years older than she was. If anything, it gave the woman a sort of wisdom. And she never disapproved. Sometimes she disagreed, or offered advice, but often she just nodded or shrugged. Like now. Shit happened, she seemed to say. It certainly had to her. And to Mona. And that was how life was. That was OK, life went on. And sometimes, when you least expected it, it took a turn for the better.

'I don't want to shatter the illusion,' David said, sticking his head out of the back door, 'but you know what being your own boss means? No one else to blame, no one else to pick up the slack and no guaranteed payday.'

Mona stuck out her tongue. 'Sounds like my life anyway. Might as well do it my own way.'

'What's the plan?' Lynda asked.

Mona's smile faltered. 'There isn't one,' she said. 'Not yet, anyway. Just ideas. Fantasies, really.'

'What's that noise?' Lynda asked, half an hour later.

Their conversation had lulled and Mona was relishing the rare luxury of reading the Sunday papers, while Lynda sat on the floor pretending to drink plastic cups of tea.

'What noise? I can't hear anything.'

'A kind of buzzing.'

Straining to listen, Mona shook her head. All she could hear was Charlie and Harrie's chatter as they poured tea and force-fed their dolls cake. 'I don't hear anything.'

Lynda cocked her head to one side for a second and then shrugged. 'Must be hearing things,' she said. And then she grimaced. 'Old age catching up with me.'

* * *

310

'Lizzie!' Mona's voice reached her from the top of the garden. 'Is that your phone?'

Lizzie looked up from her work, dazed. She'd been so engrossed, stripping the last of the beans, wondering who to ask if now was the right time to take down their wigwams, or whether there might be one more harvest if she left it a little longer, that she hadn't heard her phone ring.

'Yes!' she yelled back. 'Sorry, miles away.'

When she reached it, the buzzing had stopped. Never mind she thought. Probably Gerry calling from the ninth hole to remind her not to be late for lunch. Shucking off one of Nicci's gardening gloves, she picked up her Nokia and peered at its screen. *Three missed calls.*

Three? God, he really didn't trust her timekeeping, did he?

But her heart had begun to beat faster, and when she scrolled down the missed call log and saw the same number recurring, she knew Gerry's was not the voice she was going to hear when she returned the call.

Few people had ever described Lizzie by the speed she moved, but the woman sprinting up the garden towards the house could only be called a streak.

'What's up?' Mona called, her voice creasing with alarm as Lizzie drew closer. 'Lizzie? You OK?'

'It's Mum,' Lizzie gasped, her bag and cardigan dragging behind her. 'The care home . . . Have to go.' She tossed the shed key at Mona as she passed. 'Lock up for me, will you? Tell David, I'm sorry . . .'

'Lizzie?' David wandered onto the terrace, two open bottles of Peroni in his hand. 'What is it? What's happened? At least let me come with you.'

But by the time he'd dumped the bottles, dashed through the house to find his car keys and opened the front door, he was just in time to see Lizzie's little Renault pull into the road and vanish.

How Lizzie didn't crash on the sixty-minute drive through Sunday lunchtime traffic, she had no idea. There'd been an accident on the M23 so she used side roads, roaring up behind elderly couples on leisurely drives to the pub and leaning on her accelerator to overtake at the slightest sign of a gap in the oncoming traffic.

Forced to halt at a red light she impatiently found Karen's number and pressed dial. The five-hour time difference was the last thing on her mind.

'Lizzie?' Her sister's voice was thick with sleep, but she regrouped quickly. 'Do you have any idea what time it is here? You do realise it's seven o'clock on Sunday morning.'

'Well, Karen,' Lizzie knew her voice was brittle but she couldn't help it, 'Mum's dying. She didn't check the time first.'

There was silence, then Lizzie heard her sister say something to her husband at the other end and there was a rustling as Karen, presumably, got out of bed and put on her dressing gown. Across the Atlantic, a door shut.

'Yelling at me's not going to change anything, is it?' her sister said.

Lizzie couldn't help it. She hung up. Then, to be sure, she switched her ring tone to silent. There were two missed calls and a *For God's sake, Lizzie, call me* text from Karen by the time Lizzie pulled into The Cedars' car park. Janet, The Cedars' manager, was waiting for her in the office.

'Thank you for coming so quickly,' she said. 'Dr Clifton's waiting for you on the personal care floor. We'd appreciate it if you'd turn off any mobile. They've been known to interfere with the machinery.' Lizzie had always thought that was an urban myth, but for once she was more than happy to oblige.

This must be what an out-of-body experience feels like, she thought as she watched herself hurtle along the corridor behind a stout grey-haired woman in a navy-blue skirt and white short-sleeved blouse. A dumpy redhead with muddy patches on the knees of her jeans. On a good day, she could be described as 'good for her age'. On a bad day, like today, 'worn' would be generous.

Knackered, if she was honest.

Despite her sister's protests Lizzie had moved her mother to this floor when The Cedars' standard care package no longer 'fitted' her. Rather than do battle with social services, or start the search for somewhere cheaper, Lizzie had raided the proceeds of her mother's house sale again. Still she was surprised by the quantity of equipment that greeted her when she opened the door to her mother's room.

'When did she—' Lizzie started.

'Your mother slipped into a coma sometime between breakfast and morning rounds. About ten o'clock.'

Lizzie nodded. Finally, the day she'd dreaded and, in her private 3 a.m. moments – moments she wouldn't share with anyone – the day she secretly prayed for was here. For the first time in months her mother's expression was peaceful. The anguish and confusion that fought a constant battle with blank incomprehension had vanished.

'Dr Clifton will talk you through the treatment options.' And Janet was gone.

Did she hate doing that? Lizzie wondered, watching her recede along the corridor. Or was it all in a day's work?

'Hello again,' Dr Clifton said, briskly shaking her hand. His face was all concern. Pasting on a smile, Lizzie watched his mouth move, heard his voiced echo around her like the teacher in *Peanuts* – *wah, wah, wah*. From what Lizzie finally understood, it didn't matter what he did. The outcome would be the same. Eventually.

'There's no chance she'll wake up?' Lizzie asked, aware she sounded like a child asking if it was really safe to bury a dead pet.

'I'm not saying there's *no* chance,' Dr Clifton said. 'For now we have her on a saline drip and we're watching her vital signs. If you wish, we can do nothing more than wait and see . . .'

'And if Mum does wake up,' Lizzie steeled herself, 'what then?'

'If,' the doctor stressed the word, 'your mother regains consciousness – and I must stress that's a big *if*, given the advanced stages of her illness – I can't promise it won't be worse than it was. I can tell you with certainty it won't be better.'

Somehow two hours passed between Lizzie arriving at The Cedars and leaving again. Two hours in which she signed papers, nodded a lot, watched people's mouths move and absorbed nothing. Other than that her mother was unconscious and would probably never wake up again. Other that that for the first time in months Mum looked at peace. Or so Lizzie preferred to think.

Resting her forehead on the steering wheel, she listened to the distant sounds of a suburban Sunday afternoon and tried to calm herself. Should she have stayed longer? Would her mother subconsciously know she'd been there when she'd been calling her younger daughter by someone else's name for over a year? Did it even matter? Was the someone being there what was important? Would this even be happening if Lizzie had been a better daughter?

Guilt overwhelmed her. But the tears that had always appeared so easily refused to come. *Breathe Lizzie*, she whispered. *Breathe.*

There were thirteen missed calls when she turned on her phone. One from Mona, one from Jo, two from David, the second with Charlie and Harrie in the background sending Auntie Lizzie their love, which made Lizzie's heart twist. Six from her sister. Increasing in fury, probably, if Lizzie could be bothered to listen, but she couldn't. Deleting the lot without so much as hearing her sister's voice. Karen could learn the details by email later. Right now, being patronised by her sister was the last thing Lizzie needed. If Karen wanted to help she could get on a plane. Or she could stay in Brooklyn and make do with email updates.

And three from Gerry.

Shit, shit, shit. Lizzie closed her eyes, hitting her forehead with the palm of her hand as she listened to his first message. She'd forgotten all about Gerry and lunch at the golf club. In her hurry to get to her mother, she hadn't even thought to call him.

The first, left at one twenty was fine. All, *See you soon. We have a table in the bar. Don't forget to put on some makeup.*

The second, half an hour later, was left in a hissed tone she recognised as being on just the safe side of fury. *Where are you? Call me when you get this. We'll give you another fifteen minutes and then we're going to order. Don't make me look like a fool, Liz.*

He actually said that. She played it back, just to make sure she hadn't imagined it. *Don't make me look like a fool, Liz.* While she was in her mother's hospital room listening to the doctor talk about vital signs and nil by mouth, her husband was worrying about being made to look like a fool.

Be fair, she told herself. How was he supposed to know?

Lizzie caught her reflection in the rear-view mirror. Pale and freckly, purple shadows under her eyes. With no makeup, her eyelashes vanished into her face.

The third message was ice cold. *I don't know what you think you're doing, Liz. You made me look an idiot in front of my friends. We'll talk about this later. I don't know what time I'll be home. Not that I expect that to bother you.*

Finger poised over number three to delete, Lizzie paused. It would be worse later if she took the easy option now. Two deep breaths and she pressed to return his call.

'Where the fuck were you?' The sound of a chair being scraped back, raised voices, laughter.

His voice was tight with fury over.

You can't blame him, Lizzie told herself. It's your own fault. He doesn't know because you didn't tell him. Apologise and make it better.

'I'm sorry, Gerry,' she started. 'So, so sorry. I'd never dream of standing you up.'

'You did, though, didn't you? I should have known better than to even invite you. You always show me up. Just this once, don't you think you could have—'

'Gerry, I'm sorry,' Lizzie repeated. 'I know I should have called. I wasn't thinking str—'

'Clearly.' he said. She could hear the alcohol in his voice.

'Just let me explain.'

'It had better be good.'

'Good?' *Breathe, Lizzie breathe.* 'That depends on your definition of the word "good".' *No, Lizzie, breathe!*

'If by *good* you mean happy, then no. If by *good* you mean dramatic enough to justify making you "look a fool in front of your friends", then, yes, I think I can manage that.' Lizzie didn't recognise the anger in her own voice. 'My mother's dying, Gerry. She's unconscious and hooked up to machines, and Dr Clifton doesn't think she'll wake up. I've been at The Cedars for the last two hours. Longer. Is that *good* enough for you?'

Silence. *Nicely done, Lizzie*, she thought. *Well handled.* But at least she had his attention.

'Gerry,' she said, her voice calmer, 'don't you get it, love? Mum's not just ill, she's dying. I'm sorry I didn't call you. I know I should have, but they made me turn off my phone in the wards. This isn't about you or me, or me showing you up. It's about Mum. You could have called the others. They'd have told you.'

'You told them?' Gerry said. 'Let me get this straight. Your mother's dying and you called your friends and not me?'

'No,' Lizzie cried. 'I didn't call *anyone*. I told you, my phone was off and I was in too much of a state. I was gardening when I got the call. I just yelled something to David about Mum and hospital and ran. If you'd called him—'

'David?' Gerry's voice was cold, a mixture of hurt and barely contained fury.

'Yes, David. I was in the garden, like I told you I was going to be, and . . . Gerry? *Gerry*?'

Lizzie stared at her phone for what felt like minutes. Square fingers, tipped with mud that had worked its way under her nails, wrapped around an obsolete Nokia handset. When it was obvious that the only person left on the line was her, Lizzie clicked the off button and stared at her reflection in its scratched screen. She knew this woman, and yet she didn't.

This woman's mother was unconscious, a shrunken silent

317

figure in a room full of machines. Her sister was screaming abuse into her voicemail from three thousand miles away. And her husband had just hung up on her.

This woman wasn't even sure she cared.

FORTY

The chrysanthemums were aflame; like a reflection of the autumn sunset behind them. How clever Nicci was, Lizzie thought, planning the garden like this so it was in bloom all year. How had she been so blind to it before? Always just taking the view from the window for granted as she chopped vegetables or uncorked another bottle. Now she knew the effort that had gone into it.

Three weeks, that was how long it had been since she was last here. It felt more like three months. Three weeks of driving to Croydon every evening to sit beside the bed of a woman who didn't know Lizzie was there.

Who didn't, Lizzie was increasingly sure, know anyone was there.

The first time, Gerry had gone with her; even offered to drive. His way of apologising, she supposed. It was only the once, though. So he obviously considered that apology enough. Not that Lizzie minded. To be honest, she preferred to be alone with her thoughts in the car, relying on the drive each way to clear her head.

The garden had changed in that time. Nicci always used

to say it had a life of its own and now Lizzie believed her. Such a short time and she'd become an outsider again.

In a handful of months the garden had started to feel, if not like hers, then like it knew her, was waiting for her. Almost as if it was looking forward to her visits. Of course, it was ridiculous to assume plants had . . . Oh, Lizzie didn't know what. If not feelings, then senses. Although when she'd first taken over the garden it was as if it knew she wasn't Nicci.

Don't be ridiculous, Lizzie told herself, pushing open the unlocked back door and unhooking the shed keys from where David had promised to leave them. From upstairs she could hear splashing, Charlie and Harrie shrieking, the low timbre of David's voice and then more shrieking. The sound of bathtime. The sound of family.

Quietly, Lizzie crept down the garden to the shed, unlocked it and dropped her coat on the old leather chair. Picking up her trowel and secateurs, she set to work. She loved it here. Engrossed in her plants, in the methodical movements of weeding and pruning, she could forget – for a moment – her mother kept alive by machines forty miles away; the brittle calls with her sister, inevitably followed by angry three-page emails; the long silent nights lying awake in the dark beside a sleeping Gerry.

Her sister had approved of Gerry. His suits, his smart car and his easy manners impressed her mother as well. The day Lizzie married, her mother had been so proud. It was only later Lizzie realised her mother's joy when she became engaged was because Gerry had proposed. She and Karen had worried he might not. That Lizzie would accept had never been in doubt.

And, thinking back, it wasn't.

Gerry said he loved her, her mother and sister liked him. It would have been enough for Lizzie. Even if she hadn't been swept away by his self-confidence and ambition. *God,* Lizzie thought, *what kind of person does that make you?*

'Coffee?' said a voice behind her. 'Or can I tempt you with something stronger?'

Spinning round, Lizzie blushed at being caught in her thoughts. She forced a smile. 'Sorry, David. I hope you didn't mind me sneaking in. I didn't want to interrupt bathtime.'

'You didn't sneak. I was expecting you. You called, remember? Wine? I've got a bottle of rosé open.'

Lizzie hesitated. 'I shouldn't. It's a school night. I can't stay long. I'm bunking off as it is.'

'I don't think it's bunking off, do you? You've been there every day for three weeks. One day off won't kill anyone.' David stopped. 'Sorry, that was clumsy.'

'Don't be daft. And you're right, it won't. And nor will one glass of rosé. Yes, please.'

'Great, I'll bring it down.'

He was off before Lizzie could tell him not to go to any trouble.

Five minutes later David reappeared with a cold bottle of something pink, two glasses and an empty flower pot. Lizzie eyed the full bottle. 'I thought you said you had some open.'

He grinned. 'I do now. I was just looking for an excuse. Thanks for providing it.'

Rolling her eyes, Lizzie smiled back. 'Consider yourself enabled,' she said, as he upended the pot, set the glasses on it and poured.

'Mind if I keep you company?'

'Not at all,' Lizzie shrugged. 'If you really have nothing better to do than watch me weed.'

Being here, in this garden, made her feel calm, as if other senses kicked in and gave her panicked thoughts a break. Here she could feel, hear, touch, smell, and not think too

321

much. And she liked that. Liked the breeze in the trees, the soft coo of pigeons settling to roost, the rustle of night creatures coming alive at the bottom of the garden as the light fell, the deep note of a plane overhead, a procession of bedtime choruses from the houses around her.

Did life sound like this in her own garden?

She knew the answer to that.

Darkness was easing in, but Lizzie was still warm in her T-shirt, the long sleeves pushed up to her elbows. The whole month had been warm; September had had the weather that rightfully belonged to August, and now October was mild. Not that she'd seen much of it, other than through her car window.

'How are you?' David asked, after he'd sat in silence for a few minutes, watching Lizzie weeding and trimming. He sipped his rosé in the fading light.

'Oh, I'm fine,' she said. 'I'm sorry I haven't been in touch.'

'Don't worry about it. You've had your mother on your mind.'

Every mention of her mother brought a rush of tears to her eyes, but they never broke through. She'd always been such a crybaby, she didn't know what was wrong with her.

'What are you going to do?' David asked.

'I don't know. Watch, wait, see.'

'I hardly dare ask, but what does Karen think?'

'How long have you got?' Lizzie dropped back on her haunches. 'Pass me that drink, would you?'

David laughed. 'That bad?'

'Worse.'

'When's she arriving?'

The cold pink liquid slid down Lizzie's throat and she closed her eyes gratefully. When she opened them again, David was looking right at her, his head on one side. 'Looks like you needed that.'

'You could say that.'

'Top up?' He waved the bottle at her.

'I shouldn't. Driving,' she said, but held out her glass anyway. She could always walk and pick up the car in the morning. 'Karen isn't arriving,' she said. 'Well, there's no sign of it so far. Do I realise how much it costs to fly four people three thousand miles? She and Pat only get two weeks' holiday a year and they've already used it. If Mum's in a coma she won't know Karen's there anyway . . . All inarguable, of course. Still, it doesn't stop her thinking that what she says should go.'

Lizzie stopped, caught herself. 'Sorry,' she said, embarrassed. 'That was bitchy. It's just getting me down a bit.'

'A bit? A lot, I should imagine. What *does* Karen think should go?'

Taking another sip, Lizzie said, 'She thinks we should stop treatment.'

'And you?' David's voice was gentle. 'What do *you* think?'

Lizzie let herself drop back onto the dewy grass, her jeans feeling instantly damp. 'I don't know,' she said, looking up at him. 'I really don't. I'm torn. Part of me agrees. Even if Mum does come round, which no one thinks she will, it can only get worse. I know that's what Dr Clifton thinks; he said as much. But part of me suspects her motives. It's a terrible thing to think, let alone say, but I don't know if she really does think that's best for Mum. If she gave a toss about Mum she'd have got on a plane again the moment I phoned her.'

David nodded.

'And part of me suspects my own motives, too. Do I want what's best for Mum or do I just want an easier life?'

'Is that wrong?' David asked gently.

'Yes,' Lizzie said forcefully. 'Yes. This is Mum's *life* we're talking about.'

'And Karen? What about her? Surely she doesn't want an easier life? She has a pretty easy one as it is, if you ask me.'

'Everyday Mum's being kept alive costs,' Lizzie whispered. 'Part of me thinks Karen only wants what's best for her inheritance.' Falling silent, she stared at the dew forming on the grass around her. 'I'm sorry,' she whispered, more to the night than David. 'I can't believe I just said that out loud. I can't believe I just said that.'

'It's OK,' David said, climbing to his feet and pulling her up. 'Everyone needs someone they can say the bad stuff to. And it's not that bad, if you ask me. I promise I've thought worse in the last year.

'I'm starving,' he added, suddenly side-swerving. 'Don't suppose you fancy keeping me company with some pasta? You can't have had time to eat and I've got to open a packet so I'll only end up chucking half of it away.'

Lizzie looked at him, suddenly aware that her hand was still in his. Self-consciously she extracted it. 'OK,' she said hesitantly. 'Yes, yes, please. If you'd really be cooking anyway.'

They ate outside at the metal table on the rough stone terrace, as they had eaten so many times before – fresh penne and spicy fresh tomato sauce with chillis added, after David checked Lizzie didn't object, a green salad bowl sat between them – by the glow of the patio heater and the light that leaked from kitchen windows left open so David could hear the no-longer-baby monitors.

'I know it's stupid,' he said. 'They're three now, it's more for my benefit than theirs.'

'That was delicious,' Lizzie said, as she scraped the last of the arrabiatta from her bowl. 'If I'd known you were such a good cook, I'd have hung around in your garden more often.'

324

'I'd like to take the credit,' David grinned, dropping his own fork onto his plate, but I had help from a Mr Oliver.'

'Well, thank you, Mr Oliver,' said Lizzie, raising her glass. 'You're good. You should think of going into business.'

Glancing at her watch, Lizzie wished she hadn't. Ten o'clock. It was like a spell was broken. 'God, is that the time?' she said. 'I had no idea. I'm sorry I stayed so long, I should go.'

'You don't have to,' David said. 'It's been nice.'

Lizzie smiled. For the first time in months she felt . . . not spirit soaringly happy, but content. 'It has, hasn't it? It's such a long time since I've been able to – I don't know – be off duty, I suppose. Thank you.' She got to her feet. 'I really appreciate it. Do you mind if I leave the car outside and pop back in the morning? You won't know it's there.'

'Of course not. You can stay if you want?'

'Thanks, but I don't want to put you to any more trouble. And there's school tomorrow, I need to get home, all the homework's there, my school clothes, you know . . .' Embarrassed suddenly, she started down his garden towards the shed, to collect her belongings. Solar lights hidden in flowerbeds faintly lit her path.

'I'd walk you home,' David said, falling into step beside her, 'but I can't leave the girls.'

'I'll be fine. It's not too far. I'll text you when I get home, if you want.'

'Do. I'd feel terrible if something happened to you on my watch.'

At the open shed door, Lizzie turned. 'You would? Really?'

David frowned. 'Of course I would. What's so strange about that?'

Standing on tiptoe, Lizzie touched her lips to his cheek. 'Thank you,' she said, falling back on her heels as she felt the errant tears prick the back of her eyes. She knew they'd come no further. 'That's the nicest thing anyone's said to me for . . .' she hesitated, '. . . years. Even if I don't deserve it.'

He took a step towards her. 'That,' he said, and he was so close Lizzie could feel his breath warm against her ear, 'is ridiculous. Worse than ridiculous, it's complete crap.' He kissed the top of her head. 'You do deserve it.'

Lizzie held her breath. Her heart was pounding and her stomach contracted in a way she couldn't remember. The feeling warmed her, but scared her too. Leave now, she told herself. Leave now while you can, but her feet weren't moving.

'Lizzie . . .' David started.

Slowly she raised her head to look at him. As she did, the little that came through the shed windows from the solar garden lights vanished. His stubble was rough against her forehead, then her cheek as his face dipped to meet hers. His fingers were gentle, stroking her cheek so she could feel rough skin at the tips.

Then all she could feel was him. His lips soft on hers, his arms tight around her, his fingers in her hair. Their bodies pressed hard together and Lizzie was falling.

She gasped.

'I'm sorry.' David pulled his face away. 'That was wrong.' He stopped, but his arms stayed tight around her, one hand still tangled in her curls. 'Wasn't it?'

'Yes,' she murmured.

Although the voice didn't sound like hers.

It was another woman, one Lizzie couldn't remember ever being. Folding her body against his, she reached up, gently pulling his head towards hers and kissed him again. Tentatively. As if expecting rejection.

His lips moved against hers. Once, twice, three times, at first speculative, as if each thought the other might pull away, then longer, their breath mingling.

'David, I . . .' Lizzie tried to gather her thoughts over the sound of her heart racing. *What are you doing?* screamed a voice in the back of her head. *I love him*, screamed a voice at the front.

And then he was kissing her, and there were no voices and no thoughts, but the taste of his mouth and the way his hands left a trail of heat across her body, making the unfamiliar churning in her gut creep lower.

In the end they chose together.

He dropped into the old leather chair, pulling Lizzie down on top of him. But she kicked the door shut with her heel as she let herself be pulled. He slid cool hands under her T-shirt and gently tugged aside her bra, letting his fingers cup her breast and caress her nipple, but she unbuttoned his shirt and wondered at the goosebumps beneath her hands.

Tugging off her top, she dropped it on the floor, wrapping her fingers into his hair as his mouth moved to kiss her breasts. And as he did she wanted nothing more than to be here. David's hands, his skin, his lips on her.

So this is what it was meant to feel like.

With his tongue burning a path on her skin, Lizzie did something she'd never done before. She slid onto the floor and pulled a man down on top of her.

FORTY-ONE

'You don't have to go.' His voice, soft, came out of near darkness as their breathing slowed. The churning inside had passed.

'I do, David,' she said, feeling his back tense under her hands and instantly regretting her words. 'You know I do.'

'You could stay.'

She looked at him, hovering above her. Just able to make out the lines of his face in the moonlight, Lizzie wondered if he could see the confusion in her eyes or whether she was, just for the moment, safe. 'I couldn't.'

'I didn't mean with me . . . The girls would—'

Her laugh was sad. 'I know that.'

'It's not that they'd mind – they love you – although they might be a bit confused. It's just they crawl all over me at six o'clock, earlier some days. I wouldn't wish it on you.' He kissed her face before easing himself off to lie by her side. Skin sparked where their bodies still touched.

Lizzie felt torn. She didn't want to leave. Ever.

'It's late,' David said. 'Let me make up a spare bed.'

Propping herself up on one elbow, she reached out her other hand to stroke his face. Eyelashes, cheekbones, stubble.

A small scar to the left of his chin from a childhood accident. As her finger crossed his lip, he put his hand up to catch it and kissed softly. The moment felt stolen. Touching him was like touching something precious that belonged to someone else. But then it did. It always had.

'I . . .' Lizzie said. *I what?* What was she going to say? *I love you? I'm married? I've never done anything like this before, even when I wasn't married? I'm not the kind of woman who has sex with other people's husbands? Not even when I've loved them since the moment I met them?*

'I have school tomorrow.' Forcing herself to release his hand she stumbled to her feet, groping in the near-darkness for her T-shirt and struggling into it. Glad of the darkness when she realised her bra was still caught in the sleeve. 'I really do have to go.'

Behind her, the sound of movement. David gathering his clothes, zipping his jeans, buttoning his shirt. 'It's too late to walk home alone and you shouldn't drive.' He sounded regretful.

Afraid he was, Lizzie panicked. What if, missing Nicci, he now thought he'd made a dreadful mistake?

'At least,' he said, 'let me call you a cab.'

The beeping pierced her head as well as her sleep. On the far side of a door, a loo flushed and there was the sound of water running, Lizzie opened one eye and sunlight razored through half-open curtains.

In a book she would have said she didn't know where she was, couldn't remember what had happened. But she did and she could.

'You were dead to the world when I got in,' Gerry said, coming out of the bathroom, a towel wrapped around him. 'Didn't want to wake you. Those hospital visits are doing you in. You're going to have to ease up, you know. I don't know why you bother going every night anyway. It's not as if she knows you're there. Ask the doctors. I bet they say a couple of times a week will do.'

'Hmm,' Lizzie groaned. Why did he have to pick now to be all concerned about her welfare? 'You're probably right.' Her head hurt. It wasn't just the alcohol.

Hangers rattled as Gerry riffled through his suits. 'Damn, is my Hugo Boss still at the dry cleaners?'

'What time was it?' Lizzie said, ignoring the question. 'When you got home, I mean?'

'Gone midnight,' he said dismissively. 'Entertaining the Japanese again. I told you yesterday morning.'

'Yes, I remember now. I just forgot for a moment. Still asleep.'

Gerry threw her a glance. 'Clearly. If you don't haul arse you'll be late for school. I'm done in there now, if you want it.'

'Thanks,' Lizzie slid from the duvet, tugging her nightie down over the tops of her thighs as she did so.

'Might be gone when you get out,' he said, pecking her cheek. 'Will you be home for supper or are you going to hospital again?'

'Hospital. Should be home by nine. Maybe earlier. You don't mind, do you?'

He shrugged. 'Not much choice, is there?' But there was no malice in his voice. 'I'll get a takeaway. Shall I get you some while I'm at it?'

Shit, shit, shit. Lizzie locked the bathroom door behind her and leant against it, trying to still her breathing. *Calm,* she urged herself. *Be calm.*

She'd driven home in the end.

David tried to stop her, but she insisted on leaving and took the car with her. She had to. There was no way she could face going back this morning to collect it. And how would she explain to Gerry where she'd left it?

What would have been the most natural thing in the world – a cab home from an old friend's house after too much to drink – had suddenly become evidence of a crime in the first degree. So she'd crawled along the side streets, at fifteen miles an hour, and felt like an even bigger hypocrite because of it. All those years of giving Gerry grief for drinking and driving, and she was doing it herself. As if he'd give a shit about that. That was the least of her sins last night.

Thank God for the Japanese.

She'd forgotten Gerry's dinner until she got home and found the house dark, the garage empty. There was still no sign of him when she'd showered and gone to bed. No sound of his key in the lock when she fell into a fretful sleep, her dreams a mixture of euphoric teenage fantasy and guilt-infused nightmare.

What have you done? she thought. *You've lost a friend and cheated on your husband in one evening.* Swiping away the condensation on the mirror, she forced herself to look herself hard in the face. Her confusion didn't show there. It was the same face she usually saw: pale, heart-shaped, with a smattering of freckles, purple shadows beneath eyes puffy from lack of sleep and too much junk food consumed on the way to or from her mother's bedside. All of it surrounded by a halo of frizzy auburn hair. But her eyes looked different. Their blue-grey flecks alive with fear and longing. Lizzie's memories drifted to the previous night and for a second she was lying on a shed floor with David inside her. Her groin clenched and she heard herself groan softly.

What now?

Keep away. It was her only option. This wasn't who she was.

You're married, she whispered, turning on the tap to ensure Gerry, if he was still on the other side, couldn't hear. *To Gerry. Till death us do part.*

She'd said it aloud. In front of everyone. Said it in front of David, in front of Nicci. Not to mention her mother, whose smile had told Lizzie that for once in her life she had done something to be proud of.

And she'd meant it. This was what her life was and she was lucky to have it.

As Lizzie washed and cleaned her teeth, she mentally ticked off all the things she had to be grateful for. The things her teenage self would think herself lucky to have.

A good job.

A lovely home.

A husband who provided for her. Who would like nothing more than for her to resign her job and start a family. Something she'd always wanted for herself, even back then, when it couldn't have been less cool.

How many women could say that?

And Lizzie had responsibilities. To that husband. To her mother, lying in a coma forty miles away. She had ties that didn't allow for . . . Well, didn't allow for what she'd done last night.

How could she – who'd only ever slept with two men; an ill-advised boyfriend in the second term at uni she'd only gone with because Nicci, Mona and Jo had *done it* and Lizzie worried she was a freak, and Gerry – suddenly become someone who'd cheat?

Lizzie ran her hands through her hair in anxiety. Three lovers, now. And the third . . . She closed her eyes, seeing David's face above her, imprinted for ever on the inside of her lids. The third was . . . wonderful, unexpected, special.

The third changed everything.

He'd touched her as if she was beautiful and he wanted

nothing more than to hold her in his arms. She had come last night, not for the first time, but for the first time like that. With her body and heart and mind in unison. For the first time, without making an effort, just because it would make Gerry happy.

Catching sight of herself as she massaged moisturiser into her wan face, Lizzie shook the memory from her head. She wasn't a cheat. She wasn't the kind of woman who had affairs. Not the kind who had sex with her best friend's husband, widower or not. Not the kind who wanted a man liked by another of her friends.

Nausea overwhelmed her.

Oh God, how on earth was she going to tell Mona?

By the time Lizzie was dressed and downstairs she knew the answer to that one. She wasn't. She wasn't going to tell anyone. Not Jo, not Mona. Nobody. She was sure David was feeling the same right now.

It would be as if it had never happened. She'd keep away from David's, for a bit, and it would all blow over. It wouldn't look strange to the others; not while she had to visit her mother every day. David would probably be relieved. And Gerry would never have to know.

When she hadn't answered his first text, David hadn't been surprised. OK, so she'd promised to text when she got home, but it was late and they were both tired. Probably, she'd got home and Gerry had been there and . . .

Ah shit, David thought, flicking off the bedside lamp and staring at the streetlight striping the ceiling. *What the fuck were you thinking, Morrison?*

What was it Nicci would have said? You weren't thinking, you were drinking? *Times about ten*, he thought. *Times about ten.*

All the same, he went to sleep thinking about Lizzie, and woke to the memory of the taste of her mouth under his, the feel of his fingers as they found unexpected tears and kissed them dry.

But when the second text, sent at six a.m. after the girls had jumped on his head, went unanswered, and a third, sent two hours later on his way to work, David started to worry. What if Lizzie hadn't got home? What if somewhere between here and there, that hunk of junk she called a car had wrapped itself around a lamppost? It was irrational, he knew, but he still had to stop himself retracing the route he thought she would have taken.

He timed his call for her morning coffee break, and dialled from his office reception so she wouldn't be able to screen his call. He didn't know why he thought she might, it was just . . .

'Hello?'

His spirits soared as he heard her voice. She was fine.

'Lizzie, it's me!' he said. 'Are you OK? When I didn't hear from you, I was worried.'

'Um, David, hi,' her voice was tentative. In all honesty he couldn't say she sounded as happy to hear from him. 'Um . . . sorry I didn't text you, it's been a bit chaotic this morning.'

'That's all right. I just wanted to make sure you got home safely.'

'I did. Thank you for checking, that's kind. I'm sorry, I've got to go. Year Four is calling.'

'OK.' David could feel his confidence ebbing away. It was a long time since he'd heard one, but unless he was mistaken, this was the sound of a brush-off. 'Um, Lizzie, can I just—'

But her mobile had gone dead.

David stared at the receiver.

He'd been afraid of this since he'd watched her stumble to

her feet, searching frantically for her clothes, but he'd hoped otherwise. Selfishly, naïvely, stupidly, he'd hoped . . .

It didn't matter what he'd hoped. Because Lizzie had confirmed it for him, unequivocally. Last night had been a mistake. A lovely mistake, as far as David was concerned. But a mistake all the same.

FORTY-TWO

The coven was in his kitchen again. Well, two-thirds of it. It was always in his kitchen. Mind you, it always had been. He just hadn't seemed to notice before Nicci died. Or if he did, he didn't mind.

'Shoo, David,' Jo said, lifting his jacket from the back of a kitchen chair and pushing it into his hand. 'Don't you have a pub to go to?'

'As it happens, I do,' he said. *But I'll go in my own time*, he thought. *When I'm ready, not when you tell me*. He glanced at the clock over Mona's head. She was taking two glasses from the dishwasher and putting them on a tray, digging around in his cupboard for a bowl to put wasabi peas in. Fewer calories than Bombay Mix, apparently. Beside her, Jo was opening a bottle of Rioja.

Red? David frowned. He thought Lizzie didn't like red.

'Lizzie's late,' he said casually. 'That's not like her, she's usually Little Miss Prompt.'

'Didn't I say?' Jo said. 'She's not coming.'

'The Cedars,' Mona added.

'Again?' David frowned. 'She still going every day?'

'Yep. I'm a bit worried about her, to be honest,' Mona said.

'We haven't seen her for a couple of weeks, not properly. And last time I talked to her she sounded like a woman on the verge.'

'Really?' David rummaged in the junk drawer, looking for nothing in particular. 'What's happened?'

'Row with her bloody sister, I imagine,' Jo said, sloshing ruby liquid into a glass. 'Useless cow . . . Look, David,' she added. 'Not to be rude, it being your house and all, but if you're staying, sit down and have a drink, will you? If not, please bugger off, you're making me twitchy.'

'David was weird,' said Mona, dumping the tray on a bedside table and closing the curtains against the squally October evening.

'Makes a change from you being weird around him.'

Mona swatted her. 'I think we're over that, don't you? I've been here a few times for coffee with Lynda—' She stopped abruptly, wondering if she should quickly jam the lid back on that particular can of worms.

But Jo just nodded thoughtfully.

'And it's been –' Mona continued, 'I don't know – almost comfortable. Dan likes seeing a bit more of David, too. He misses having a bloke to talk to.'

'I don't want to tempt fate.' Jo absent-mindedly touched the windowsill. 'But it seems like we're over the worst. He's even chilling out about Charlie and Harrie. They're coming to stay overnight in a couple of weeks and I didn't even have to twist his arm.'

Kicking off her boots, Mona flung herself into the velvet chair that sat in the bay window and began massaging her toes. 'Cramp,' she explained. 'How was Si with that?'

'Fine. It's our weekend for his two. He figured two more wouldn't make any difference.'

'Wow,' Mona said, moving on to the ball of her foot. 'Four

kids under one roof aged between three and ten? Rather you than me. Si really is one of the good guys, isn't he?'

Jo tipped her head on one side to examine her friend, but Mona didn't look up. 'He is. But what makes you say that?'

'Oh, I was just thinking about my friends' marriages. You and Si – you have your ups and downs but you're a team. Like Nicci and David were. One of those couples who are greater than the sum of their parts.'

Jo laughed. 'Brad and Angelina, Victoria and David Beckham, Samantha and David Cameron . . . Me and Si! Yep, I can see that.'

'You know what I mean.'

Jo stopped laughing, her gaze wistful. 'I do. Sorry if this sounds soppy, but I knew Si was a keeper from the first night we spent together.'

'Sex that good, huh?' Mona said.

Grabbing the nearest pillow, Jo threw it at Mona. 'Oops, sorry. No, it wasn't the sex. Although that was great. It was next morning.'

'Huh?' Mona dropped the pillow onto the floor beside her. 'Next morning?'

'You remember what Nicci always said? It's not Saturday night, it's Sunday morning that matters? Life's not about Saturday nights. It's about Sunday mornings. A guy who's great on Saturday night is all well and good, but does he know what to do on a Sunday? Si does. I realised that when we woke up together and he didn't bolt for the door. Well, he did, but only to buy bread, milk, bacon and the Sunday papers.' She blushed. 'That's probably where my passion for Sunday papers in bed comes from.'

Mona sipped her wine thoughtfully. Jo could almost see the thoughts moving behind her eyes. If only she could read them. 'Sounds good,' Mona said finally. 'Not that I've ever met anyone like that. But I can definitely see the attraction.'

'What on earth is this?' Mona held up a piece of white broderie anglaise dragged from Nicci's wardrobe. From the look on Mona's face, she found it almost as repellent as the rabbit-fur shrug they'd discovered on the first evening they'd gathered to sort their way through Nicci's collection of clothes.

'From where I'm sitting it looks like a pillow case,' Jo said. 'Where did you find it?'

'Halfway back, left-hand side. It can't be Nicci's, surely? She wouldn't be seen dead in something like this.' Mona stopped. 'Sorry, I've got to stop saying that.'

'Chuck it here.' Jo caught the soft white fabric and turned it over in her hand before looking inside the neck for the label. 'I knew it!' she said triumphantly. 'Chloé.'

'Chloé?' Mona looked blank. 'You mean *that* cost several hundred quid?'

Ignoring her, Jo said, 'Are there some flared jeans in there, next hanger along, maybe?'

'Flares? Nicci didn't wear . . . God, so there are. How did you know? And, let me guess, do these go with them?' Mona emerged from the wardrobe, a pair of cork platform sandals hooked over her thumbs.

'Yep, that's the entire outfit. You must remember it; you were here for the christening, weren't you?'

'Yes!' Mona said crossly. Just because she'd missed the wedding, didn't mean she'd missed everything. The truth was she remembered it vividly for all the wrong reasons. Neil had just dumped her.

'Then if you remember the christening, you remember this,' Jo was saying. 'The Chloé smock top. It was *the* piece of the season. The only time I remember Nicci buying – and

339

wearing – a whole look, head to toe, straight off the catwalk. She must have been suffering from preg-head. Made me laugh, because the only time Nicci looked remotely pregnant was three months later, at the christening, when she wore this thing.'

Seeing Mona's stare, Jo pasted on a smile. Thank God Mona was short-sighted and too vain to wear her glasses. Because Jo was pretty sure the smile didn't reach her eyes.

FORTY-THREE

The Chloé Smock
2006

'Jo, my love, please come out. We have to get moving or we're going to be late. And you can't be late. You're the godmother.' In typical fashion, Si corrected himself for accuracy. 'Well, one of them.'

His face was just inches from hers, separated by the wood of the bathroom door, just as it had been for most of the last hour. About half as long as Jo had been sitting on the cold ceramic tiles, her baggy old sleep T-shirt forming a tent over her knees. Every ten seconds or so she glanced at the white stick lying beside her and willed it to say something different.

For the first hour he'd left her, giving her the space to cry herself out – that was Si's style – but now time was running out. 'Joey . . .'

'I'm not going.'

'You have to.'

'Si, I can't . . . I can't face . . .'

'Jo darling,' his voice was patient, 'at least let me in.'

Reaching up, Jo slid the bolt back, then shunted away on her bottom, leaving just enough room for Si to push the door open and slide his hand through.

'Let me see it, sweetheart.'

'I know what it says. I know how to read it. I've read enough of them in the last year . . .' Her voice broke up.

'Shhh, shhh. Joey, it's OK. I know you do, I just want to see it for myself. Please.'

The white stick skidded across the tiles, stopping just short of his hand. Spiderlike, tan fingers scrambled to pick it up and his hand vanished behind the door again. All he'd wanted to do was get the damn pregnancy test away from her. She knew that.

'See?' she said. 'It didn't work. I'm not pregnant.'

Si was quiet for a moment, composing himself, trying to be sure his own voice would not choke up before he spoke. 'They told us,' he said gently. 'The doctor said this might happen. Probably would happen. Remember what she said? Only twenty per cent of couples conceive the first time they have IVF. That . . .' he paused, making himself add, 'many couples never conceive at all.'

Her wail cut him off and Si took advantage of the distraction to push the door open wide enough to slide through. 'We'll get there, my love, I promise.' He wrapped his arms tight around her.

'Will we?' she sobbed into the box-fresh shirt he'd put on an hour early to go with his new Autograph suit. 'How do you know?' she gasped. 'What if we don't?'

The truth was, Si didn't know.

Like her, he could only hope. And pray. And offer to sell his soul to the highest bidder. She knew that and he knew that. They'd been trying for a baby for a year before they dropped £3,800 they didn't have on their first round of IVF, the joy having ebbed out of sex with every monthly bleed.

Three shots at IVF they'd promised themselves. Three and no more. They wouldn't go on for ever, like some people. Seven, eight, nine tries with no success. Hearts broken, marriages crushed, lives destroyed. They wouldn't let that happen to them.

Three strikes and they were out. That was the deal.

And now they were one strike down. How easy would it be to

342

stick to the deal if Jo was sitting there, sobbing, on the floor, on the other side of the bathroom door, after three?

Si felt his stomach knot. Why did she have to do the test this morning? Stroking her hair, he felt her sobs shudder to stillness in his arms. Why hadn't she waited until tonight or tomorrow, when they'd have time to cope with the disappointment? But Si knew the answer, and he understood. Because if the result had been different Jo could have sailed through the christening with a smile in her heart as well as on her face, a secret growing in her belly, instead of feeling what she'd been feeling ever since Nicci had told Jo she was pregnant.

She'd come home and locked herself in the bathroom for several hours that day, too.

'I can't go, Si. I can't. You go without me.' Jo looked up at him, eyes red and pleading. 'Please . . .' She'd been crying so hard the blood vessels under her eyes had broken. It would take serious concealer to hide that.

'You have to, my love, 'Si said, easing her to her feet and propping her against the basin, as he put in the plug and flicked on the taps. 'You don't have a choice. You're a godmother.'

His heart sank as her face began to crumple. He wanted a baby as much as she did. Possibly more. Secretly he suspected she might have embarked on this whole thing for him. But he didn't want this. He'd rather have her, his Jo, his love, his second chance, than this.

'Nicci has two others,' she wept. 'She won't miss me.'

'You know that's not true, Joey. You're chief godmother.' He swept her hair back from her face. 'You're the important one. The show can't go on without you.'

Her crying stopped and he could feel her taking his words on board.

'Come on,' he coaxed, wetting her flannel, squeezing it out and pushing it into her hand. 'Wash your face and put on some makeup.' He kissed her forehead, then her nose, then her lips. 'And some concealer. Lots and lots of concealer.'

Was that a smile? Yes, he thought, maybe the slightest flicker of a smile.

They made it by the skin of their teeth. And then only because he texted Nicci to say they were stuck in traffic (he didn't say it was an emotional blockade) and she insisted on delaying the ceremony for them.

Lizzie was pacing the church porch, waiting. 'Oh my God, where have you been?' She ran towards them when she spotted them coming from the car park at a trot.

'Sorry, something come up,' Si said, staring meaningfully at Lizzie. She raised her eyebrows questioningly. Had it . . . ? Were they . . . ? Was it good news? Si shook his head, making a cutting motion at his neck as Jo entered the church in front of him.

Lizzie's face drooped. 'I'm so sorry,' she mouthed, and followed them inside.

Only Lizzie looked even remotely happy, Si thought, sitting in the second pew between Dan on a PSP and Gerry on a BlackBerry, watching the godmothers gather around the font. And even Lizzie . . . well, she wasn't one for emotional extremes, so far as he could tell, but she didn't look unhappy. Not by the others' standards, at least.

Mona was wearing dark glasses. In church, for crying out loud. If it had been down to him he'd have taken them from her as she passed. He didn't say anything; it wasn't his place. Anyway, they all knew why. It was one of those open secrets the women's friendship seemed to thrive on.

He kept out of all that stuff as far as possible, but hadn't she broken up with a married guy she'd been seeing? It was her call, Jo had said (not that Si really listened, just nodded in the places he thought apt). To judge by her face, whether or not it was her call, she wasn't exactly thrilled about it.

Standing by the altar, Jo was holding it together pretty well, Si thought, in the circumstances. The Touche Éclat had worked its magic, and the black Armani suit he'd shoved her into looked a bit business-meetingy but it did the job. She'd stumbled over the oaths, studiously avoiding his gaze. Somehow, though, through sheer force of will she'd got through. He was proud of her standing up there, vowing to care for the spiritual and emotional welfare of someone else's babies without her voice breaking, even though, inside, he knew her heart was shattered.

And Nicci . . . well . . .

Si was the first to admit she was the authority on fashion around here, but . . . He looked again. Maybe he was missing something, but really, what did she look like?

Nicci was small, birdlike. Not his type — way too bony — but she usually looked stylish. In that way women liked other women to look and men didn't get. According to David, who got that from Nicci, he assumed. But what Nicci was wearing today swamped her. A smocky thing that looked like she'd made it from a sheet.

The smock was part of a flares-and-cork-wedges combo. He'd seen his six-year-old niece raid a dressing-up box and look less ridiculous. If Nicci had been going for a part in a Flake ad, he might have understood. Although she didn't have the hair for it; that was Lizzie's domain. But Nicci looked awful. And knackered.

Mind you, that was what having kids did to you. They turned your life upside down, emptied your bank account and raided your sleep. And that was just for starters.

Si already knew that. It lay at the heart of Si and Jo's problem: that Si did have kids — with someone else — he just couldn't have them with Jo.

Nicci felt wrecked. She looked wrecked too. She must do, or people wouldn't be staring at her the way they were. And not in a good way. Si particularly; his gaze kept flicking from her to Jo and back again.

Swallowing, Nicci closed her eyes and felt herself sway, so she opened them again but the church didn't come into focus. She had a feeling she knew why Si was staring, just as she knew why Si and Jo had been really late. Poor, poor Jo. And poor Si, for that matter. OK, so he already had two gorgeous boys of his own, but that didn't make it any easier.

Beside her, Harrie slept in David's arms; against her own breast Charlie snuffled and Nicci felt her heart swell. So this was how it felt being a mother: exhausting, exhilarating, earth-shattering . . .

Nicci tried to stop the thoughts from going where she knew they wanted to take her, but they had ideas of their own.

She would do anything for Charlie and Harrie. Anything. Killing for them didn't seem too extreme. From the moment they'd been handed to her after the C-section, two tiny red bundles, their features subsumed by wrinkles, she'd known that without question. Nothing, no one, would be allowed to come between her and her girls. Not even David, and until she gave birth she had thought nothing could surpass her love for him.

Then why?

Stop it, Nicci, she thought, hearing the vicar's voice in the distance, aware of Jo, Lizzie and Mona, each swearing to protect her babies in their turn.

Then how?

How could her mother have done it? Left her, for him.

It wasn't the first time her thoughts had taken this turn in the past nine months. When Nicci found out she was pregnant. When they were told it was twins. Every time she bought a Babygro. Whenever she changed a nappy. Each time she sat up in the dark, feeding and rocking her daughters to sleep. Whenever she had a question she couldn't answer, or the terror that she wasn't going to be able to cope became overwhelming. All those times and more, Nicci had longed for her own mother.

Someone to stroke her hair, to tell her everyone struggled with breast-feeding, to reassure her all women shared these fears.

To tell her that everything would be OK: that being a bad mother didn't run in the Webster genes.

346

David's mother had been amazing; would do more if Nicci let her, but it wasn't the same.

'Nic.' David's voice was soft in her ear. 'Nic? Are you in there, my love?'

Nicci snapped to, and Jo and Lizzie's concerned faces came into focus. Mona's mouth was set in a firm line below her dark glasses.

'Is there a problem, Mrs Morrison?' the vicar asked, his hand poised over the font. 'Is something wrong?'

Pasting on a smile, Nicci shook her head and bent to touch her lips first to the baby in her arms, and then to the sleeping daughter David held out to her.

Her babies would never have to feel the way Nicci had. Nicci would see to that. If it was the last thing she ever did, Nicci would make sure there was never any shortage of people to love them.

FORTY-FOUR

'You sure you're OK?' Jo watched David prowl the kitchen, stopping every so often to peer down his garden. What on earth was he looking for? Could he see something down there that she couldn't? Jo stood beside him and looked out, but she was damned if she could see what he was staring at.

This was the second time she'd seen David in the last ten days, and both times he'd been a bit out of sorts. He hadn't been this distracted since the weeks before Nicci's death. In those painful months he'd had to sit in silence and watch his wife insist on undergoing treatment they all knew in their hearts wasn't going to work.

Maybe she'd overstepped the mark, Jo thought anxiously, asking him to let the girls stay over. Maybe this was too much too soon.

'I don't have to take the girls,' she said tentatively. 'Not if you've got cold feet.'

'For the last time,' David said. 'I haven't—'

Instinctively, Jo took a step back.

'Sorry, sorry, sorry,' he said, holding up his hands. 'It's nothing to do with that, honestly. Bad week, that's all. I shouldn't take

348

it out on you. Look, I said Charlie and Harrie could have a sleepover and I meant it. Apart from anything else they've been looking forward to this for weeks. There'd be a knee-high riot if I changed my mind. Their Peppa Pig cases have been packed since yesterday morning.'

Jo smiled. She guessed as much. She'd seen them lined up at the bottom of the stairs. Two little pink cases, two matching pink rucksacks. And a navy holdall, presumably packed by David, containing the genuinely useful stuff, like toothbrushes and pyjamas. So like their mother. They were going away overnight, wouldn't even be out of the house twenty-four hours, and between them Charlie and Harrie had enough luggage to open a toyshop.

'Don't worry about me, if that's what this is about,' David said, touching her arm as he passed. 'I have loads of work to do. A new bank complex. I could work solidly for the next seventy-two hours and it wouldn't even scratch the surface.'

Somehow Jo didn't believe him.

'How's Lizzie?' David asked, as they were buckling Charlie and Harrie into the booster seats he'd just removed from the back of his people carrier and installed in Jo's red Golf for the journey.

Jo shrugged. 'Not great, so far as I know. Haven't seen much of her lately. She popped by for a coffee last weekend on the way back from seeing her mum. She wasn't herself, but then who would be with their mother on her deathbed? Why?'

'No reason,' David said. 'She just hasn't been round much lately. Wondered if she was all right.'

'She hasn't been round to tidy the garden?' Jo sounded surprised. 'That's odd. I just assumed if anyone had seen her it would be you.'

David shook his head. 'Too busy, I expect. If she's driving to Croydon every night and twice at weekends.'

'She loves that garden, though, I'd have thought she'd make time to do that, if nothing else.' Jo laughed. 'Never thought I'd see the day I said that.'

Mind you, she thought, looking at Charlie and Harrie sitting in the back of her Golf, kicking their little Converse in enthusiasm to get going, never thought I'd see the day of most things that have happened this last year.

'It's autumn now,' David said. 'It's not like much needs doing.'

David kissed Charlie and Harrie on the head. 'Love you, monsters. Be good for Auntie Jo.' Turning to Jo, he pecked her cheek. 'Guess Lizzie's got more on her mind than a few dead runner beans.'

Si, Sam and Tom were in the kitchen when Jo unlocked the front door and herded the girls inside. The unmistakable smell of pizza wafted along the hall. *Toy Story 2* was playing in the living room.

'Hello my lovelies!' Si cried, scooping them up, one under each arm, and spinning them round until they shrieked.

'Watch it, Si,' Jo said. 'You'll make them puke.'

'Puke!' yelled Charlie.

'Jo-o.' Tom rolled his eyes, as he'd seen Si do many times when Jo had opened her mouth and put her foot in it, unintentionally teaching his children words he'd rather they didn't know. 'Watch what you say.'

'Yes, boss.' Jo swatted her elder stepson's head fondly. He was ten going on forty, some days.

'What are you up to?' she asked, seeing empty supermarket pizza boxes on the side, scrunched-up blue and white carrier bags on the floor, a sure sign Si was 'cooking'.

'Making lunch,' Si said. 'What else? We did a hit and run

on Tesco while you were out, didn't we, boys? And Sam's on pizza face duty, aren't you, mate?'

'Yes,' Sam said proudly. 'Cucumber eyes, tomato mouths and red pepper for noses. We got a great big tomato specially so I can do teeth.'

'Excellent,' Jo said. 'That's perfect. Charlie and Harrie will love them.'

Pizza faces were a Si thing, one of a dozen ruses he'd invented for making vegetables fun or, if not fun, almost invisible. He'd been making them for the boys since Jo first met him. It touched her that he'd think to make them for Charlie and Harrie, without her asking. Just as well: she'd been so preoccupied with not upsetting David she hadn't got as far as thinking about food, let alone buying any.

Coiling her arms around Si from behind, she reached up to kiss the back of his neck in the gap where his hair met his collar. 'Thank you,' she whispered.

The pizza faces went down a storm, but pizza paled into insignificance beside the pink ice cream Si, Sam and Tom put in individual bowls cut into the shape of a pig's face – sort of – using an ice-cream scoop.

'It's Peppa!' the girls squealed, eating their cartoon friend without a second thought.

'I didn't know we even owned an ice-cream scoop,' Jo muttered as she tidied the chaos that littered the worktops. Si stacked the dishwasher, while Tom and Sam, rather than get roped into washing up, took Charlie and Harrie outside to play in the garden.

'We didn't,' Si said. 'Just like we didn't have pink ice cream.'

Jo grinned. Typical of him to pick up the ball and run with it before she even knew she'd dropped it. Mona was right. They were a team. 'Any more surprises up your sleeve?'

'As it happens . . .' Si spun round. In his hand was a sparkly DVD.

'*Beverly Hills Chihuahua*?' Jo said. 'You're kidding me. How did you swing *that* past Sam and Tom?'

'Like this.' Si whipped out his other hand from behind his back. In it was a Harry Potter.

'It's a skill,' he said. 'It's called common or garden bribery. Great place, Tesco Metro. Sells everything.'

'And where did you learn that skill?' Jo asked. 'At parent school?'

Si stopped and looked at her. Putting the DVDs on the worktop, he stepped towards her. 'I'm sorry,' he said. 'I didn't mean—'

'Hey,' Jo stepped into his arms, 'I didn't either. It's fine, I promise. And look.' They both turned to the kitchen window.

Sam and Tom were teaching the two small girls, who didn't come up to their waists, to play football. Or trying. Even Tom laughed as Charlie bent down to pick up the ball and started to run away, her little legs motoring up the garden like pistons. 'It's *FOOT. BALL*,' Sam yelled. 'You use your feet.'

'Kick it,' shouted Tom, running his hands through his hair in frustration and looking more like Si than ever. '*KICK. IT.*'

'Wow, she's fast for a tiddler,' Si said. 'No catching her.'

'They're good boys,' Jo said.

'They're trying.'

'I know. They're doing brilliantly. I'll buy them something, a present, to say thank you. Something for the DS, maybe?'

'No need,' Si said, turning serious. 'They're doing it for you. You love Charlie and Harrie, they're part of your life, therefore they're part of our family.'

Jo looked at him questioningly.

Where had this come from? They hadn't even discussed her responsibilities to Charlie and Harrie in any depth since she finally told him – way later than she should have done – about Nicci's letter.

'They love you, Joey. Like I do. You've been great for them, and they know it. They love being here and that's down to you—'

'But it's their home.' Jo interrupted.

Si held up his hand. 'Let me finish,' he said. 'I've wanted to say this for ages. But with everything being the way it's been, well, there's never a right time.'

She held her breath.

'You've worked hard with them. Played with them, done homework with them, fed them junk food and snuck in vegetables. You've put up with them treating you like chief cook and bed maker. And you've let them beat you at football.'

'Er, Si, I didn't *let* them. They beat me fair and square. I'm crap at football.'

'You played it, that's the point. You also taught them the word "crap". And many other excellent forbidden words besides.'

'Oops.' Smiling, Jo put her fingers on her lips.

'They love you. I can't tell you how grateful I am for that.'

'To me? But I—' Jo started.

Sam's face suddenly appeared on the far side of the kitchen window. 'Get a room!' he yelled, and stuck out his tongue.

Si and Jo leapt apart. 'He didn't get *that* from me,' Jo said.

'Again!' Harrie cried, the second the credits began to roll on *Beverly Hills Chihuahua*.

'Again!' Charlie agreed.

'No, Dad!' Sam yelled. 'Please!'

'No way,' Tom grumbled. 'Talking dogs. It was crap the first time.'

'Tom . . .' Si said warningly.

'Bathtime!' Jo said brightly. 'Not for you,' she added, heading off Sam's protests before he had time to open his mouth. 'You, Dad and Tom watch *Harry Potter*, or find some other crap . . . I mean, find something educational, while I scrub mud off these two.'

'Can I at least have a drink now?' Si said, as she passed, ushering two small girls singing the *Beverly Hills Chihuahua* theme tune in front of her. The tune would be rattling around in her head for weeks to come.

'If you want. And pour me one while you're at it. Who was it said two more wouldn't make any difference?'

'Not me,' said Si. 'Must have been some bloke who didn't have the faintest idea what he was on about.'

It took two hours to get Charlie and Harrie bathed and into bed, then Jo had read *Peppa Goes Swimming* twice before they crashed out. In revenge, Tom and Sam refused to go to bed until ten. Tom even tried to stay up for *Match of the Day*, but to Jo's huge relief, Si vetoed that.

'Bed?' Jo said, downing the last of her wine and easing herself off the sofa. It wasn't yet eleven, but she could barely keep her eyes open. Too tired even to consider a second glass. Unknown Facts About Kids No. 96: they were great for keeping your alcohol consumption in check. Who knew?

'Is that bed? Or *bed*?' Si asked. 'Because frankly if it's *bed*, I'm not sure I'm up to much this evening.'

'You should be so lucky,' Jo laughed. Sex had been the last thing on her mind, so she was surprised to feel a ground-swell of disappointment in her belly. Sex had been good from the start with her and Si. OK, they had their off times, like all couples, when one or the other was too stressed or tired. Or, the unsayable, simply didn't fancy it. Then, for a while, it became compulsory. Just another thing to tick off her internal to-do list. The last couple of months it was back to being something she looked forward to.

Double-locking the back door, Jo checked the windows were shut and stubbed her toe on something, small, sharp and plastic. A toy gun or Dinky car probably.

Jo could hardly remember how the baby thing started now. How having one of their own became so important it was worth risking everything for. It wasn't to do with Nicci having Charlie and Harrie. That came later. Jo and Si had been trying for a year when Nicci announced she was pregnant, with twins. Just like that. Or so it seemed to Jo at the time.

To begin with, trying had been fun. 'Oh dear, we'd better go home and have sex,' they used to say whenever they got bored at a work do, or one of their families' houses. Sometimes they hadn't bothered to go home. Just snuck off to the bathroom or drove to a secluded spot. But her periods kept coming and suddenly it wasn't fun any more. It became compulsory. No longer making love, but making babies. Or not.

They found out their third attempt at IVF had failed the week Nicci told them she had cancer. It had started in her right breast, but the doctors said it had spread. Suddenly, whether or not Jo got pregnant seemed less significant. Her friend was dying, that was all that mattered. Then Nicci died and Jo had been so caught up in saving Capsule Wardrobe that she and Si stopped talking, stopped making love, stopped doing anything that was about them. So they had never had the conversation . . . the one about whether to stick to their deal, that three strikes meant they were out. Because if they did, they were out already.

Too much had been about Nicci, for too long. Jo could see that now: Nicci's side of the business, Nicci's style, Nicci's husband, Nicci's babies, how Jo was going to manage without Nicci. When all along she'd had Si. Sitting there, waiting for her to come back to him. What if he hadn't waited? What if she'd pushed him beyond his patience? Jo couldn't bear to think how close she might have come to that.

'Si . . .' Padding into the bedroom as he was closing the shutters, she watched him stretch up to reveal the tan flesh around his still firm middle. She shut the bedroom door, then remembered Charlie and Harrie, and opened it again slightly, just enough to hear the girls if they woke, but not be heard by Sam and Tom at the other end of the corridor. If there was anything for them to hear.

'Uh-huh?' He turned towards her as she flicked off the bedroom light and reached around him to open one side of the shutters. 'That thing you said about not being up to much . . .' Her fingers slid under his shirt, followed the trail of hair that led down his stomach, and found their way into his jeans. A moan escaped him as her hand worked its way down and she felt him grow hard. 'You didn't mean that, did you?'

'Who, me?' he gasped as her fingers curled around him. 'Didn't say a word. Must be that other bloke.' Turning, his hands slipped inside her sweatshirt. Finding her bra-less, he grinned and pulled her sweatshirt over her head, burying his face between her breasts. Only removing it long enough to say, 'The same idiot who thought four kids were no more exhausting than two.'

'I've been thinking,' Jo said, curling her naked body around his.

'Don't think, Joey,' Si said sleepily, stroking her arm with his hand. 'Just sleep.'

356

Smiling, she kissed his chest, and lazily flicked her tongue over his nipple. 'Uunngh,' he groaned, and tangled his fingers in her hair. 'What have I done to deserve this?'

'Everything,' she said. 'Everything. I just sometimes – often – forget to say.'

'I'm here, Jo,' he said. Jo could tell he was suddenly wide awake in the dark. 'I've always been here. Always will be.'

She crept up to kiss him. 'I know,' she said softly. 'At least, I do now. And I'm sorry.' She took a deep breath, resting her hand on his chest. 'I love you, Si. I love the boys. I . . . I know they're not mine, but I love them anyway.'

'And they love you.'

Jo smiled. 'Thank you. I can't tell you how much that means to me. They don't have to; I know that. They choose to. I'm not their mum, after all.'

'Joey . . .' Si started.

She put her fingers on his lips to hush him. 'Not their real mum, I mean. They have one of those, and it's not me. I'm Jo. Just Jo. But they're still my family. You're my family. And I wanted . . . I wanted to say . . .' Taking a deep breath, she ploughed on. 'I don't *need* to be a mum, Si. I don't *need* us to have children of our own. It would have been nice. But it wouldn't make us any better than we are.'

'You mean that?' Si's voice was serious.

'I do. I really do.' Jo sat up, trying to see his face in the light through the open shutters. 'Let's stop trying,' she said, her voice earnest. 'Three strikes, that was the deal. We've had three tries and it hasn't worked. We mustn't let it destroy us. What if it doesn't work a fourth time? What if it doesn't work a fifth?'

Fingers tracing his cheeks, she realised they'd grown damp since she started speaking. Guilt twisted inside her.

She hadn't once thought, what about Si? What was this doing to him?

'I don't need a baby with you to know I love you. You, the boys, my goddaughters. That's my family.'

She couldn't see Si's face, but in the darkness, Jo felt him smile.

FORTY-FIVE

'Mrs O'Hara? Mrs O'Hara?'

For a second Lizzie didn't know who the voice was talking to, she just wished whoever Mrs O'Hara was she'd answer them so they'd stop disturbing Lizzie.

'Mrs O'Hara?' There was a hand on her shoulder. 'You need to come now. We think it's going to be soon.'

Opening her eyes, Lizzie saw the visitors room come into focus. Magnolia walls, three-for-two framed prints of water-colour flowers, a pine-effect coffee table with its piles of years-old magazines, matching brown two-seater sofas. One of which she was lying on.

'What time is it?' she murmured, rubbing her eyes to see what was left of her mascara come away on her knuckles.

'Five a.m.,' the nurse said. 'Nearly dawn. We were going to let you sleep, but . . .' she paused.

'It's OK,' Lizzie nodded. 'I understand.' They weren't sure her mother would make it to dawn, she wasn't stupid.

Glancing at her mobile, she debated calling Gerry or texting her sister. But what would she say? It's nearly time? What was the point of that? It had been nearly time since they stopped the drip feed five days earlier. If Karen had chosen not to get on a plane then, she was hardly going to do so now. At the time Lizzie had been angry, but now she felt strangely sorry for her sister. If she really couldn't take a week off to be with her mother when she died because she wouldn't have any compassionate leave left for the funeral, then what sort of life was it anyway?

In a drab little visitors' toilet – more magnolia, no framed prints – Lizzie splashed her face with cold water and dried it on a coarse paper towel from the dispenser. She tried not to look at herself in the mirror. One way and another, she had long since ceased to like what she saw.

'Morning, Mum,' she whispered, slipping into a room that was empty but for what was left of her mother, lying in a bed next to a heart monitor that beeped softly.

'Well, it's not really morning,' Lizzie said in the conversational tone she'd adopted in the two months since her mother lost consciousness. Lizzie had never been good at small talk. That, at least, she'd got from her mother. Lately, however, she'd become an expert at talking endlessly and saying nothing. She hoped she hadn't been driving her mother to distraction with her inane chitchat about work, the weather and whichever celebrity was in the news. How typical would it be if, even on her deathbed, Lizzie had been a disappointment to her mother?

'Let's open the curtains, shall we?' Lizzie said. 'We'll be able to see the sunrise, assuming there is one.'

There wasn't. It was too early. And even if it wasn't, the sun would have been hidden by the thick autumn mist that shrouded The Cedars and the trees that surrounded it. So Lizzie sat in the armchair beside her mother's bed, held her frail hand and talked about mist and trees and how chilly it was even for November, instead.

She'd thought something would change when it happened. A presence, or absence, in the room. Maybe the atmosphere would shift or the air still. At the very least, the machines would go nuts and previously unseen scores of medical staff come running. But there was none of that. Not even a tiny exhalation of breath. Just a drop in the tone of the machine as the green line flattened and Lizzie looked at her mother's face and knew – or thought she knew – she was now an orphan.

Reaching out to push the button that would summon the staff, she hesitated.

Through the mist beyond the window a faint yellow glow told her dawn had come, and the distant buzz of engines on the M23 said another rush hour had begun. *What now?* Lizzie thought, gazing at nothing much. What now that she couldn't hide behind her sick mother any more?

'So, how long's Karen staying then?' Gerry asked without looking up from his paper.

'As little as possible, I expect,' Lizzie shrugged, pushing soggy Special K around her bowl. 'She's arriving the day after tomorrow and I imagine she'll leave after the funeral.'

'That's barely forty-eight hours.' Gerry rattled his paper irritably. 'What about all the stuff that needs doing?'

'What stuff?' Lizzie shrugged. 'The funeral's organised. We agreed all that on the phone. I've called everyone I can think of. The solicitor who handled Mum's house sale is doing the probate. And it's not as if there's a house that needs clearing. I did that three years ago.'

There it was. Sixty-eight years of her mother's life dismissed in a few phone calls, some paperwork and four platters of M&S sandwiches.

'. . . About that,' Gerry said.

Lizzie jumped. She'd been drifting. She did that a lot lately. 'About what?'

'The will. I've been thinking.'

'Gerry!'

'Ah, come on, Liz. The funeral, the will, and then we're done. Don't pretend it's not a relief that all this is nearly over.'

Lizzie stared at her cereal. It had disintegrated, leaving the milk a grubby beige. Gerry was right, it *was* a relief. She just didn't like the way he kept saying it. The first time was when she called him from The Cedars to say it was over. 'Thank God for that.' He'd actually said that, after he'd made the appropriate noises, of course. Not the first thing he'd said, but he was clearly thinking it: *Thank God for that.*

All right, so he hadn't seen that much of Lizzie for a few months. But it wasn't as if all the toing and froing had been a hardship for him. He'd only set foot in The Cedars twice, and the second time was because he was atoning for hanging up on her.

In one way he was right. What Lizzie was feeling wasn't sorrow or grief, it was relief. Ninety per cent relief with ten per cent guilt. But she really, really didn't need her husband pointing that out. Not yet.

'More coffee?' Lizzie asked, getting up. Normally, at this point in a conversation, on the cusp of a row, Lizzie would have left. Not stormed out, just wandered off. It was the way it had always been. Not in the very beginning – they didn't row in the beginning – but certainly since they'd moved in here. It was almost a routine. He'd hold forth and she'd say, 'I'm off to Nicci's. See you there after golf?' And that would be that. Even after Nicci died Lizzie would have done that. But now, she didn't have that option. She hadn't been round to Nicci's house since that night. Hadn't seen David once, despite his many texts. She had to keep away.

'Nah, I'm good thanks. Actually, Liz, can we talk?' Gerry's face was serious. He folded the paper and pushed it away from him.

Thwarted, Lizzie sat back down.

'We do need to talk about the will, what happens now.'

'No, Gerry!' Lizzie leapt up. 'I will not talk about my mother's estate, such as it is, less than a week after she died.'

'It's not the estate,' Gerry said, leaning back in his chair. 'It's us.'

'Us?'

'Yes, I've been thinking. We've discussed starting a family. And I was talking to Michael and Lianne . . .'

At the mention of Gerry's boss and his wife, Lizzie's heart sank. 'About families?'

Gerry nodded. 'Having a family grounds you. Gives you stability. Now you've inherited we can make it happen.' His face was alight with an enthusiasm Lizzie usually associated with his work.

'Go on,' she said cautiously.

'We'll move,' Gerry said. 'Face it, Liz, I'm not being mean when I say you're knocking on a bit on the baby front. And we haven't needed your salary for a few years now. We can easily manage a bigger mortgage without.'

Leaning across the table, he clasped her hands and pulled them to his lips.

'Let's find a bigger house, Liz. A *family* house. It's what you've always wanted. You put in your mum's money and I'll do the rest. Then you can give up your job and have babies.'

Sharp wind whipped Lizzie's damp hair into her face. It was only drizzle, but the squall felt like a thousand little needles. And the weather was fierce enough to see off the cluster of small children and their takeaway-coffee-hugging parents, who had filled the playground when Lizzie first arrived. They were gone now. Back home, to friends' houses, to piles of newspapers and kitchens full of friends and family, already warm with the sound of chatter and the scent of Sunday roast. The way Sundays used to be at Nicci's.

Soggy leaves squelched underfoot, and the disintegrating corpse of a dead firework rolled away as she walked to the now empty swings. Sweeping rainwater from a red plastic seat, she dried her hand on her coat and sat down.

With rain dimpling the puddle in front of her feet, Lizzie began to sway, Gerry's words echoing in her head. *Give up your job . . . have babies . . . it's what you've always wanted.*

I don't want to give up my job, she'd wanted to yell. I don't want your babies.

But instead she'd said, 'I'll think about it, Gerry. Give me some time.' Thinking that would be enough. It would buy her a few days. At least until after the funeral.

But he'd looked at her like she imagined he looked at his underlings at work, impatience mingled with irritation, and issued what sounded a lot like her first verbal warning.

'Don't think too long,' he'd said. He'd looked pointedly at her belly. If he'd made ticking noises with his tongue it wouldn't have surprised her. 'Don't think too long.'

Pushing back her chair, Lizzie had heard it scrape on the cream tiles, before taking her coffee cup to the sink and rinsing it, putting the dessicated remains of her Special K down the waste-disposal unit and headed for the door.

'Where are you going?' Gerry had asked.

She'd turned. Smiled. 'To think.'

She'd debated going to Jo's. Even Mona's. Although that was a trek, and Mona wouldn't be there anyway. She'd be at work, and if she wasn't, she'd be at David's house, putting the world to rights with Lynda. It was uncanny the way she'd hit it off with Lynda.

And if she went to see Jo . . . ? Then Jo would ask too many questions. No, Lizzie had to get her ducks in a row, as

Gerry would say. Not that she even knew where her bloody ducks were right now. Or even how many she had.

I don't want babies, she thought, swinging a little higher. Hearing the chains groan under her weight as she gained speed and height. *I don't want babies, I don't want babies.* The wind picked up the rhythm and it became a vicious chant in time to the creaking of the chains. *I don't want babies, I don't want his babies.*

She stopped abruptly.

But we've always wanted babies, said a small voice in the back of her head. Lizzie aged eleven, Lizzie aged fifteen, Lizzie aged nineteen, biting her tongue when Jo and Mona ranted about motherhood being tantamount to slavery. Lizzie, aged twenty-five, in bed with Gerry. The Lizzie she remembered being. *We always pictured us, roses round the door, two kids, maybe three. Didn't we? You're thirty-six Lizzie; time's running out. That's the only thing he said that's true. What if it's too late? What if you can't? What if you're like Jo?*

It was true. Lizzie let the swing slow as the truth sank in. She did want children. She'd always wanted to be a mother. She just didn't want to have them with Gerry.

When she got back Gerry was in the living room, a glass of viscous red by his right hand, television tuned to Sky Sports. It felt like only minutes, but there were already Sunday afternoon football results running along the bottom of the screen like ticker tape. She must have been gone hours.

'Thought?' he said, without looking up.

'Yes,' she said, surprised at the certainty in her own voice. 'I have.'

'And . . . ?' Fingers working the remote, he lowered the sound, but didn't turn his head to face her.

Afterwards, Lizzie supposed that made it easier; that Gerry couldn't even be bothered to look at her. She liked to think she could have looked him in the eye and said it. But this way she never had to find out if she'd have had the courage.

Steeling herself, Lizzie balled her hands into fists in her pockets and felt her chewed nails cut ragged half-moons in the flesh of her palms. 'I'm leaving you.'

Just like that. *I'm leaving you.*

'You're what?' He did turn then. Surprise and fury mingled on his face. '*You're* leaving *me*?'

Lizzie nodded. She'd hardly believed it herself until she said it. *She* was leaving *him*.

She expected to feel panic, to hyperventilate; to have all those little critics in her head – her mother, her sister, her teachers – shrieking warnings, telling her not to be an idiot. Not to trash the one thing in life she'd achieved that made everyone happy.

Just not her. Not any more.

But the voices were quiet. As if her mother's death had silenced them.

'You're just upset about your mum, Liz,' Gerry said. 'You'll get over it in a few weeks, you'll see.'

'It's not that,' Lizzie said calmly. 'I'm leaving.' And she knew with absolute clarity it was true.

Gerry stared at her in disbelief, as if seeing her for the first time. 'Oh, I see,' he spat. Suddenly, his eyes were blazing, his lips pulled back. 'You come into some money and now I'm disposable, am I? You have your mother's money now so you don't need me bankrolling you any more?'

Bankrolling? Don't rise to it, Lizzie told herself. He's in shock. Let him say what he wants to say. Just get this over with.

'It's not like that,' she said. Lizzie was still standing at the living-room door, ready to back away if he tried to stop her. Not that she thought he would. He wasn't a bad man, she just didn't love him any more. If she ever had.

366

The thought rolled in like a wave, swallowing her thoughts. It was her mother who'd thought Gerry was the best thing that had ever happened to her. And her sister. They loved his ambition, his guts and his confidence, and all the material things that went with them. Lizzie had been transfixed by that too, in the beginning. And when the doubts had set in, longer ago than Lizzie dared admit, she'd pushed them aside, not wanting to add her marriage to her list of failures.

'There's not much money left after The Cedars, you know that.'

'Oh, come off it, Liz. Do I look like I just got off the boat?'

Lizzie winced. 'Gerry, don't be racist.'

'Don't take the high ground with me,' he snapped. 'I'm not the one walking out on eight years of marriage. Who is he? Come on, I'm not a fool. I know there's someone else.'

'There isn't,' Lizzie said.

And her voice was clear, unwavering, because it was true. She wasn't leaving him for David. David didn't know she was leaving. Nor did Mona. Nor did Jo. She wasn't even sure she was going to tell them – any of them – not yet, at least. A bit of her, the biggest bit, wanted to walk away from everything and everyone that had gone before and not look back.

'I'm not leaving you for anyone else, Gerry. And I'm sorry, I really am. The only person I'm leaving you for is me.'

From the look on his face, she realised, too late, that this was worse. If she'd been leaving for another man he could have understood, railed against it. But to be left for no one . . . ?

'I don't believe you,' he said finally. 'You've got someone else. I know it. You just think you'll get more out of me if you pretend you haven't. Well, go, if you want to. But if you think you're taking anything from this house you've got another think coming. I'm not giving you a penny.'

Lizzie looked around the room: Gerry's favourite room, in the house Gerry chose. A huge flatscreen TV, a Blu-ray player, surround-sound speakers, the largest Bose iPod dock available, two cream sofas without so much as a cushion to soften their edges.

Gerry's house.

On a smoked-glass coffee table in the far corner was a small pile of half-read paperbacks, a couple of gardening books, and a fruit bowl with four tangerines. Under the tangerines were a red elastic band and a stray button. Lizzie knew, because she'd put them there.

Three years they'd been in this house and, in the main room, those few things were the only sign she lived here.

'Don't worry,' she said, turning back to the hall and heading for the stairs. 'There's nothing here I need.'

FORTY-SIX

There was a train strike. And engineering works. It was, she decided later, just as well, since taking an intercity express nowhere in particular wasn't one of her brighter ideas. OK, so she could have driven nowhere in particular, but her little Renault was almost out of petrol. Plus she was crying so much she couldn't face driving for long. Finally, the tears had broken through. That was something, Lizzie supposed.

'Please be in, please be in, please be in,' Lizzie repeated the words like a mantra as she stood on Jo's doorstep, only partially shielded from the rain by the open porch. If Jo wasn't in, she didn't know what she'd do. She couldn't go to Mona's; her flat was the size of a shoebox. And there was no way she could face David. Not now. And it wasn't as if she could have gone back to her mum's with this news, even if she had still had a mum . . .

'Jo,' she cried, as the door opened.

It wasn't Jo who stood in the doorway, it was Si. 'Lizzie, hi, we weren't . . . Were we expecting you?' He looked dishevelled.

Suddenly Lizzie was conscious of her sodden hair, the small suitcase by her feet. Si peered around her at her Renault parked in the street. From where he stood, Lizzie was sure he couldn't see the four carrier bags of school work and cardboard box of books piled on the back seat.

'No Gerry?' he asked.

'N-no Gerry,' Lizzie stammered, the hugeness of what she'd done crippling her. 'I . . . Si . . . I need to speak to Jo.'

'She's in the bath,' he said, stepping aside so Lizzie could pass. 'I'll go and get her.' Without a word, he reached for her case. The gesture made Lizzie burst into tears all over again.

Sitting at their kitchen table, a steaming cup of tea and a glass of brandy in front of her, Lizzie dabbed ineffectively at her puffy face with a balled-up piece of kitchen roll.

'I left him,' she sobbed when she saw Jo hovering in the doorway in her dressing gown. 'Gerry . . . he was talking about using Mum's money to help buy a better house. Saying I had to give up my job, and it was getting too late for me to have babies . . .' she gasped, 'and I left him.'

Crossing the room, Jo wrapped her arms tight around her friend. 'Really?'

Lizzie nodded.

'About time.'

'About . . . ?' Lizzie couldn't even begin to think about that. 'I'm sorry I got you out of the bath.'

Smiling Jo pulled out a chair. 'Is *that* what Si told you? He's so modest. You got us out of bed. Be grateful to Si. If it was down to me you'd still be on the doorstep.'

'But it's five o'clock!'

'Oh, Lizzie,' Jo stroked her friend's damp hair, 'grown-ups in bed in the middle of the afternoon shocker! And not to sleep, double shocker! But who's to know if we sneak off to bed on a Sunday afternoon, except us? And now you, of course.'

370

As Lizzie looked at her, her face crumpled. 'Gerry and I never went to bed on a Sunday afternoon.'

'Not ever?' Jo asked in surprise.

Bottom lip wobbling, Lizzie shook her head, the tears tumbling down. 'Never,' she sobbed. 'Not once. Not even before we were married.'

It took Jo an hour to get the full story out of Lizzie, and even then she wasn't sure her friend was being entirely straight with her. 'You'll stay here, of course,' Jo said when it became obvious Lizzie had said all she was going to.

'Can I? Just for a day or two. Until I sort myself out?'

'Indefinitely,' Jo said. Over Lizzie's head, Si nodded his agreement. 'Where else would you go? Do you even have any money?'

'I have my salary. It's a couple of weeks till payday. I'll make sure it's not paid into our joint account. I imagine Gerry will be onto the bank to lock that. And there's Mum's money. What's left is to be split between me and Karen.'

'How did your mother leave it, precisely?' Jo asked.

'Split down the middle. After solicitors and estate agents, The Cedars was eating its way through it. There's maybe sixty grand left, perhaps a little more.'

'OK,' said Jo. 'You need a solicitor to sort that, and extract your share of your and Gerry's joint savings.' She put up her hand to silence Lizzie. 'Don't. You might say you don't want anything but don't be a mug. You're entitled to your half of that, if nothing else. If you can get that, then you'll have enough for a deposit on a new place.'

Lizzie sniffed into what was left of her tissue.

'Right,' Jo said. 'This calls for a council of war. I'm going to call Mona and David and get them round here now.'

'No!' Lizzie leapt from her chair, almost sending her tea flying. 'You can't!'

371

'Lizzie . . .'

'All right, you can tell Mona. Not David. Let's keep this between us for now. And Si. Please. Just while I get everything sorted.'

Lizzie's pleading gaze flicked from Jo to Si and back again. 'Please?' she begged. 'Do this one thing for me? One more thing, I mean.'

Jo and Si exchanged glances. 'All right,' Jo said, 'but I don't get it, Lizzie. And, to be frank, I don't think it's fair. David's one of us. It's not right to exclude him.'

'I'll tell him,' Lizzie promised. 'After the funeral . . .'

'Funeral? Oh, Lizzie,' Jo said. Si was already heading for the brandy. 'When is the funeral?'

'Tuesday,' Lizzie said. Her eyes were dry now.

'But I'm at work, I've got some big meetings. You should have warned us.' Jo was already scrolling through diary entries in her head, working out what could be cancelled.

'I didn't warn you because you're not coming.'

It was Lizzie's turn to silence a hail of protests from Si and Jo.

'I mean it, she said. 'Two funerals in one year – I wouldn't wish that on anyone.'

'You're kidding!' Mona's shriek echoed down the line.

'Shhh. Keep your voice down,' Jo hissed. 'Yell like that and she'll hear you.'

It was an exaggeration. There was no way Lizzie would hear Mona. She was unpacking her case in Jo's spare room.

'Way to go, girl. About bloody time,' said Mona, as Jo held the receiver away from her ear.

'That's exactly what I said.'

'Hang on. Let me go into the back office. I'm getting strange looks from the customers.' There was a crashing as Mona's voice vanished for a few seconds while doors opened and shut again.

'Nicci would have cracked open the pink champagne,' Mona said when she returned. 'She always said Gerry was wrong for Lizzie.'

Jo raised her eyebrows. It wasn't like Mona to talk about that. She hadn't been too chuffed when Nicci cracked open the pink champagne for her.

'How long's Lizzie staying?'

'She says two days, I say indefinitely.'

'I say you'll win,' Mona said. 'Where else is she going to go?'

'I don't know. She says she could rent a spare room from someone at school for a bit, while she gets her hands on enough cash to rent somewhere bigger.'

'And you believed that?' Mona laughed. 'She's just trying not to be a burden. She hasn't got any friends at school. Not proper ones, like us.'

'She must have. Everyone has friends at work,' said Jo, and then laughed. 'Except me. Colleagues, employees, but no friends.'

'Exactly,' said Mona. 'Me neither. Do you think there's a man involved?'

'A man?' Jo snorted. 'Don't be ridiculous. This is Lizzie we're talking about here Mo, not you.'

'Oi!'

'You know what I mean. Anyway, she'd have told us. Wouldn't she?'

'She'd have told you, probably,' Mona said. 'Or David. They've been pretty tight lately. Have you asked him?'

'No,' said Jo, thoughtfully. 'That's the weird thing. Lizzie expressly said not to. Said she wanted to keep it between us for now. And Si. I pointed out David is *us*, but she got so stressed I let it go.'

Frowning, Jo replayed the conversation, pinning down what bugged her most. Lizzie and David had been such good friends. If anything, through the hideousness with her mother, Jo would have said Lizzie talked to David more than the rest of them, until the other day, when he mentioned that he hadn't seen her for a few weeks.

'Has Gerry called yet?' Mona asked.

'Hardly,' Jo said. 'Gerry's never been my biggest fan. And vice versa. I'm hardly going to march Lizzie home with her tail between her legs, am I?'

'Where else is she going to go, though? Surely you're the first place he'll look? Try to talk her round?'

'You'd think. But from the sound of it his ego's pretty wounded.'

'Not surprised,' Mona said. 'I know we all think he's a dickhead, but he did love her, in his way.'

'Did,' Jo muttered.

But Mona ignored her. 'Maybe he'll call Si instead.'

'Good luck to him. No love lost there either. Si only ever put up with him because he was part of the package with Lizzie.'

'Really?' Mona was silent for a moment. 'I'd never have known.'

Jo shrugged. 'That's because Si's polite.'

On the far end of the phone, Jo heard a door open and somebody ask a question. Muffled by her hand over the receiver, Mona's reply sounded efficient and knowledgeable.

'What about the funeral?' Mona asked, coming back on the line.

'Tuesday afternoon.'

'Oh God. This is messing with my head. First, she leaves Gerry. And who saw that coming? Second, she does it two days before her mum's funeral. And third, she doesn't give us any warning of the first or invite us to the second. What's going on, Jo, seriously? This is Lizzie we're talking about. It's not you, or me, or Nicci. Lizzie can't do this without us. We're family. She needs us.'

'She went to the station.'

'She what?'

'I know. She was going to catch a train. I'm not even sure she knew where she was going. Luckily, she forgot about the strike. And I told her she needs us there on Tuesday, but she said one funeral a year is enough for anyone. Something like that, anyway.'

'Fair point,' Mona said. 'Can't say I want to set foot in another church this year. Or next. Keep expecting to go up in flames.'

'Be serious, Mo,'

'I am.'

'I'm worried about her,' Jo said, lowering her voice as a door opened at the top of the house. 'I think Nicci, then her mum dying, all this with Gerry . . . I don't know . . . I'm worried Gerry's right and she is having a breakdown.'

FORTY-SEVEN

December was usually David's favourite month of the year, November a close second. Nicci had been wild for Christmas, her enthusiasm infectious. From the moment the last Guy Fawkes firework fell from the sky, life was all about log fires and long walks, mulled wine and twinkling lights, parties and presents.

The tree always had to be real – an eight-foot Norwegian spruce that scraped the ceiling – and if she'd had her way the decorations would have gone up the day the bonfire burnt down.

There were boxes and boxes of tree decorations stashed in the eaves. She'd started buying them their first Christmas together and added to the collection each year. A gaudy Indian bauble, a bone snowflake, Italian glass teardrops, black glass balls from Heals, even a Santa Russian doll. A chaos of clashing colours, wooden and glitter, vintage and modern, cheap and expensive. Their tree always looked more like it had been decorated by a five-year-old than a woman whose middle name was style.

It was the weirdest thing. Nicci was so scrupulously, aggressively stylish, yet in this one thing, she threw taste to the wind and trampled all over it. But now, having learnt what he had, David was beginning to understand. Like most things in her life, Nicci had wanted to own Christmas; to grasp the fantasy holiday of other people's childhoods and make it hers.

Even last year, when it became traumatically clear that, unlike everyone else, her cancer wasn't planning to see things Nicci's way, she'd thrown herself into Christmas. Well, thrown David into it. Machine-gunning instructions at him from the bed, maxing out both their credit cards without ever leaving the sofa. She'd bought the food, everyone's presents – including hers from him – on the internet. Knees up, her MacBook balanced precariously on top.

'Louboutins? Are you sure?' he'd said when she pointed them out online, ostentatiously adding them to her wish list.

Her brow had creased, a sure sign of displeasure. 'Why not?' she demanded, daring him to say it. Knowing all the while he wouldn't. After all, they wouldn't be the only unworn pair of shoes in her closet.

'Just checking you wouldn't rather have a new dishwasher,' he said. And ducked to avoid a half-heartedly hurled pillow.

The Louboutins were here beside him now. Untarnished red soles, uncreased leather. First he'd salvaged three boxes of Nicci's decorations from the attic, then something had drawn him to her wardrobe. He'd steered clear of it until now. Obeying her strict instructions to leave it to Jo, Mona and Lizzie. The Chuck, Cherish, Charity committee, she'd called them in her letter. But somehow, today, the first of December – officially the start of Nicci's Christmas – he couldn't keep away.

*   *   *

The Louboutins
Last Christmas

The Snowman *soundtrack was playing on the iPod. They'd watched every possible permutation of* A Christmas Carol, *the last two, thankfully, on mute. And if he ate one more mince pie, David was sure he would wake up to find he had currants for eyes. Certainly none of his jeans would fit by tomorrow. Everything was perfect.*

Harrie and Charlie sprawled across him in a carbohydrate coma, overcome with excitement, pigged out on chocolate, and bemused that a fat man with a beard would come down the chimney tonight and, for some perverse reason, that was OK. In fact, it was so OK they had to leave him mince pies and Baileys. In return he would fill a pillowcase for them with toys. Run that by me again, *said their faces, as they snuggled, deceptively angelic, in their matching check flannel pyjamas. Two and a half years old and already as cynical as their mother.*

Beside him, in the Eames-alike recliner he'd bought to make her as comfortable as possible, their mother dozed. Watching her chest rise and fall, her eyelids flicker, Albert Finney doing an ill-advised jig on the screen behind her, David felt his eyes well up. For a second, he allowed himself to think the thing he knew he shouldn't. Not if he wanted to get through the next forty-eight hours in one piece.

Not wanting to disturb Nicci, but desperate to feel the life still pulsing in her flesh, he reached out and ran one finger along her hand.

Her lids flickered open. 'You OK, babe?' *she whispered.*

'Couldn't be better,' *he said.* 'Go back to sleep.'

And her eyes closed again.

This, he allowed himself to think – just once, just tonight – was what their last Christmas together looked like.

'Go on, open it,' *David urged.*

Nicci smiled.

'Don't tell me it's a surprise,' Jo laughed. 'If that's a surprise, there really is a first time for everything.' She was right, of course. Cancer or no cancer, everything was organised with military precision right down to the last detail.

David and Nicci exchanged conspiratorial glances.

Honestly,' Mona said, half exasperated, 'there's no stopping you, is there? I bet you've shopped the internet dry.'

David pasted a smile onto his face and held it. Because I could not stop for death . . . The quote sprang into his head all the time now. Unbidden and unwanted. . . . He kindly stopped for me.

'They're incredible!' Lizzie exclaimed, as Nicci pulled five-inch black studded heels from a caramel-coloured box laced with extravagant white script.

'Hooker shoes,' David heard Gerry mutter.

'So what?' Nicci turned on him.

Uh-oh, David thought.

'These . . .' she said, in her best 'here comes a fashion lecture' voice.

'Here we go!' Mona laughed, but Nicci ignored her.

'These,' she repeated, 'are a design classic. A collector's piece. These babies are just one of my babies' heirlooms.'

She reached down to take off her shoes, then flinched. A flash of pain crossing her face. 'Hey, babe,' she turned to David, her smile tight. In her eyes he could see an echo of anguish. 'Help me put these on, would you?'

Kneeling at his wife's feet, he unzipped first one biker boot then the other, before carefully buckling on the Louboutin stilts he knew would make Nicci almost as tall as him. David forced on a brave face. Everything was right, everyone was here, everything was as it should be. Presents piled obscenely high under the tree, lights sparkled on every available surface, mulled wine flowed, and the turkey slowly basted. Charlie and Harrie, already in their second outfit of the day, were torn between fighting over

379

identical toys and stage diving from a Moroccan leather pouf into a mound of cushions and discarded wrapping paper. Everything was as Nicci prescribed it.

And nothing was.

The touch of her fingers on his neck brought David back to the moment. He knelt up so his cheek was next to hers. Her newly regrown lashes brushed his cheek. Their secret sign. 'I'm OK, sweetheart,' she whispered. 'I promise. Please smile, be happy, for me. Let's make this day perfect for our babies. Their first proper Christmas. Let's give them a memory.'

So brave. He was so proud of her.

Smiling back, David kissed her, his lips lingering on her cheek as he resisted the urge to bury his face in her cropped hair and howl.

'I love you,' he whispered.

'I know,' she said. 'And I love you. More than you can ever know.'

'Fairytale of New York' segued into Slade's 'Merry Xmas Everybody'. 'I think this calls for a dance, don't you?' Nicci announced, wobbling to her feet. David stepped forward to catch her, then stopped himself. Over her shoulder he saw Lizzie and Jo exchange glances. Catching his eye, Mona gave the slightest shake of her head. Dan and Si, playing PSP, seemed oblivious. They were all agreed: this was Nicci's day.

'Come on, babies,' she called, and Charlie and Harrie emerged from the paper, glitter stuck to their hair and faces. 'Dance with Mummy.'

Retreating to the kitchen, David watched the scene from a place of near-safety. Nicci's always skinny legs even skinnier in stratospheric heels, black leggings and a loose grey cashmere sweater, reaching down to clasp her daughters' hands. They laughed, they clapped and every so often he caught the pain that flashed across her face and twisted his heart. Because for once, there was nothing he could do to take it away.

*   *   *

It was done. Her last duty fulfilled. Give or take a few. She could rest now, for a while.

Through the regrown lashes she'd missed so much, Nicci watched her friends. Her framily. So much less happy than they deserved to be. Slumped in front of the TV, full of four courses none of them had really tasted, a drink too far in everyone's hands.

The girls were reluctantly tucked in bed, and David, Mona and Jo were pretending to watch the latest Harry Potter *on* Sky Movies. *Si read some military history book he'd been ecstatic to receive from Nicci and David (under strict instruction from Jo), Dan was plugged into his PSP, as always. Lizzie and Gerry had already gone. To Gerry's parents for Boxing Day. Nicci didn't know which was worse — it being a lie, to get away, or, if it were true, Gerry planning to drive two hundred miles with that much booze in his system.*

Lizzie, Lizzie, Lizzie, *she thought.*

Nicci worried about Lizzie more than the rest put together. So kind, so beautiful, so much nicer than she was herself. And so unhappy. How had she ended up with Gerry, a man who thought he was God's gift to women when, to Nicci's mind at least, Lizzie was God's gift to him?

Did he ever touch her? He must, in private. After all, Lizzie was a private kind of person. But still, it bothered Nicci, the public lack of passing casual intimacies. All she could remember was the kiss on their wedding day, and Gerry placing his hand in the small of Lizzie's back to usher her away. Always ushering her away.

Nicci had a vision of how Lizzie's life should be. A vision Lizzie had conjured and drunkenly shared with her, long ago at uni. One Nicci had never forgotten, although it seemed Lizzie had. Of children, and pets and roses around the door. As far as Nicci could see, she'd never have that with Gerry. Gerry's visions would be altogether grander.

'You OK in there?' David leant over and whispered. 'Anything

I can get you? Wine, vodka, morphine? All three?'

A faint smile lifted her lips. Slowly, she shook her head. 'I'm fine.'

On the far side of the room, Si stretched and put his arm around Jo, the other propping his history book on the arm of the sofa. They'd be all right, Nicci decided. They were strong, they'd make it. If they could get through the choppy waters of IVF, which had been hurling them relentlessly against the rocks right until Nicci's diagnosis threw everything off track. That was the one good thing to come of this, she thought, watching them.

Jo had always been work, work, work. Babies had never seemed to figure. And then she met Si and suddenly she was risking everything – wrecking everything – to get one. For months Nicci hadn't been able to get close enough to ask. But she wanted to. If she could find a way to remind her, maybe she could make them stop.

And Mona, so fiercely independent, and still searching.

If only Nicci could work out for what. So tall, so striking. When Mona walked down the street men stopped and turned to stare at her. She didn't see them, she never really had. If Nicci hadn't known better she might have wondered if Mona even liked them.

As sleep took her, Nicci started to plan the first letter. She had things to say, important things, and time was not on her side.

My dearest, my love, my David. My Sunday man.

Don't be angry when you read this. I know you will be, at first. But, slowly, I hope, you'll come to understand. Assume everything is not what it seems but let me do it this way. And remember this. I don't want the rest of your life to be about losing me. You're too good for that. You're a keeper.

And, if I could, I would keep you for myself for ever. But I can't.

Everyone deserves a second chance, David, everyone. Please remember that in the dark, dark days ahead . . .

FORTY-EIGHT

The sweetness of cinnamon and nutmeg, oranges and cloves seeped out into the chill air of the street as David opened the door. It was only when Jo got inside that she could smell the brandy . . .

'Wow, David,' she said, hugging him tight, 'sure smells like Christmas in here!'

'That's the plan,' he said. 'Looks like Christmas too. Si, Sam, Tom, Happy Christmas. Come in. Mona and Dan are already in the kitchen.' He was all bonhomie and smiles, clapping Si on the arm as he pushed past, but it didn't escape Jo that David was looking over her shoulder.

'Lizzie!' he said, his voice betraying his relief. 'It's so good to see you. It's been too long. I . . . the garden's missing you. And I'm so sorry about your mother . . . How are you?' He paused. 'Where's Gerry?'

'Good to see you too,' she said, freeing herself from his hug. Her eyes bulged at Jo in panic. 'Gerry's . . . at his parents.'

'At his parents?' David looked confused.

Jo tried not to catch Si's eye. And failed. *This*, Si's stare said, *has gone too far.*

384

Shrugging, Jo escaped into the sitting room. If Lizzie had won the argument she wouldn't be there at all, but Jo had refused to back down. In the end, using guilt. Lizzie was in her house and she wasn't going to leave Lizzie there alone on Christmas Day. Besides, it was the first Christmas since Nicci died, and they all *had* to be there. When Mona took Jo's side, Lizzie caved in.

Everything looked the same. Eight-foot Norwegian spruce. Kaleidoscope of mismatched ornaments that made the tree look like it had been decorated by three-year-olds. Although this year it had. Twinkling fairy lights on every surface and window. 'Fairytale of New York' on the iPod speaker, proclaiming that *the bells were ringing out on Christmas Day.*

It was one of Nicci's favourites. Swallowing hard, Jo bit back tears. She would not cry. She would get through today without crying if it killed her.

Everything looks the same, she repeated to herself.

Except, of course, there was no Nicci, which was to be expected. And no Gerry, which wasn't. Not that Nicci would have had any objection to that.

Jo was just grateful David drew the line at inviting Lynda. Not that it hadn't occurred to him.

'It's too much,' she'd said when he'd phoned to sound her out. 'Next year, maybe?' He'd backed down so fast, Jo knew his heart hadn't been in it.

'What can I do?' she asked now, walking into the kitchen and taking the mulled wine David pushed into her hand. 'Spuds to peel? Sprouts to wash? Stuffing to make?'

'Under control,' Mona said. She looked great today, in a black wrap dress and the stiletto ankle boots she'd last worn to Nicci's funeral. Her hair suited her blown out. 'David started them, I finished them. No idea what time he must have got up . . .'

'Six,' David said.

It looked like it too, Jo thought. Knackered would have been generous

'It would have been even earlier if these two had had their way. You can give them a present if you want,' David added, pushing his daughters in Jo's direction a little too enthusiastically. 'They're suffering gift withdrawal. It must be, ooh, twenty minutes since the last one.'

'Presents!' Charlie and Harrie hollered as one, galloping past Jo.

'Us too,' said Sam. 'Can I have a present? I'm desperate. We have to wait for Mum to give us our stockings tomorrow,' he explained to Mona.

'Don't fall for the sob story.' Jo tousled his hair. 'They've already had two presents when they got up.'

'But those were *books*,' Sam wailed.

'Hey, if there are presents going, I'm in,' Dan said, not as oblivious to the world as his headphones suggested.

'Presents it is then.' Picking up a tray now only half full of glasses brimming with mulled wine, David headed back into the hall.

'I'm just going out to check the garden, if that's OK with everyone.' Lizzie, who had been silent until then, took a glass from the passing tray and moved in the opposite direction.

Jo and Si exchanged glances. 'Don't get mad at me,' Jo muttered as they ushered Tom and Sam into the sitting room. 'It's not my fault.'

'I know it's not,' Si said, leaning in to kiss her. 'But I do think it's time you stopped protecting her.'

Jo opened her mouth to protest.

'Three times David's called me now to ask if I've seen Lizzie. I'm not lying to him any more,' Si whispered. 'I want to know what the hell is going on around here. Don't you?'

He obviously didn't whisper quietly enough, because Mona nodded.

'I do,' she said. 'Lynda thinks . . .'

Glancing through the window, Jo saw Lizzie heading for the shed. Her hair glowed in the mist, her body was shrouded by a chunky Stella McCartney cardigan Jo and Si had given her that morning.

She looked lost and alone. The heartbreak diet had taken pounds off her. Which would have made sense, except Lizzie's heart wasn't meant to be broken. She'd done the leaving, after all. And so far as Jo could tell, had not once looked back.

'I don't really care what Lynda thinks right now,' Jo told Mona, 'but I do want to know why Lizzie still won't let us tell David.'

'Make a wish,' David said to Sam, handing him two crackers, one for each hand. 'Pull it hard, and whoever gets the fat end gets their wish granted.'

The large refectory table was strewn with the debris of enough food to feed an entire town. Turkey and nut roast, roast parsnips and potatoes, four different vegetables, two kinds of stuffing, gravy and cranberry sauce. David had put on an amazing spread, but staunchly refused to take the credit. 'Don't thank me, thank M&S,' was all he said.

Turning to Mona on one side, and Harrie on the other, Sam pulled hard. When he came away with two small sides his lips began to wobble.

'Don't worry,' Jo said, homing in like emergency services. She handed him her cracker, tearing slightly at her end so the other end – the big one – would come away in his hand. 'What's your wish?'

'For Chelsea to win the cup.'

'Bor-ing!' Tom said. 'And unlikely.'

'Not!' Sam said.

'What about you, Mum?' Dan asked. 'What's yours?'

387

'We-ell . . .' Mona hesitated.

'I know what Mona's wish is!' Jo said. 'Well, I know what my wish is for her. This is the year we find your mum a new man!'

Mona smiled. 'That's your wish used up then,' she said. 'Although judging by the last lot you tried to fix me up with—'

'Do you mind?' David laughed. 'That's my friends you're talking about. Don't worry, I learnt my lesson last time. I won't be setting myself up like that again. You have no idea how many pints that cost me.'

'Sorry,' Mona said unconvincingly. 'This year, I'm not wasting any more time on men. You three excepted.' She turned to Si, David and Dan, then spotted Sam and Tom. 'Sorry, you *five* excepted. They never fail to let you down. No, this year, I have a better wish.' Mona's face turned serious. 'I have a deal for you: I'll find *myself* someone new, if you write me a business plan.'

Over the children's head the adults fell silent. Dan took off his headphones and even Lizzie looked up from her plate. 'A business plan?' Jo said.

'Yes,' Mona nodded. 'I've got it all worked out. I'm fed up with slaving twenty-four hours a day, seven days a week to line someone else's pockets. Nobody ever got rich working for someone else. Isn't that what they say? I mean, look at you two.'

Her eyes flicked between David and Jo.

'I've got all the skills necessary to run a restaurant. I've been doing it for other people for years. All it takes is an idea, management skills, contacts and bloody hard work. I've been researching the area and there's a real gap in the market. You know how Nicci was always saying that restaurant in Piccadilly, The Wolseley, is busy whatever time of day you're there; breakfast, elevensies, lunch, afternoon tea, pre-theatre dinner, supper . . . ? Breakfast in particular is lacking around here. And I've found the perfect location. There's enough of a local community to get a coffee morning crowd and I'll install Wi-fi for business breakfasts.'

Her confidence carried the entire table with her.

'Set-up costs shouldn't be too high. There's already a kitchen, and it won't cost much to kit out the dining room with second-hand stuff. I'm thinking a fifties, sixties vibe. I've found a great vintage market down in Sussex. And I know just the chef. I've sounded her out and, potentially, she's interested. Although she'll cost me. I've got it all planned. There's just this one, small problem.'

'Let me guess,' Jo said, puncturing the balloon.

'Money,' Si, Lizzie and David agreed.

'That's where you come in.'

'Oh, surprise me,' Jo said.

'Seriously, I need a business plan. And maybe you could come and do some pitches with me? You're impressive, you know you are. You had those money guys eating out of your hand for Capsule Wardrobe. And before you say, "That was Nicci", it wasn't, it was you. Anyway, I only need a fraction of the set-up costs of Capsule Wardrobe. There's little stock, for a start, and you know I'll work all the hours of the day myself to pay back any loan you can arrange. Call it my Christmas present?'

'In that case I'll have my Wright & Teague bracelet back.'

Snatching her arm away, Mona waited. 'Will you?'

All eyes around the table were on Jo, even Charlie and Harrie's, although Jo was sure they didn't know why. 'Of course I will,' she said. 'After all, now we actually have some staff at Capsule Wardrobe, what else am I going to do?'

Si squeezed her hand.

Mona grinned.

'Way to go, Mum,' Dan said, his face glowing with pride. 'Way to go.'

Lizzie, Jo and Mona had barely finished drying up when Lizzie pulled on her cardigan. 'Going for a walk?' Mona asked. 'I'll come with you. I could do with burning off some of those roast potatoes.' She patted a barely visible stomach.

'Er, no,' Lizzie said, ignoring Jo's glare. 'I think I'll head off now. I'm tired and it all feels a bit weird, you know, no Nicci, no . . .'

'No Gerry,' Jo said pointedly. 'On the subject of which—'

'Not now, Jo,' Lizzie groaned. 'I'm tired.'

Two goblets of mulled wine, a glass of champagne, two glasses of Chablis and the heavily laced brandy butter had got to Jo. 'I'm tired too, Lizzie,' she said, folding the damp tea towel onto the back of a chair. 'We're all *tired*.'

'Well,' Lizzie turned on her, 'I'm sorry to be such a burden. I'll move out in New Year. I told you that already.'

'Lizzie!' Mona said. 'Stop it, both of you. You know Jo didn't mean that.'

'Who knows what she means?' Lizzie said, wrapping the cardigan tight around herself. 'And I'm not ready to talk about this. I can't tell David and I can't pretend nothing's happened, I just can't.' She glared at Jo and Mona who looked at each other in despair. 'I've had enough of this. Just leave me alone.'

At the sound of a door slamming, David looked up from his book. 'Has Lizzie gone for a walk?' he asked Si, who was sitting with Dan, his own two and the girls. Even Dan was watching *Spirited Away*.

'Sounds like it.' Si said, getting up. 'I'll be right back.'

Si entered the kitchen just as Jo was about to come out. Turning her round, he herded her back inside and shut the door firmly. 'What the hell is going on now?' he demanded.

'Lizzie's gone,' Mona said.

'For a walk?'

'No, *gone* gone,' said Jo. 'We tried to stop her.'

'It's not Jo's fault,' Mona said. 'Lizzie wouldn't listen.'

'Oh, for fuck's sake,' Si sighed. 'I've had enough of this. I know she's upset. Obviously, she's upset. Her mother's dead and it must be hard not to be relieved it's all over. And I imagine she feels guilty about that. And Gerry's being a bastard about the divorce, which hardly comes as a surprise. But why the hell are we supposed to keep the divorce a secret from David? It doesn't make sense.'

'I don't know,' Jo said. 'Really, I don't.'

'Actually,' said Mona. 'It might do. Speaking as someone who's kept her share of secrets.'

'We have to tell him.' Si's hand was on the kitchen door handle.

'No.' Jo put herself between Si and the door. 'We can't,' she pleaded. 'We promised. It's not our secret to tell.'

'Si's right, Jo,' Mona said. 'He has to know.'

'We can't.' Jo was panic-stricken.

'Well, if you two won't tell David,' Si said, folding his arms, 'I will.'

'Tell David what?'

In the furore, none of them had heard David open the kitchen door behind them. They moved back to allow him in. David shut the door quietly and leant against it.

'Tell David what?' he repeated. His voice was steely. 'Come on. I'm fed up with being kept in the dark and fed shit in my own house. What's going on?'

Jo's eyes shot wildly from Si to Mona. 'You do it then,' she said. 'At least that way I won't have broken my promise.'

'What promise?' David said, irritation rising.

'Well . . .' Si hesitated, 'Lizzie and Gerry broke up. Six, seven weeks ago now. Right after her mother died. She left him. He wanted to use her mother's money to buy a bigger house, Lizzie to give up her job, have babies. She didn't want to, or so she says. Jo thinks there's way more to it than that.'

David turned to stare at Jo.

'I'm so sorry, David,' she whispered. 'Lizzie's been living with us since the middle of November and she wouldn't let me tell you. I tried to make her do it herself. She kept saying she would . . .' Her voice trailed away.

'That's why I'm telling you now,' Si finished. 'Because it's stopped being a lie of omission and started being an outright lie. Today was the final straw. Whatever happened – and I'm fucked if I know – Lizzie's hurting. And it's about more than moving bloody house.'

'And I reckon,' Mona said, turning to David, 'you might know the answer.'

David was glad he'd leant against the door. It saved him having to find a chair. 'Run that by me again?' he said, his fury ebbing away as quickly as it had surged in.

'I think you might be able to tell us,' Mona said.

'No,' David said ignoring the curiosity on Mona's face. 'All the stuff that went before.'

While Si gave him the full story in as much detail as he knew, Jo made tea and Mona, reluctantly, went to check on the children.

'She left him six weeks ago?' David repeated.

Si nodded.

'Why would she do that and not want you to know?' Jo asked.

'I don't know,' David shrugged.

But he did know. Or thought he did. What else could it

be? But was that night's secret his to tell? Obviously Lizzie didn't think so.

She'd left Gerry.

Right now David didn't even know what he was feeling. Other than that he was on the verge of throwing up, although he wasn't sure whether that was from guilt or euphoria or too much Christmas lunch. His spirits soared, and at the same time he felt crushed. If he'd made a wish over his cracker he wouldn't have dared wish for this. It would have been for Lizzie just to speak to him again; to take his calls, return his texts as she had before that night in the shed.

Just to be his friend. To sit in his garden and talk to him. That would have been enough. This was better and worse. Lizzie was free now, and yet she so obviously wasn't.

Was this his fault? Had he broken up her marriage by taking advantage of her when she was vulnerable? Surely if Lizzie had left Gerry because of that night she'd have told him? Wouldn't she?

He cleared his throat. 'Did Lizzie tell you why she left? Why she *really* left, I mean?'

Jo gave him a strange look.

'I don't believe Gerry wanting to spend her mother's money on a new house is the reason,' he said carefully. 'Well, not the only reason.'

'Nor do I,' said Si.

'She said she wasn't leaving for someone else, she was leaving for her,' Jo said. 'It was something she had to do. Something like that, anyway.'

That sounded more like Mona than Lizzie.

'David,' Jo said, '*do* you know why she wouldn't let me tell you?'

As he opened his mouth to speak, the kitchen door handle turned.

They watched Mona come in and shut the door firmly

393

behind her. 'I've put Dan in charge. He's got Sam and Tom taking turns on his PSP and he's playing something horsy that seems to involve Harrie and Charlie climbing all over him. He's even taken off his precious headphones. It'll cost me later, but I'm not missing this for anything.'

David looked at them. He felt ecstatic, guilty, confused. Like Judas, he'd betrayed Nicci by sleeping with Lizzie, and now he was about to betray Lizzie by telling the others he'd done it. And then there was Mona. Oh shit, he'd forgotten about her. Hadn't Nicci planned this for him and Mona, not him and Lizzie?

Four women, three betrayals. They deserved so much better. Nice work, David.

'All right,' he said, taking a deep breath. He was just going to say it. 'There was an evening back in October, when Lizzie's mother was first in a coma. Lizzie was in the garden. I went down to see how she was . . .'

FORTY-NINE

It had been dark for a couple of hours now. The mist had barely had a chance to lift before it descended again, but the Calor Gas heater threw enough light for the two women to see each other's faces.

'I knew it,' Mona said, chain-lighting her third Marlboro from the second. 'I knew there was a man involved.'

'No, you didn't,' Jo said protested, pouring the brandy she'd abducted from the kitchen into a mug. 'You asked if there was. I said, "Lizzie says not." And that was that. End of conversation. Anyway, there isn't. Not really. Lizzie didn't leave Gerry for David. She didn't tell him she was going, and hasn't spoken to him since she left.'

'They slept together, though,' Mona said gleefully.

Her face told Jo she was enjoying this a little too much. 'Our Lizzie had sex, with a man, not her husband, while she was married. And I bet she liked it. She must have loved it. Look at the chaos it's caused.'

'She's in pieces because she *enjoyed* it?'

'You know Lizzie. Guilt in inverse proportions to how enjoyable something is.'

'Stop it,' Jo said, but she couldn't help laughing.

With David's words everything had slotted into place. Jo was surprised to find she didn't feel angry on Nicci's behalf. Now Jo knew, it just felt . . . obvious. She just wished Lizzie had felt able to tell her. Instead of beating herself up in self-imposed isolation for weeks.

Jo looked at Mona's profile in the twilight. 'D'you mind?' she asked at last. 'That David, well, you know?'

'Fancies Lizzie more than me?' Mona smiled and shook her head. 'Not really. I mean, my ego does, a bit. But it never made any sense. I mean, me and David? It's hardly an obvious combination. I never really got Nicci's logic where that was concerned.'

'Me neither,' Jo said. 'I remember when you called me, you know, after we got the letters. I couldn't believe it. It was so . . . *unlikely*. I kept thinking over and over, David and Mona, Mona and David? Trying to think myself into Nicci's head. It made no sense at all. Mind you, Lizzie and the garden was just as mad.'

Cigarette halfway to her mouth, Mona stopped. 'Doesn't seem mad now, though, does it?' she said. 'Nicci knew Lizzie, of all of us, would do what she asked, within reason. And she put her right in David's path. In his line of sight out of his office window, out of the kitchen, under his feet and into his head . . .'

'And she put David right in front of Lizzie,' Jo finished. 'A decent guy, who had loved and had been loved, who would talk and listen and care.'

Jo ran her fingers through her hair. 'So many secrets,' she said. 'I'm not sure I can take any more. Give me one of those, will you?'

Pulling a Marlboro from her packet, Mona lit it from hers and handed it over. 'While we're on the subjects of secrets,' she said. 'I'm afraid you're going to have to cope with one more.'

396

Jo's head shot up. 'About Lizzie?'

'About me. But I want to tell you. Since today's turned into show-and-tell day. We can start the restaurant idea with a clean slate. New Year, New Me and all that. All right?'

'Is it bad?' Jo sounded nervous.

Mona shrugged, took a drag. 'Give me a sip of that, will you?' she said, taking Jo's mug from her and half emptying it before handing it back. 'You'll think so, probably. But that's nothing new where I'm concerned, is it? So I apologise in advance.' Taking a deep breath, Mona balanced her cigarette on a shelf. Finding her free hands a liability, she picked it up again.

'I lied, Jo,' she said. 'I lied to you, Nicci, Lizzie, David and Si, all of you. And Dan. That's the worst thing of all. At the very least, I let you think something that wasn't true and kept letting you think it for a long time.'

'How long?'

'Three years.'

'*Three . . . ?*'

'But that stops today. Actually, the whole thing stops now. Bear with me . . .' Mona inhaled and blew a smoke ring at the ceiling. 'I forgot how much I love smoking,' she said. And then she produced her mobile, looked at her watch and smiled bitterly. After minutes tapping at the keys she pressed Send.

'Right, where were we?'

'You were about to reveal your big secret.'

'That guy, the one you saw in the City?' Mona said. 'Neil? The married one?'

It was rhetorical, but Mona nodded. 'I wasn't well out of it.' She looked at her mobile. 'Although I imagine I am now.'

'You mean . . . ?'

'Uh-huh.'

'Shit,' Jo said. 'I'm so sorry. I'd never have . . . If I'd

397

known . . . I mean, I would have told you, obviously. Just not like that.'

''—s' all right.' In the half-light Mona's face was sad. 'I'm over him. Or I will be, soon. It was the wake-up call I needed, to be honest. I was getting there – slowly, admittedly. You seeing him was the final push. Next year, is the year of me.'

Jo stared at her friend. 'You told us . . . You said . . . You finished with him . . . Nicci cracked open the pink champagne.'

'I lied,' Mona shrugged. 'After a while I got used to it. Lying gets, if not easy, then instinctive. And it's not like I saw him that often anyway. Before the christening he'd finished with me, Yes, I know I told you it was the other way round. And then he came back. Said he'd made a mistake, begged me to take him back. And I fell straight back into bed.'

Seeing Jo's face, she smiled bleakly. 'I loved him once,' she said. 'Well, I thought I did. And the sex . . . It's all right for you, with your Sunday man. And Nicci, with David. You got the Holy Grail – great sex with people who loved you.'

'And Lizzie?'

'Well,' Mona said, 'as far as I can tell she had not very much, not very good sex with a man she didn't fancy anyway.'

Jo snorted.

'Lizzie's never seemed very interested in sex, has she?' said Mona. 'Even at uni. Mind you, having met her family . . . But me, I think I'm a bloke in that respect. I need sex. I've just never met a man I liked enough to want to live with,' she paused. 'Except Greg. And look where that got me.'

'Is that true?'

Mona nodded. 'And if there's one thing Neil's good at – was

good at – it's commitment-free sex. He's not even up to scratch on that front any more.'

Jo didn't know what Mona was seeing in her mind's eye, but she knew she didn't want to see it too. 'No wonder you didn't fancy any of David's mates,' she said. 'Poor sods didn't stand a chance.'

'To be honest, I'm not sure I'd have been interested anyway. I know it's not very PC – Lizzie won't approve – but nice guys don't really do it for me.'

'So,' Jo said. 'Do I get to know what you said in your text?'

Pulling her mobile out of her bag, Mona passed it across. 'He's with his in-laws,' she said. 'They should be eating dinner around now.'

Happy Christmas. You're dumped. This time don't bother coming back.

Jo burst out laughing.

'In the meantime,' said Jo. 'What are we going to do about Lizzie and David? 'Because somebody's got to do something.'

'D'you think they're in love?' Mona asked. 'Lynda does.'

'Lynda? What's she got to do with anything?'

'I kept trying to tell you,' Mona said. 'That last time Lizzie was round, you know, when her mother went into a coma, Lynda just said, right out of the blue, "Nice girl, that. For what it's worth, I approve."'

'You what?'

'I know. Funny how someone who'd only met Lizzie two or three times could see clear as day what her best friends couldn't.'

Jo looked thoughtful. 'Then I think she's right. They are. In love, I mean. Well, David is, for sure. And Lizzie . . . I've certainly never seen her in a state like this before. I think it's Nicci that's stopping her. Nicci – and you.'

'Me?' Mona laughed out loud. 'Well, she can stop worrying

about that. It makes a million times more sense for them to be together than David and me. Nicci wasn't stupid, she *must* have known that.'

For a moment Mona looked thoughtful. 'Put yourself in Nicci's shoes,' she said slowly. 'Lizzie worshipped her. But Lizzie was married – would she leave Gerry just because Nicci asked her? Even Lizzie wouldn't do that. But this way, well, Lizzie's free now. And she got there on her own, albeit with a bit of manoeuvring. If you think about it, that's not much short of genius. Manipulative as hell, but genius all the same.'

Unable to fault Mona's logic, Jo asked, 'So, what are you thinking?'

Mona grinned and took one last puff before getting up and tossing her cigarette out into the night. 'Think we can handle one more little white lie?'

FIFTY

The lock on David's side gate was stiff from months of disuse. The wood had expanded with the damp and frost had rusted its hinges. Where the ivy had been left unpruned it had grown over the hinges and held the gate shut.

Using all her weight, Lizzie threw herself against it and felt the wood give. There was less of her, Lizzie thought, although she could stand to lose a little more. It was the alcohol that ruined the diet. Since she'd moved in with Jo and Si, the three of them had been clearing a couple of bottles a night. Christmas had been even worse.

After last night, Lizzie could almost hear her liver begging for mercy.

New Year's resolution number 354: give up drinking.

Or at least have a couple of nights off a week. Mind you, that wouldn't be so hard when she moved into her new flat at the end of January. The rent was so extortionate, she wouldn't be able to afford to eat, let alone drink.

Jo and Si had been great. But, saintly as they were, it was obvious they couldn't wait to get their house back. And since Christmas, well, Si had clearly had enough. Lizzie couldn't say she blamed him. Even she could see she'd blown it. But what was she supposed to do, when she couldn't even be in the same house as David without wanting to touch him?

Slowly the gate gave enough for her to get her fingers into the opening. With one last heave she was in.

David's people carrier wasn't in the road outside. She hadn't expected it to be. To be safe, she parked her old Renault round the corner, well out of sight. Thanks to Jo she knew he'd taken the girls to their grandparents for New Year and wouldn't be back until tomorrow. That gave Lizzie plenty of time to make amends to the garden. And to Nicci, for letting her down on just about every level.

This time, when Lizzie left, it would be for good. She would post the keys through the letterbox, for David to find on his return. David would understand. Lizzie just hoped Nicci would.

New Year's Eve with Si and Jo and Jools Holland had felt wrong. No kissing and hugging, no declaring undying love and swearing to be together for ever. No drunkenly opening pink champagne at midnight, no appalling hangovers, getting worse with every passing year. No full English, David-style.

But then everything felt wrong this Christmas. And who did Lizzie have to blame for that? Nobody but herself.

The garden was dank, leaves and stalks black with mould, the lawn boggy under her wellies. In the months since she'd last worked on it, everything had gone into hibernation. But it looked bedraggled and unloved, as if it had crashed out in its summer clothes, teeth unbrushed, makeup still on.

It had to be even longer since she'd sat here properly, pruning and weeding, wondering whether to take those runner bean wigwams down, minding her own business, oblivious to her phone ringing, the grim reaper waiting on the other end. Four months, she guessed, in which her life had changed so irrevocably she hardly recognised herself.

Down in the shed she'd come to think of her own, Lizzie made a cup of rosehip tea – what was left of Nicci's teabags – and slumped in Nicci's old leather chair, with its view through the shed door, right up the garden to the kitchen window. She'd grown used to seeing David's head bent over the worktop, scrutinising architectural drawings, a cup of coffee in his hand, a pair of reading glasses he pretended not to need unless he thought no one was looking perched on the end of his nose. The affectation surprised her. It seemed so unlike David to put what other people saw above being able to see himself.

Closing her eyes, Lizzie steadied herself, swallowed back the tears that were already threatening. Oh, how she'd missed it: the shed, the garden, the peace and quiet . . . How she'd missed David.

Stop it, she told herself, *he's not yours to miss. He's Nicci's, and Mona's . . . maybe. Whoever he belongs to, it's not you. Enough with the crying and the moping. Enough.*

Poor Gerry, she still felt bad about that. Or she would have done, if he wasn't refusing to speak to her except through a 'boutique solicitor' in Chancery Lane, who was all out to stop Lizzie taking even a fraction of the money in their joint savings account.

He'd find someone more . . . groomed. Better suited to the life he aspired to live. A woman who wasn't constantly showing him up and letting him down. Someone *blond*, Lizzie thought with a flash of cynicism. Someone who liked coffee mornings and didn't regard his work dos as torture. Someone who could laugh along to his boss's jokes, because that was her *job*.

A sudden memory of the last night in the shed hit her and propelled her from the armchair in search of something else to occupy her mind. For a second, arms and lips and hands held her as she fought the memory and made herself reach for a refuse sack. It was a memory. A memory was all it would ever be.

She didn't regret it. Quite the reverse.

But Lizzie couldn't let herself think about that right now. So many days and nights spent thinking about not thinking about David. If she could go back and change it she wasn't sure she would. And she wasn't sure she shouldn't, if only to avoid losing what she'd lost because of it. Not Gerry, not their house, not their life's savings; but her friends, her self-made family, who now seemed all but lost to her.

She'd never known what it meant to be torn; to turn one way and be afraid she should have turned another. To hurt so badly, and not know what to do to make things better. But now she felt *torn* like she'd ripped herself in two.

Escaping the shed with black refuse sack in hand, Lizzie headed for the vegetable patch, and began ripping down runner bean wigwams left over from that Sunday morning back in September.

Shutting the front door behind him, David closed his eyes and leaned back, feeling the wood solid behind him. Silence. Total and absolute silence. Except for pipes creaking and floorboards easing, the hum of the boiler and the kitchen clock slowly ticking. That was what passed for silence in this house. What he meant was, no people.

Thank God that was over, David thought. Christmas, New Year, all of it. No more enforced jollity and bonhomie. No more feeling obliged to put a brave face on it – at least until tomorrow tea time, when his parents brought Charlie and Harrie back. Twenty-seven hours to decompress.

He headed up the stairs, going first to his bedroom to dump the overnight bag, then wandering into his office. The answerphone showed fresh messages. A click of the space bar on his keyboard revealed a dozen new emails, none of which he could be bothered to answer.

What a fucking mess, he thought, throwing himself into his chair and spinning it round to face a montage of photographs of Nicci and the girls. 'What a fucking mess,' he repeated aloud, the echo muffled by the books lining the walls. Leaning back, hands in his hair, he stared at the ceiling

If only he could turn back the clock . . .

How many idiots who'd let the moment run away with them had thought that before him? But if he could, what would he turn it back to? The point she'd scrambled from the floor, so he could stop her? The call to her school so he could say something different . . . ? Or before that?

No. What he wanted was for that night to have happened again and again. Lizzie not to have run away like a frightened rabbit, his budding happiness collapsing like a house of cards behind her.

In a strange way the loss of Nicci had pulled them altogether. But this, the loss of Lizzie, David was afraid it had begun to tear them apart. He certainly felt as if he'd ripped himself in two.

He had to find her, David decided. He needed one last shot at changing her mind. So what, if she thought he was an idiot? So what, if she didn't love him the way he loved her? And if she wouldn't, he wanted peace. A truce, at least. They couldn't go back, but maybe they could find a way to go forwards. There was nothing to lose, after all. He'd agree to her terms, whatever they were. Just to get his framily back. But mostly, he just wanted her friendship.

First, he'd drop round to Si and Jo's, not that he was keen to see Jo again, just yet. The look on her face on Christmas Day when he admitted he'd slept with Lizzie would stay with him for a while yet. Or maybe Lizzie was at the cemetery? He hadn't a clue where Lizzie's mother was buried, but he was sure he could find out easily enough. How far away could it be? He could get there and back before dark.

He'd start with Jo and Si. Full of renewed energy, David tapped out a text to Si on his iPhone and pressed Send. *Don't tell Jo I asked, but is Lizzie there?* Then he turned to face his desk and fired up Google, ready to search for cemeteries if Si's answer was *No*.

The sound of wood cracking in the garden beneath his window made David freeze. There was nothing visible beyond the window but the dank, fetid remains of the vegetable patch, and a mulched pile of leaves he'd got as far as sweeping up in November and then abandoned in the middle of the lawn. Tom and Sam had used it as a goalpost last time they were round before Christmas.

Another crack. This time David's head shot up from his keyboard, in time to see one of the runner bean wigwams tumble to the ground. A flash of red hair appeared behind it before vanishing again.

David did a double take.

There it was again. He was sure. A streak of auburn.

She was here. He'd been about to go driving around Surrey looking for her, and Lizzie was here. Twenty yards away, in his back garden.

In his pocket, he felt his iPhone vibrate.

Not here. There, said the reply. *Don't tell Jo I blew the plot or I'm dead meat. Now delete.*

Not with Si, but already here, at his house. And if Jo had hatched some plot to bang their heads together, that meant there was hope. For a moment David was transfixed by the sight of Lizzie's auburn head bent over the bare earth. Just as the sight of her by the flowerbeds had comforted him through the long Sunday mornings of summer. He was surprised to find how easy her presence made him feel in his own home.

'I'm so glad you're back.'

Heart lurching, Lizzie dropped her secateurs and spun round. She was so shocked she felt her stomach plummet.

'David, shit, I . . . I thought, I'm sorry, I wouldn't, I was tol— I thought you were away.'

'Nope,' said David. 'Most definitely here.' Inclining his head towards an upended flower pot, he said, 'Mind if I join you?'

'No, of course not.' Lizzie's heart was pounding. 'Your garden. Your flower pot. You sit, you know, wherever you want to.'

Smiling, he bent to pick up her secateurs and handed them to her. 'Here's good.'

'I'm sorry,' she paused. 'Jo told me you were at your parents, otherwise I wouldn't have . . .'

He nodded. 'I was. The girls still are. Si told me you were here.'

'Ah.' She looked at him nervously. Did that mean he knew she was here? Had come back specially?

'It's a stitch-up,' he said.

Oh.

'Looks like it,' she said, spare hand fidgeting with her cardigan. 'I won't be under your feet for long. I just noticed, you know, last week . . .' Lizzie stopped, aware she was blushing furiously. The way David was looking right at her, his head on one side, was making her nervous.

'Noticed what?'

'That I'd left it in a state. I thought I should tidy it up, before . . . But I didn't want to disturb you.'

What does he want? Lizzie wondered, not daring to look straight at him, not daring to hope David wanted what she wanted. He couldn't, wouldn't. He loved Nicci. They all did. That was the problem. Or one of them.

'Si told me,' he said.

'That I was here? Yes, you said.' Then realisation dawned. 'Ah, you mean about Gerry. Yes, Jo told me. Si's a bit pissed off with me.' Lizzie ventured a smile. And the telltale crinkles of an answering smile radiated from David's brown eyes. 'He's right to be. I should have told you I'd left Gerry myself, I'm sorry.' Lizzie stopped. 'God, sorry seems to be all I say these days.'

'Always was,' David smiled. 'You've been apologising as long as I've known you. Usually for things that aren't your fault.'

'Have I?'

David nodded. 'So, if you're planning to say sorry for anything else, please don't.' He took a deep breath. 'Because, a) you don't have anything to apologise for. It wasn't your fault, it was mine, and, b) I'm not sorry.'

'David.'

'I refuse to be sorry,' he said. 'Are you sorry?'

Lizzie looked at him, really looked at him.

It was the first time she'd dared in months. She used to watch him, without thinking, without anyone noticing or caring less. She looked at his eyes, the warmth in them, the way they crinkled when he looked at her. The way he looked right at her. Like he really saw her.

Slight lines ran from his nose to his mouth, where it turned up when he smiled. His face had lost its youthful softness. But he was still the boy standing next to the kegs of cooking lager at that student party.

She shook her head. 'Never,' she whispered.

'Now what?' He looked suddenly anxious.

'I'm sorry I've spoiled everything between us.'

What did David see when he looked at her? If even half

of what Lizzie felt showed on her face she was in deep trouble. It hardly mattered, she was in deep trouble already. She'd gone too far to stop now.

'You haven't,' he started.

'I . . . I tried to stay away,' she said at the same time, 'to give you a chance to get on with your life. That's why I didn't tell you about Gerry. I didn't want you to think . . . to feel obliged.'

'Obliged? I don't feel obliged.'

'You don't?'

David shook his head. 'I feel fortunate.'

Risking a glance into his eyes, Lizzie sought doubt. But all she saw was what he told her. He felt fortunate.

'Can I offer you a drink?' he said, the smile breaking out of his eyes and reaching his lips. 'Tea, coffee . . . or something stronger?'

Getting up, he held out his hand. For a moment, Lizzie hesitated, glanced behind her, at the shed Nicci left her, at the garden Nicci had entrusted to her, then she took David's hand. 'Only if you have something open,' she said.

He was back within a minute, a bottle of pink champagne and two glasses in his hand. 'I do now,' he said.

EPILOGUE

Six Months Later

There was blue sky, there was sun, there was champagne. Pink, of course. And there was juice for the birthday girls, plus all the E numbers they were never usually allowed to eat. There were all the people Lizzie loved and who loved each other – friends, lovers, children, godmothers, grandpa and grannies – sprawled on tartan blankets laid over the shingle in front of the newly painted pistachio-green beach hut.

The windbreaks were redundant. For once there was no icy east wind blowing off the North Sea. Children shrieked and splashed, seagulls screamed as they wheeled overhead. And, just where the shingle tipped downhill towards the water's edge, she could see two small blonde girls in Hello Kitty T-shirts trying valiantly to build a dolls' house with dry grit and gravel.

As Lizzie watched, their sandless castle began to crumble. 'Lizzieeeeee!' Charlie and Harrie squealed in unison. 'Help us!'

'I'm making lunch!' Lizzie called back. 'Ask Granny Lynda.'

'Granneeeeee!

'You look good,' Jo said, padding barefoot into the beach hut and wrapping her friend in a hug. 'Great, in fact.' Stepping back, she took another look and said, 'Have you had your hair cut?'

'A bit.' Lizzie fiddled self-consciously with her red curls. Three inches wasn't a lot when you had as much hair as she did, but it still felt weird. The difference between long and shoulder-length. But it went with her new, thinner face. 'Lost some weight too.' She did a twirl.

'Lost more weight,' Jo said pointedly. 'Didn't know you were on a diet.'

'I'm not. Just eating less and moving more.' There was more to it than that, of course. Lizzie was happy too. 'Sick, isn't it?' she said. 'All those years of calorie-counting, and then it comes off without my trying.'

'All right for some,' Jo said, looking at her friend with real affection. 'You look fab. Really happy. Happier, I think, than I've ever seen you . . .' She paused, not sure what she was allowed to say, even now. Lizzie blushed.

'You too,' Lizzie said hastily. 'Lots better.'

'I am. We are.' Jo glanced over to where Si and David were trying to persuade a barbecue to light. Precariously close to their open canister of paraffin, one teenager and two smaller boys kicked a football furiously.

'Daniel! For God's sake!'

They couldn't see Mona but they could hear her, as her son kicked the ball wide and it soared past David's ear.

Mona's restaurant was opening the following week. Lizzie was surprised she'd agreed to skive the Sunday before, but India had persuaded her. India was small, dark-haired, a few years younger than they were. She was Mona's chef and had arrived with Dan and Mona, nervously clutching a bottle of pink champagne. If Mona had mentioned she was bringing her, no one had told Lizzie.

412

'What d'you get?' Lizzie asked, nodding at a blue and white icebox Jo had dumped on the table earlier.

Pulling a large cake in the shape of a pig's face from the top of the box, Jo said. 'This OK?' It was covered in pink icing. 'It's Percy. They won't notice the difference, will they?'

Lizzie rolled her eyes. 'Well, it's pink. Apart from that, it looks nothing like Peppa. They're never going to fall for it, not in a million.'

Jo shrugged. 'Worth a try.'

'Not interrupting anything, am I?' David appeared around the door. His cheeks were pink from the sun; by tomorrow his skin would have turned a healthy sun-burnished brown. Life was unfair like that.

In one step he crossed the hut, wrapped his arms around Lizzie and buried his face in her hair.

'Gerroff,' she said, making zero effort to disentangle herself. 'We're discussing pigs.'

David laughed. 'Granny says it's champagne o'clock. And the girls are gasping.'

'Which Granny?' Jo asked.

David raised his eyebrows. 'The Granny Mafia are as one on this particular subject. Grandpa will have a gin. Two cubes of ice. Light on the tonic.'

'Presents!' Charlie shouted.

'Cake!' Harrie joined in.

'Burfday!'

'Shhh,' Lizzie said. 'In a second. Daddy wants to say something first.'

'It's all right,' David said, passing the last of the champagne flutes to Dan, despite Mona's disapproving glare. 'I've been surrounded by women for the last twenty years. I'm used to not being able to get a word in edgeways.'

'Here, here.' Si said, ducking as Jo mock slapped him.

'I feel we should stand,' David said. 'Given the formality of the occasion. After all, a fourth birthday is a very big thing. And this fourth birthday even more so. Not because it's Charlie and Harrie's first since they lost their mother. And I – we – lost Nicci. That birthday, as we know, was last June. A bleak time in our lives that I think we'd all rather forget.'

Glancing around, he avoided catching anyone's eye.

'So, I have two toasts to make. No, make that three. The first, of course, is to the birthday girls. My babies are big girls now. Charlie and Harrie are four. Who can believe it? And, in a minute, I think, Auntie Jo might have a few hidden presents. Happy Birthday, big girls!'

'Happy Birthday, big girls!' everyone chorused.

'Presents!' Charlie and Harrie echoed.

They might as well have added, 'Sod the cake,' Lizzie thought happily. *After all, their mother would.*

'My second is to all of you. Nicci's closest friends. *My* closest friends. I couldn't have got through these past eighteen months without you, despite occasional appearances to the contrary.' He winked at Mona, who glanced nervously at the woman beside her.

'So,' said David. 'Jo, Mona, and Lizzie, for your love and support. For being there and refusing to go away, even when I told you to F off. And for coming back again when you did. Thank you.'

Laughter rang out and the adults raised their glasses.

'To us.'

'Jo, Mona, Lizzie.'

When the glasses were lowered and the laughter had subsided, David took a deep breath. Now came the serious bit. 'And last, but very much not least,' he said, 'to Nicci. My wife, my first real love, mother of my babies, my friend and yours. We miss you so very much. I know I speak for

414

us all when I say life is not the same without you. It's been tough, it's been dark. There have been days when, for me at least, it's been close to unbearable. But we've made it. We're here, sitting in the sun. Friends, old and new, and family, old and new, and lovers . . .'

He hesitated, his eyes locked with Lizzie's. And for a split second they might as well have been alone on the shingle.

Then he whispered, 'Ditto.'

Glancing around, David smiled. 'To Nicci. We're here because of you. Even if we didn't get here quite the way you intended.'

'Or maybe we did,' said Mona. 'I wouldn't put it past her.'

ACKNOWLEDGEMENTS

To My Best Friends owes its existence to many people, some of whom I'm bound to forget to credit here. If you're one of those, I apologise. To the rest, in no particular order:
I read several books in the course of my research, most notably, *Keeper* by Andrea Gillies and *Take Off Your Party Dress* by Dina Rabinovitch.

My inimitable agent, Jonny Geller. Thanks for keeping the faith (and getting me all those deadline extensions). Pretty sure I owe you a drink. And the team at Curtis Brown who put up with my (many and ongoing) stupid questions.

My wonderful editor, Lynne Drew, and her partner-in-crime, Sarah Ritherdon. With hindsight that suggestion was a touch radical, but you were totally right, as usual. From now on, I will always think of the credits rolling. Also, digital Kate and the production, design, marketing and publicity teams at HarperCollins who made this happen.

Team Red, indisputably the best in the business; and my boss, Kevin, for allowing me the time off to finish this book, just a teensy bit behind schedule.

All my followers/followees on twitter (I'm @samatredmag). I've never met a bigger bunch of malingerers in my life. OK, so my 20,100 tweets (at time of going to press!) translate into 2.8 million characters – and a helluva lot of words that might have been better used elsewhere – but it wouldn't have been half as much fun. Particular love and thanks to Jojo, Sali, Viv, Sarra and Kath. You are enablers extra-ordinaire and you should be proud of yourselves.

Marian, who so generously supported my books when, frankly, she had more important things on her mind. Get well soon.

Café Nero, Winchester, for letting us camp in the corner for an entire rainy August when our new house was a building site, and the decorator was singing along to Barry Manilow.

And Jon. Who knew you'd still be putting up with me after all these years? I count myself very lucky that you are.

The Stepmothers' Support Group

'Eve never expected to fall for a married man. Well, widowed, to be more accurate. It just hadn't occurred to her this was something she'd do.'

Ian is grown-up, sophisticated and successful. But he comes with kids attached, and, just as difficult, he still hasn't got over his wife. Fortunately Eve has friends – some new, some old, but all there for her.

Eve, Clare, Lily, Mel and Mandy share coffee, wine and the hopes, dreams and troubles we all have: love, work, not to mention, of course, family. But, as their friendships deepen, tensions surface. How will Eve and her friends cope where there are serious choices that have to be made?

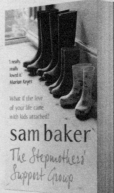

'I loved it… all the women's different stories [are] engaging and entertaining… a really good read'
Jane Fallon

'I really, really loved it'
Marian Keyes

A stepmother is not a mother. She can help you with your homework and make dinner, but she should not be able to decide when you should go to bed.

Delia Ephron

Read on for a glimpse inside

The Stepmothers' Support Group

The Stepmothers' Support Group

Even in a café full of brunch-seeking tourists, there was no missing them. The round table by the window looked like an accident in a cake factory. Eve took in the mix of Power Rangers, Spider Man and My Little Ponies using an assortment of cream slices, éclairs and croissants as barricades, jumps and stable walls, and grinned.

'Eve!' Ian shouted the second he saw her. His voice was loud, too loud. His nerves radiated around the room like static, drawing the attention of a couple on the next table. One of them started whispering.

Pushing back his chair, he knocked a plastic figure from the table. Three pairs of long-lashed blue eyes swivelled in Eve's direction.

'You made it!'

'I'm not late, am I?' Eve said, although she knew she wasn't. She'd set two alarm clocks and left her flat in Kentish Town half an hour early to make sure she arrived on time.

Ian glanced at his watch, shook his head. 'Bang on time.'

'Hannah, Sophie, Alfie, this is Eve Owen, the friend I've told you about.'

Eve smiled.

'Eve, this is my eldest, Hannah, she's twelve, Sophie is

eight. And Alfie, he's five.'

'And two months,' Alfie said firmly. The matter corrected, he returned to twisting Spiderman's leg to see how far it would turn before dislocating at the hip.

Smiling inanely, Eve felt like a children's TV presenter.

'Hello,' she said.

Three faces stared at her.

'I'm Eve,' she added unnecessarily, putting out a hand to the girl sitting nearest. Hannah might be twelve, but she looked older. Already teenage inside her head. And way taller than four feet. She exuded confidence. 'Hannah, really nice to meet you.'

'Hi.' Hannah raised one hand, in token greeting, then used it to flick long, shiny golden hair over her shoulder, before reaching pointedly for her cappuccino.

'And you must be Sophie.'

The child in the middle was a smaller, slightly prettier and much girlier version of her sister. Except for Levi jeans, there was nothing she wore, from Converse boots to Barbie hair slides that wasn't pink.

'How do you do?' Sophie said carefully. She shook Eve's hand, before glancing at her father for approval. He nodded.

'I'm Alfie,' the boy said.

'Hello Alfie.'

'Do you like Spiderman or Power Rangers? I like Power Rangers, but Spiderman is all right. You can be Venom.' Recovering a plastic figure from the floor, he shoved it into Eve's outstretched hand.

'That's kind,' she said, feeling stupidly grateful.

'Don't be so sure,' said Ian, tousling the boy's hair until the tufts stuck up even more. 'All that means is your figure gets bashed.'

'Venom's the baddie,' said Alfie, as if it was the most obvious thing in the world. 'He has to lose, it's the law. Can we eat our cakes now, Dad?'

Without waiting for permission, he grabbed the nearest éclair, one twice as big as his hand, and thrust it mouthwards, decorating his face, Joker-style, with chocolate and cream.

'Sit, sit, sit,' Ian said, pulling out the empty chair between his own and Hannah's. 'I'll get you a coffee. Black, isn't it?'

You know it's black, she wanted to say. When has it ever been anything else?

She didn't say it, though. And she resisted the urge to touch his hand to tell him everything would be all right. Hand squeezing was out of bounds. As was reassuring arm touching and even the most formal of pecks on the cheek. They'd been lovers for nine months, but this was something new and Eve was still learning the rules.

This was more than girl meets boy, girl fancies boy, girl goes out with boy, falls in love, etc . . . This was girl meets boy, girl fancies boy, girl goes out with boy, girl discovers boy has already gone out with another girl, girl meets boy's children.

In other words, this was serious.

WIN A LUXURY HOLIDAY FOR 4
WITH PREMIER COTTAGES

To let your friends know how special they are
to you, we're offering you the chance to win
an exquisite break with Premier Cottages.

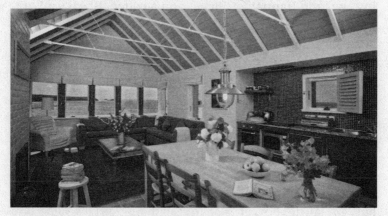

The prize, for up to four people, includes a week's stay in a
stunning holiday cottage. There is a fantastic collection
of properties to choose from across the UK, all of which
are 4 and 5 star tourist board graded.

Whether you want to relax by the Cornish coast, explore picturesque
Ireland or unwind in the breathtaking Cotswolds, Premier Cottages will
ensure you find the right cottage holiday for you and your friends.

Log onto **www.harpercollins.co.uk/premier** to enter

For more information on Premier Cottages and their outstanding
self-catering accommodation visit **www.premiercottages.co.uk**